Handbook of
Community-Based
and
Home Health
Nursing Practice

Tools for Assessment, Intervention, and Education

DATE

5-7-02

I0619607

GAYLORD

PRINTED IN U.S.A.

Handbook of
Community-Based
and
Home Health
Nursing Practice

Tools for Assessment, Intervention, and Education

Marcia Stanhope, RN, DSN, FAAN, c
Professor and Associate Dean
College of Nursing
University of Kentucky
Lexington, Kentucky

Ruth N. Knollmueller, RN, PhD
Clinical Associate
School of Nursing
University of Connecticut
Storrs, Connecticut

Third Edition
122 illustrations

St. Louis Baltimore Boston Carlsbad Chicago Naples New York
Philadelphia Portland London Madrid Mexico City Singapore
Sydney Tokyo Toronto Wiesbaden

Editor-In-Chief: Sally Schrefer
Executive Editor: June D. Thompson
Senior Developmental Editor: Linda Caldwell
Project Manager: John Rogers
Cover Art: Kathi Gosche

3rd EDITION
Copyright © 2000 by Mosby, Inc.
Previous editions copyrighted 1992, 1996

NOTICE
Pharmacology is an ever-changing field. Standard safety precautions must be followed, but as new research and clinical experience broaden our knowledge, changes in treatment and drug therapy may become necessary or appropriate. Readers are advised to check the most current product information provided by the manufacturer of each drug to be administered to verify the recommended dose, the method and duration of administration, and contraindications. It is the responsibility of the appropriately licensed health care provider, relying on experience and knowledge of the patient, to determine dosages and the best treatment for each individual patient. Neither the publisher nor the editor assumes any liability for any injury and/or damage to persons or property arising from this publication.

Mosby, Inc.
A Harcourt Health Sciences Company
11830 Westline Industrial Drive
St. Louis, Missouri 63146

Printed in the United States of America

ISBN 0-323-00875-5

99 00 01 02 03 CA/FF 9 8 7 6 5 4 3 2 1

REVIEWERS

Lorraine Noll, MSN, RNC
Associate Professor
Professional Nursing Program
University of Wisconsin—Green Bay
Green Bay, Wisconsin

Fatma Youssef, DNSc, RN
Professor
School of Nursing
Marymount University
Arlington, Virginia

PREFACE

This work is a compilation of practical instruments, guidelines, hints, and charts that can be used to aid public health, community nursing, community-based, and home health nurses in implementing care plans and intervening with clients, whether families or individuals. Use of these tools will also aid the nurse in collecting information that can be used to evaluate health care outcomes. The tools are not exhaustive in identifying problems or strategies that may be useful in community and home settings. However, they do offer practical guidance for dealing with many of the problems community-based and home health nurses typically face.

The guidelines presented are general. Agency policies and procedures and client mix will dictate the specific strategies used for applying the nursing process to client care in the community. This handbook provides the nurse with a ready reference for reviewing pertinent nursing knowledge at the time of providing care. This information will also assist faculty and students by providing structure for the students' synthesis of knowledge related to all areas of practice in nursing. In addition, researchers may apply these tools to the study of problems encountered in the community.

We wish to thank those who have permitted their work to be shared and acknowledge their expertise and the contributions they have made to promoting the health of communities, families, and individuals.

Marcia Stanhope   **Ruth N. Knollmueller**

CONTENTS

Tools and Measurements   290
Pain Measurement   290

Other Measurements   298

PART FOUR: NUTRITION GUIDELINES

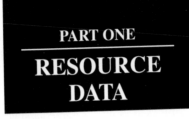

QUICK REFERENCE INFORMATION

The context of the home visit and safety guidelines are elements of the nurse's daily life in the field. Proper bag technique, essential supplies and equipment, and tips for improvising care in the home are all necessary to provide safe, quality care in an efficient manner.

Safety Guidelines

Procedure
Take the following precautions before visits:

Appearance
1. Wear a name badge and uniform that clearly identify you as a representative of the home health agency.
2. Call clients in advance and alert them to the approximate time of your visit. Confirm directions to the residence.
3. Request that unruly or overly friendly pets be properly secured before making visits. Back away, never run from a dog. Walk slowly around farm animals so as not to frighten them.
4. Keep change for a phone call in your shoe or pocket; **do not** carry a purse. Before leaving the agency, lock your purse in the car's trunk; otherwise, cover your purse with a blanket if the purse will be visible.

Precautions when traveling
Car
1. Keep your car in good working order and with a full tank of fuel. Obtain an automobile club membership for assistance with car problems.
2. Consider using a personal cellular phone to maximize communication and personal safety.

Modified from Rice R: *Manual of home health nursing procedures,* St. Louis, 1995, Mosby.

1

3. Store a blanket in the car in the winter and a thermos of cool water in the summer. Keep a snack in the glove compartment.
4. If your car fails, turn on emergency flashers, put a **Call Police** sign in the window, and wait for the police. Do not accept rides from strangers.
5. Keep your car locked when it is parked and when you are driving. Keep the windows rolled up if possible.
6. Park in full view of the client's residence. (Avoid parking in alleys or on deserted side streets.)

Walking on the street

1. Have the nursing bag and equipment ready when exiting from the car. Keep one arm free.
2. Walk in a professional, businesslike manner and walk directly to the client's residence.
3. When passing a group of strangers, cross to the other side of the street, as appropriate.
4. When leaving the client's residence, carry car keys in your hand. (Pointed ends of keys between fingers may make an effective weapon.)

Precautions during visits

In the home environment

1. Use common walkways in buildings. Avoid isolated stairs or darkened (unlit) areas.
2. Always knock on the door before entering a client's home.
3. If relatives or neighbors become a safety problem, consider the following:

    Discuss the problem with the client and schedule a visit time when the relative or neighborhood is quiet.

    Make joint visits with another home health nurse or arrange for escort services.

    Close the case if the client, physician, and you are unable to resolve the problem.
4. Request escort services, as appropriate, for night visits.

Defense techniques

1. Run.
2. Scream and yell, **"fire."**
3. Kick shins, instep, or groin.
4. Bite and scratch.
5. For defense use a whistle attached to your key ring, use chemical sprays, or use your nursing bag.

Consult with the home health agency's clinical service manager and administration regarding notification of violation of personal safety to the appropriate public officials.

Nursing Considerations

Visit neighborhoods with questionable safety or gang- or drug-related problems in the morning.

Some areas may have to be declared unsafe and therefore cannot be serviced by your home health agency.

Do not make home visits when guns or drugs are present.

Regard uniforms and agency identification badges as an important part of identification to the public and your personal safety.

In the event of robbery, never resist the assailant's attempt to take your nursing bag. It can easily be replaced.

When you are on duty, notify the home health agency clinical service manager of car trouble, auto accident, or other incident for further instructions when personal safety is in question.

Never go into or stay in a home if you feel your personal safety is in question. Always respect and listen to your *gut feelings*.

Phases and Activities of a Home Visit	
Phase	**Activity**
I Initiation phase	Clarify source of referral for visit
	Clarify purpose for home visit
	Share information on reason and purpose of home visit with family
II Previsit phase	Initiate contact with family
	Establish shared perception of purpose with family
	Determine family's willingness for home visit
	Schedule home visit
	Review referral and family record
III In-home phase	Introduction of self and professional identity
	Social interaction to establish rapport
	Establish nurse-client relationship
	Implement nursing process
IV Termination phase	Review visit with family
	Plan for future visits
V Postvisit phase	Record visit
	Plan for next visit

From Stanhope M, Lancaster J: *Community health nursing*, ed 3, St. Louis, 1992, Mosby.

Essential Supplies and Equipment

The following checklists contain suggested supplies and equipment needed for the home visit.

Home visit bag
1. Sphygmomanometer
2. Stethoscope _____
3. Thermometer _____
   a. Oral _____
   b. Rectal _____
4. Scissors _____
5. Forceps _____
6. Soap _____
7. Towels _____
8. Apron _____
9. Antiseptic wipes _____
10. Tape measure _____
11. Penlight _____
12. Oto/Ophthalmoscope (optional) _____
13. Gloves/mask/eyeshield _____
14. Tuning fork _____
15. Reflex hammer _____
16. CPR mask _____
_____

Additional supplies/equipment for home visit
1. Wound care supplies
   a. 4 × 4 _____
   b. 2 × 2 _____
   c. Kling gauze _____
   d. Antiseptic solution _____
   e. Irrigation solution _____
   f. Other _____ _____
2. Asepto syringe _____
3. Intravenous therapy setup _____
4. Catheter equipment _____
5. Suction catheter _____
6. Irrigation setup _____
7. Enema _____
8. Ace bandages _____
9. Slings _____
10. Splints _____
11. Other _____ _____
_____

Bag Technique

Equipment

1. Nursing bag
2. Paper towels
3. Fresh newspapers or suitable barrier
4. Liquid soap (bar soap can be a haven for bacteria) Note: Antiseptic hand cleanser may be used instead of liquid soap

Procedure

1. Observe principles of universal precautions and body substance isolation at all times. The inside of the nursing bag shall be regarded and maintained as a clean area.
2. Transport the nursing bag in the car on top of a supply of fresh newspapers.
3. Once in the client's home, select the cleanest or most convenient work area and spread the newspaper.
4. Place the bag on the newspaper.
5. Prepare a receptacle (plastic trash bag for disposable items).
6. Open the nursing bag and remove items that are needed to wash the hands. Handwashing supplies should be kept at the top of the bag. Close the bag. Open and close the nursing bag as few times as possible.
7. Take items to wash the hands (liquid soap, paper towels) to the sink area. Spread out one paper towel on which to place other items. A second and third towel are used for washing and drying the hands before and after care has been given. Follow manufacturer recommendations for use of antiseptic hand cleanser.
8. Wash and dry hands.
9. After the hands have been dried, turn the water faucet off with a paper towel. Return liquid soap to the nursing bag after care has been given.
10. Open the nursing bag again and remove items necessary for the visit. Apply personal protective equipment. Keep the bag closed during the visit. Leave all plastic containers in the bag. If additional equipment or supplies are needed from the bag during the home visit, the handwashing procedure must be repeated.
11. Discard disposable personal protective equipment in the plastic trash bag. To discard a disposable gown or plastic apron, remove

Modified from Rice R: *Manual of home health nursing procedures,* St. Louis, 1995, Mosby.

the apron by folding the exposed side inward. Clean all equipment with soap and water or home health agency–approved disinfectant when providing client care.

Contaminated equipment or equipment that cannot be cleaned may be transported to the agency in a sealed plastic bag for disinfection. Never place used needles, soiled equipment, or dressings in the nursing bag.

12. Discard newspaper, paper towels, and any remaining disposable items in a plastic trash bag at the end of the visit. Secure the trash bag, and place it in the family trash. Review local and state ordinances regarding disposal of infectious waste in the home.

13. Wash hands. Close bag and fasten.

Nursing Considerations

The nursing bag should not be exposed to extreme temperatures or left in the car for long periods of time.

The nursing bag should be cleaned, disinfected, and restocked weekly at the home health agency.

The following information should be considered when selecting work areas in the client's home:

- Adequate work space, preferably a clean surface
- Protection of the client's property
- Protection of the nursing bag: place in a safe place away from children or animals
- Proximity of water

Tips About Documentation

- Write legibly or print neatly. The record must be readable.
- Use permanent ink.
- Identify the time and date for every entry, sign the entry, and include your title.
- Describe care or interventions provided and client's response or mark appropriate box on flow sheet.
- Write objectively when describing findings (e.g., behaviors).
- Document in consecutive and chronological order with no skipped areas.

Modified from Marrelli TM: *Handbook of home health standards and documentation guidelines for reimbursement,* ed 3, St. Louis, 1998, Mosby.

- Document or enter information either at the client's home (if safe and appropriate) or as soon as possible after care is provided.
- Be factual and specific.
- Use the client's name (e.g., "Mr. Smith").
- Use client, family, or caregiver quotes that are in response to instruction or any other care intervention.
- Document client complaints or needs and their resolutions. (Remember to also discuss the complaints with your manager, who may document them in the complaint log and note the resolution or follow-up actions taken and any trends.)
- Make sure the client's name is listed correctly on the visit record, daily note, or other form.
- Be accurate, complete, and thorough.
- Write out what you are saying if anything is questionable. (Avoid potentially confusing abbreviations.)
- Chart only the care that you provided.
- Promptly document any change in the client's condition and the actions taken based on that change.
- Document the client's, family's, or caregiver's response to teaching or any other care intervention.
- To correct an error: (1) draw a line through the erroneous entry, (2) briefly describe the error (e.g., "wrong date," "spilled coffee on visit record"), and (3) add your signature and the date and time (per organizational policy).

Try to avoid
- Relying on memory
- Whiting out or erasing entries, which may appear to be an attempt to cover up incriminating entries
- Crossing out words beyond recognition
- Making assumptions, drawing conclusions, or blaming
- Leaving blank spaces between entries and your signature
- Waiting too long to record entries
- Leaving gaps in documentation
- Using abbreviations unless they are clear and appear on the organization's list of approved abbreviations

Home Care Nurse's Checklist for Effective Documentation

- Recognize that at the first visit the nurse initiates the process of claims payment (or denial) with the initial Health Care Financing Administration (HCFA) form 485.
- Try to read your documentation objectively. Ask yourself if the HCFA form 485 or visit record reflects why the client is homebound (if the client has Medicare or another insurance that has that criterion) and how the skills of a nurse or therapist are needed. (Many home health agencies have a peer review process that significantly helps home care nurses objectively review and create documentation.)
- Emphasize (1) why the care was initiated, (2) what the skilled nursing interventions are, (3) where the client's plan is going (client-centered goals), and (4) what the plans are for discharge (rehabilitation potential).
- Try to complete your client documentation as soon as possible. Try to document in the client's home when safe. Explain to your clients that the last few moments of every visit are for completing the documentation required by Medicare or another payer. Clients and their families understand. In fact, during this quiet time the clients may think of questions and save your getting calls once out of the home. This is of particular importance when working with new admissions because of all the associated forms that the clients must sign, the information you need for the completion of the HCFA form 485, and the initial and daily visit notes. Relying on memory or rough notes after seeing many clients at the end of a long day can be difficult and often unsafe.
- Remember that the plan of care (POC) is the most important part of the home care clinical record. All other information flows from the skilled nursing needs ordered on the plan. The POC must be complete, and the content must be clear. The POC can have no gaps.
- Make sure your client meets the organization's and insurance program's admission criteria. This is important from both risk management and reimbursement perspectives. Be able to clearly identify the skilled, covered service. In addition, although the client may not meet a particular insurer's requirements, the client may still have needs that another program can safely provide.

Modified from Marrelli TM: *Handbook of home health standards and documentation guidelines for reimbursement,* ed 3, St. Louis, 1998, Mosby.

- Focus on the client's problems in your documentation. They are the reason home care is being provided, and the payers must see evidence of such to justify reimbursement.
- Demonstrate through your documentation that the care provided is client centered. For example, make your client goals quantifiable and your outcomes realistic and specific to the client's unique problems and needs.
- Remember that anyone else who picks up your client's clinical record does not have the depth of knowledge that you have gained from actually being there and seeing the client in the home setting. Because of this, document information that is objective and clearly paints a picture of the client, the relevant problems and needs, and how the care is directed for goal achievement and discharge.
- Remember that effective documentation does not have to be wordy. However, it should convey to any reader, such as your manager or a state surveyor nurse, the status of your client, the adherence to the ordered POC, and the consistent movement toward predetermined client-centered goals.
- Check that the information in the clinical record flows well and that you can tell, by objective evidence, what is happening with the client. This includes the problems and the skilled services that are needed, again based on the clear picture presented in the documentation.
- Remember that the clinical record's entries need to be legible, neat, and consistently organized. How the clinical record looks may be seen as an indicator of care and the quality of the organization.
- Try to look at the documentation objectively. Does it tell the story of the client's progress (or lack of progress) and the interventions implemented based on the initial assessment and POC?
- Make sure telephone calls and other communications with physicians, community agencies, and other team members are documented. Include interdisciplinary team conferences and discussions. Does the documentation explain what occured with the client; what actions were ordered, modified, and implemented; and what the client's response was to these interventions?
- Demonstrate the nursing process in the record. Look for the nursing diagnoses, the assessment, evidence of care planning, implementation of ordered interventions and actions, movements toward client-centered goals, assessment of the client's response, and continued evaluation.
- Document goal achievement and/or progress toward goals and outcomes. Are the goals realistic, quantifiable, and client centered?

- If progress has not occurred as planned, explain the reasons in the documentation. If a client is too ill for a rehabilitation service or refuses the service, is written communication with the doctor about this included? Has an order been made to place the service on hold or to discharge the client from that service?
- Documentation should include family/caregiver teaching and their responses to, and demonstration of, learning.
- Document the client's response to care interventions and other nursing actions.
- Modify the interventions based on the client's response, where appropriate.
- Document evidence of interdisciplinary team conferences and discussions.
- The chart should show continuity of care planning goals and consistent movement toward outcomes/goal achievement by all members of the team.
- Generally, the record should tell the story of the client's care, needs, and progress while receiving home care services.
- The nursing entries and overall information are to reflect the level of care expected by today's health care consumers and their families.
- The clinical documentation should demonstrate compliance with regulatory, licensure, and quality standards.

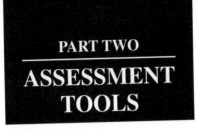

PART TWO

ASSESSMENT TOOLS

ENVIRONMENTAL ASSESSMENT: HOME

Healthy populations are active and reach out to various community groups. Individuals and families who function in a healthy way think of themselves as being part of a larger community. Part of successful coping is the ability to seek, receive, or accept appropriate resources to meet the need for a safe environment in which to live. The following assessment tools provide the structure for gathering valuable data related to the home.

Home Assessment Checklist

General household

1. Is there good lighting available, especially around stairwells?
2. Are there handrails (which can be easily grasped) on both sides of the staircases, designed to indicate when top and bottom steps have been reached?
3. Are top and bottom steps painted in easily seen colors? Are non-skid treads used?
4. Are the edges of rugs tacked down? (Suggest the use of wall-to-wall carpeting.)
5. Is a telephone present? Does the telephone have a dial that is easily readable? Are emergency numbers written in large print and kept near the telephone?
6. Are electrical cords, footstools, and other low-lying objects kept out of walkways?
7. Are electrical cords in good condition?

Modified from Tideiksaar R: *Home assessment checklist,* New York, 1983, Ritter Department of Geriatrics and Adult Development, The Mount Sinai Medical Center.

8. Is furniture arranged to allow for free movement in heavily traveled areas?
9. Is furniture sturdy enough to give support?
10. Is furniture designed to accommodate easy transfers on and off?
11. Is the temperature of the home within a comfortable range?
12. If fireplaces or other heating devices are present, do they have protective screens?
13. Are smoke detectors present (especially in the kitchen and bedroom)?
14. Are rapidly closing doors eliminated?
15. Are there alternative exits from the house?
16. Are basements and attics easy to get to, well lighted, and well ventilated?
17. Are slippers and shoes in good repair? Do they fit properly and have nonskid soles?

Kitchen

18. Are there loose extension cords, small sliding rugs, slippery linoleum tiles present? (Suggest the use of rubber-backed, nonskid rugs and nonskid floor wax.)
19. Is the cooking stove gas or electric?
20. Are there large, easily readable dials present on the stove or other appliances, with the "on" and "off" positions clearly marked?
21. Are refrigerators in good working order? Are refrigerators placed on 18-inch platforms so the client will not have to bend over?
22. Are spaces for food storage adequate? Are shelves at eye level and easily reachable?
23. Is a sturdy stepladder present for reaching?
24. Are electrical circuits overloaded with too many appliances?
25. Are electrical appliances disconnected when not in use?
26. Are sharp objects (such as carving knives) kept in special holders?
27. Are cleaning fluids, polishes, bleaches, detergents, and all poisons stored separately and clearly marked?
28. Are kitchen chairs sturdy, with arm rests and high backs?
29. Is stove free from flammable objects?
30. Are pot holders available for removing pots and pans from the stove?
31. Is baking soda available in case of fire?

Bathroom

32. Are there grab bars in the bath, in the shower, and around the toilet?
33. Are toilet seats high enough to get on and off of without difficulty?

34. Can the bathroom door be easily closed to ensure privacy? (Avoid locks.)
35. Are bathroom doorways wide enough for easy wheelchair and walker access?
36. Are there nonskid rubber mats in the bath, in the shower, and on the floor?
37. Is there good lighting in the area of the medicine cabinet?
38. Are internal and external medications stored separately? Are they stored safely (especially important with young grandchildren present in the house)?
39. Do medication containers have childproof tops? Are they labeled in large print? Is a magnifying glass present for reading medication instructions?
40. Have all outdated medications been discarded?
41. Do you notice any medications (both prescription and over-the-counter) that could cause adverse side effects or drug-drug interactions that the client is unaware of?
42. Can the water temperature be easily regulated?
43. Are electrical cords, outlets, and appliances a safe distance from the tub?
44. Are razor blades kept in a safe place?
45. Is a first-aid kit available?

Bedroom

46. Is there adequate lighting from the bedside to the bathroom?
47. Are lights easily accessible? (If not, suggest keeping a flashlight by the bedside or using a flashlight for entry into dark rooms if light switch is not within easy reach.)
48. Are beds in good repair?
49. Are beds at the proper height to allow for easy transfer on and off without difficulty?
50. Do bedroom rugs have nonskid rubber backings?

Guidelines for Home Safety Assessment

	Okay (y/n)	Plan to improve
Basic structure		
Intact roof		
Solid floors and stairs		
Functioning toilet (or outhouse)		
Source of fresh water		
Wheelchair ramp		
Temperature control		
Fan/air conditioner		
Proper use of heating pads		
Proper water heater temperature		
Adequate heat/insulation		
Nutrition		
Kitchen condition/food storage		
Evidence of alcohol use		
Pests		
Fire prevention and response		
Use of kerosene heaters		
Use of open gas burners on stove for heat		
Smoking in bed		
Use of oxygen		
Dangerous electrical wiring		
Smoke alarms		
Exit plans in case of fire		
Self-injury/violence prevention		
Locks		
Method of calling for help		
Proximity of neighbors		
Surrounding criminal activity		
Emergency phone numbers by telephone		
Loaded guns/knives		
Household toxins		
Water/bathtub		
Power tools		
Medication management		
Duplicate medicines, outdated drugs, pill box		
Correct labeling		
Storage safety, accessibility, refrigeration		
Caregiver familiarity		
Wandering control (for confused clients)		
Doortop latches, special locks		
Fenced yards with hidden latches		
Identification bracelets		
Electronic wandering alarms		

Modified from Yoshikawa TAT, Cobbs EL, Brummel-Smith K: *Ambulatory geriatric care,* St. Louis, 1993, Mosby.

Environmental Assessment for the Elderly

1. How many rooms are available to client?

   Own bedroom _____   If shared, with whom? _____

   Bathroom _____

   Kitchen _____

   Living/sitting room _____

2. Must client climb stairs to enter or leave house?

   Yes _____   No _____

   If yes, are they well lit and in good repair?

   Yes _____   No _____

3. Is neighborhood dangerous?

   Yes _____   No _____

4. Is house clean?

   Yes _____   No _____

5. Does house seem adequately insulated and ventilated?

   Yes _____   No _____

6. Are there signs of neglect?

   Old food in refrigerator _____

   Unwashed dishes _____

   Accumulated dirty clothing _____

   Other (describe): _____

7. Is there a sufficient supply of food for at least several days?

   Yes _____   No _____

8. Safety checklist

   a. Can the client:

	Yes	No
Lock and unlock the door	____	____
Reach light switches	____	____
Call for help (telephone and numbers accessible)	____	____
Safely transfer from bed, chair, toilet, tub	____	____

   b. Are there obvious dangers:

	Yes	No
Overloaded electrical outlets	____	____
Frayed electrical wires	____	____
Poor lighting	____	____
Cluttered furniture	____	____
Unsafe furniture	____	____
Frayed carpets or broken floors	____	____
Missing or broken smoke alarm	____	____

From Kane R, Ouslander J, Abrass I: *Essentials of clinical geriatrics,* ed 3, New York, 1994, McGraw-Hill.

9. Fall hazard checklist (after *Clinical Report on Aging,* Volume 1, Number 5, 1987)

a. Throughout the household, check that the following are in order:

_____ **1.** Flooring and carpeting are in good condition without protruding obstacles that may cause tripping and falling.

_____ **2.** Lighting is bright and without glare.

_____ **3.** Nightlights are strategically placed throughout the house, especially on stairways and along routes between bedroom and bathroom. Illuminated light switches are used when possible in similar high-risk locations.

_____ **4.** Telephones are positioned so that persons do not have to hurry to answer a ringing telephone.

_____ **5.** Electric cords are not located in walkways. When possible, they are shortened and tacked down to baseboards.

_____ **6.** Clutter does not obstruct walkways.

b. Bathroom

_____ **7.** Railings are installed in the bathtub and toilet area and are easily accessible for use.

_____ **8.** A nonslip surface is on the floor of the tub and shower. If a bath mat is used, it is of substantial quality.

_____ **9.** If a throw rug is used, it has a nonskid rubber backing.

_____ **10.** Water drainage is appropriate to prevent the development of slippery floors after bathing.

c. Bedroom

_____ **11.** Throw rugs do not represent a slip or trip hazard, particularly those en route to the bathroom.

_____ **12.** Bedside table is present for placement of glasses and other items rather than cluttering the floor beside the bed.

d. Kitchen

_____ **13.** The floor is made of a nonslip material.

_____ **14.** Spills are cleaned up quickly to prevent slipping.

_____ **15.** Cleaning and cooking supplies are stored in locations that are not too high (for shorter persons who would otherwise climb) or too low (for persons who develop lightheadedness after stooping).

_____ **16.** A high chair is available for doing dishes.

_____ **17.** A sturdy step stool is available for reaching high places.

e. Living room

_____ **18.** Throw rugs are not present over a carpet or otherwise scattered about.

_____ **19.** Furniture is placed in positions that allow for wide walkways.

_____ **20.** Chairs and sofas are of a height sufficient to permit easy sitting and standing for elderly persons.

f. Stairways

_____ **21.** Sturdy railings are provided along both sides of stairways, including the stairway to the basement.

_____ **22.** Step surfaces are nonskid.

_____ **23.** Materials are not stored on stair landings or thresholds.

_____ **24.** When possible, bright nonskid tape is placed on the top and bottom steps to indicate where the steps begin and end.

g. Outside the house

_____ **25.** Front and back steps are in good condition. During the winter, sand (or salt) is available for slippery surfaces to ensure safety.

_____ **26.** Walkways are shoveled free of ice and snow in the winter to prevent slips and falls.

_____ **27.** Stairways and railings are sturdy.

CULTURAL ASSESSMENT

The nurse will want to learn the culture within that community before beginning any efforts at intervention or change. When assessing families, the nurse needs to be aware of the factors in the following table.

Notes

Cultural Characteristics Related to Health Care of Children and Families

Cultural group	Health beliefs	Health practices	Family relationships	Communication	Comments
Asians					
Chinese	A healthy body viewed as gift from parents and ancestors and must be cared for Health is one of the results of balance between the forces of *yin* (cold) and *yang* (hot)—energy forces that rule the world Illness caused by imbalance Believe blood is source of life and is not regenerated *Chi* is innate energy	Goal of therapy is to restore balance of yin and yang Acupuncturist applies needles to appropriate meridians identified in terms of yin and yang Acupressure and *tai chi* replacing acupuncture in some areas *Moxibustion* is application of heat to skin over specific meridians Wide use of medicinal herbs procured and applied in prescribed ways	Extended family pattern common Strong concept of loyalty of young to old Respect for elders taught at early age—acceptance without questioning or talking back Children's behavior a reflection on family Family and individual honor and "face" important Self-reliance and self-restraint highly valued; self-expression repressed	Open expression of emotions unacceptable Often smile when do not comprehend	Do not react well to painful diagnostic workup; are especially upset by drawing of blood Deep respect for their bodies and believe it best to die with bodies intact; therefore may refuse surgery Believe in reincarnation Older members fear hospitals; often believe hospital is a place to go to die Children sometimes breast-fed for up to 4 or 5 years*

18

4

1

8

	Lack of chi and blood results in deficiency that produces fatigue, poor constitution, and long illness	Folk healers are herbalist, spiritual healer, temple healer, fortune healer Meals may or may not be planned to balance hot and cold Milk intolerance relatively common Use of condiments (e.g., monosodium glutamate and soy sauce) may create difficulty with some diet regimens (e.g., low-salt diets)	Males valued more highly than females; women submissive to men in family	Generational categories: *Issei*—1st generation to live in U.S. *Nisei*—2nd generation
Japanese	Three major belief systems: *Shinto* religious influence Humans inherently good Evil caused by outside spirits	Believe evil removed by purification Energy restored by means of acupuncture, acupressure, massage, and moxibustion along affected meridians	Close intergenerational relationships Family provides anchor Family tends to keep problems to self Value self-control and self-sufficiency	Issei—born in Japan; usually speak Japanese only Nisei, Sansei, and Yonsei have few language difficulties

From Wong D: *Whaley and Wong's nursing care of infants and children*, ed 6, St. Louis, 1999, Mosby.

*Most Asian cultures consider the child 1 year old at the time of birth. Traditional Chinese custom adds 1 year on January 1 regardless of the birthday—a child born in December is 2 years old the next January.

Continued.

Cultural Characteristics Related to Health Care of Children and Families—cont'd

Cultural group	Health beliefs	Health practices	Family relationships	Communication	Comments
Japanese— cont'd	Illness caused by contact with polluting agents (e.g., blood, corpses, skin diseases) Chinese and Korean influence Health achieved through harmony and balance between self and society Disease caused by disharmony with society and not caring for body Portuguese influence Upholds germ theory of disease	*Kampō* medicine—use of natural herbs Believe in removal of diseased parts Trend is to use both Western and Oriental healing methods Care for disabled viewed as family's responsibility Take pride in child's good health Seek preventive care, medical care for illness May avoid some food combinations (e.g., milk and cherries, watermelon and crab) and believe pickled plums to have special properties	Concept of *haji* (shame) imposes strong control; unacceptable behavior of children reflects on family Many adopt practices of contemporary middle class Concern for child's missing school may result in sending to school before fully recovered from illness	New immigrants able to read and write English better than able to speak or understand it Make significant use of nonverbal communication with subtle gestures and facial expression Tend to suppress emotions Will often wait silently	*Sansei*—3rd generation *Yonsei*—4th generation Issei and Nisei—tolerant and permissive childrearing until 5 or 6, then emphasis on emotional reserve and control Cleanliness highly valued Time considered valuable and used wisely Tendency to practice emotional control may make assessment of pain more difficult

| Vietnamese | Good health considered to be balance between yin and yang
Believe person's life has been predisposed toward certain phenomena by cosmic forces
Health believed to be result of harmony with existing universal order; harmony attained by pleasing good spirits and avoiding evil ones
Belief in *am duc*, the amount of good deeds accumulated by ancestors
Many use rituals to prevent illness | Family uses all means possible before using outside agencies for health care
Fortune-tellers determine event that caused disturbance
May visit temple to procure divine instruction
Use astrologer to calculate cyclical changes and forces
Regard health as family responsibility; outside aid sought when resources run out
Certain illnesses considered only temporary (such as pustules, open wounds) and ignored | Family is revered institution
Multigenerational families
Family is chief social network
Children highly valued
Individual needs and interests are subordinate to those of family group
Father is main decision maker
Women taught submission to men
Parents expect respect and obedience from children | Many immigrants are not proficient in speaking and understanding English
May hesitate to ask questions
Questioning authority is sign of disrespect; asking questions considered impolite
Use indirectness rather than forthrightness in expressing disagreement
May avoid eye contact with health professional as a sign of respect | Consider status more important than money
Children taught emotional control
Time concept more relaxed—consider punctuality less significant than other values (i.e., propriety)
Place high value on social harmony |

Continued.

Cultural Characteristics Related to Health Care of Children and Families—cont'd

Cultural group	Health beliefs	Health practices	Family relationships	Communication	Comments
Vietnamese—cont'd	Practice some restrictions to prevent incurring wrath of evil spirits	Seek generalist health healers May use special diets to prevent illness and promote health Lactose intolerance prevalent			
Filipinos	Believe God's will and supernatural forces govern universe Illness, accidents, and other misfortunes are God's punishment for violations of His will Widely accept "hot" and "cold" balance and imbalance as cause of health and illness	Some use amulets as a shield from witchcraft or as good luck pieces Catholics substitute religious medals and other items	Family is highly valued, with strong family ties Multigenerational family structure common, often with collateral members as well Personal interests are subordinated to family interests and needs Members avoid any behavior that would bring shame on the family	Immigrants and older persons may not be able to speak or understand English	Tend to have a fatalistic outlook on life Believe time and providence will solve all

African-American Blacks	Illness classified as: Natural—affected by forces of nature without adequate protection (e.g., cold air, pollution, food, and water) Unnatural—evil influences (e.g., witchcraft, voodoo, hoodoo, hex, fix, rootwork); symptoms often associated with eating Believe serious illness sent by God as punishment (e.g., parents punished by illness or death of child) Believe serious illness can be avoided	Self-care and folk medicine very prevalent Folk therapies usually religious in origin Attempt home remedies first; poorer people do not seek help until illness serious Usually seek help from: "Old lady"—woman in community with a common knowledge of herbs; consulted regarding pediatric care Spiritualist—has received gift from God for healing incurable diseases or solving personal problems; strongly based in Christianity	Strong kinship bonds in extended family; members come to aid of others in crisis Less likely to view illness as a burden Augmented families common (unrelated persons living in same household) Place strong emphasis on work and ambition Sex-role sharing among parents Elderly members respected Maternal grandparent strong influence	Alert to any evidence of discrimination Place importance on nonverbal behavior May use nonstandard English or "Black English" Use "testing" behavior to assess personnel in health care situations before seeking active care Best to use simple, direct, but caring approach	High level of caution and distrust of majority group Social anxiety related to tradition of humiliation, oppression, and loss of dignity Will elect to retain dignity rather than seek care if values are compromised Strong sense of peoplehood High incidence of poverty Black minister a strong influence in Black community Visits by family minister are sought, expected, and valued in helping to cope with illness and suffering

Continued.

23

Cultural Characteristics Related to Health Care of Children and Families—cont'd

Cultural group	Health beliefs	Health practices	Family relationships	Communication	Comments
African-American Blacks—cont'd	May resist health care because illness is "will of God"	Priest (voodoo priest/priestess)—most powerful healer Root doctor—meets need for herbs, oils, candles, and ointments Prayer is common means for prevention and treatment			
Haitians†	Illnesses have a supernatural or natural origin Supernatural illnesses are caused by angry voodoo spirits, enemies, or the dead, especially deceased ancestors	Health is a personal responsibility Foods have properties of "hot"/"cold" and "light"/"heavy" and must be in harmony with one's life cycle and bodily states	Maintenance of family reputation is paramount Lineal authority supreme; children in a subordinate position in family hierarchy	Recent immigrants and older persons may speak only Haitian creole May prefer family/friends to act as translators and confidants	Will use biomedical and ethnomedical (folk) systems simultaneously Resistant to dietary and work restrictions

Natural illnesses are based on conceptions of natural causation: Irregularities of blood volume, flow, purity, viscosity, color, and/or temperature (hot/cold) Gas (*gaz*) Movement and consistency of mother's milk Hot/cold imbalance in the body Bone displacement Movement of diseases Health is maintained by good dietary and hygienic habits	Natural illnesses are treated by home remedies first Supernatural illness treated by healers: voodoo priest (*houngan*) or priestess (*mambo*), midwife (*fam saj*), and herbalist or leaf doctor (*dokte fey*) Amulets and prayer used to protect against illness due to curses or willed by evil people	Children valued for parental social security in old age and expected to contribute to family welfare at an early age Children viewed as "gifts from God" and treated with indulgence and affection	Often smile and nod in agreement when do not understand Quiet and gentle communication style and lack of assertiveness lead health care providers to falsely believe they comprehend health teaching and are compliant Will not ask questions if health care provider is busy or rushed	Adherence to prescribed treatments directly related to perceived severity of illness

Continued.

†This section was written by Lydia DeSantis, RN, PhD.

Cultural Characteristics Related to Health Care of Children and Families—cont'd

Cultural group	Health beliefs	Health practices	Family relationships	Communication	Comments
Hispanics Mexicans (Latinos, Chicanos, Raza-Latinos)	Health beliefs have strong religious association Believe in body imbalance as a cause of illness, especially imbalance between *caliente* (hot) and *frio* (cold) or "wet" and "dry" Some maintain good health is a result of "good luck"—a reward for good behavior	Seek help from *curandero* or *curandera*, especially in rural areas Curandero(a) receives his/her position by birth, apprenticeship, or a "calling" via dream or vision Treatments involve use of herbs, rituals, and religious artifacts Practice for severe illness—make promises, visit shrines, offer medals and candles, offer prayers	Traditionally men considered breadwinners and key decision makers in matters outside the home; women considered homemakers Males considered big and strong (*macho*) Strong kinship; extended families include *compadres* (godparents) established by ritual kinship Children valued highly and desired, taken everywhere with family	May use nonstandard English Some bilingual; many speak only Spanish May have a strong preference for native language and revert to it in times of stress May shake hands or engage in introductory embrace Interpret prolonged eye contact as disrespectful	High degree of modesty—often a deterrent to seeking medical care and open discussions of sex Youngsters often reluctant to share communal showers in schools Relaxed concept of time—may be late for appointments More concerned with present than with future and therefore may focus on immediate solutions rather than long-term goals

Illness prevented by performing properly, eating proper foods, and working proper amount of time; accomplished through prayer, wearing religious medals or amulets, and sleeping with relics at home Illness is a punishment from God for wrongdoing, forces of nature, and the supernatural	Adhere to "hot" and "cold" food prescriptions and prohibitions for prevention and treatment of illness	Many homes contain shrines with statues and pictures of saints Elderly treated with respect		Magicoreligious practices common May view hospital as place to go to die
Puerto Ricans Subscribe to the "hot-cold" theory of causation of illness Believe some illness caused by evil spirits and forces	Infrequent use of health care systems Seek folk healers—use of herbs, rituals Consult spiritualist medium for mental disorders *Santeria* is system, and practitioners are called *santeros*	Family usually large and home centered—the core of existence Father has complete authority in family—family provider and decision maker Wife and children subordinate to father	May use nonstandard English Spanish speaking or bilingual Strong sense of family privacy—may view questions regarding family as impudent	Relaxed sense of time Pay little attention to exact time of day Suspicious and fearful of hospitals

Continued.

Cultural Characteristics Related to Health Care of Children and Families—cont'd

Cultural group	Health beliefs	Health practices	Family relationships	Communication	Comments
Puerto Ricans— cont'd		Treatments classified as "hot" or "cold"	Children valued—seen as a gift from God Children taught to obey and respect parents; corporal punishment to ensure obedience		
Cubans[‡]	Prevention and good nutrition are related to good health	Diligent users of the medical model Eclectic health-seeking practices, including preventive measures, and, in some instances, folk medicine of both religious and nonreligious origins; home remedies; in many instances seek assistance of santeros and spiritualists to complement medical treatment	Strong family ties with mother and father kinships Children supported and assisted by parents long after becoming adults Elderly cared for at home	Most are bilingual (English/Spanish) except for segments of the senior population	In less than 30 years Cubans have been able to obtain a higher standard of living than other Hispanic groups in U.S. Have been able to retain many of their former social institutions: bilingual and private schools, clinics, social clubs, the family as an extended network of support, etc.

				Nutrition is important; parents show over-concern with eating habits of their children and spend a considerable part of the budget on food; traditional Cuban diet is rich in meat and starch; consumption of fresh vegetables added in U.S.	Many do not feel discriminated against nor harbor feelings of inferiority with respect to Anglo-Americans or "mainstream" population
Native Americans (numerous tribes)	Believe health is state of harmony with nature and universe Respect of bodies through proper management All disorders believed to have aspects of supernatural	Medicine persons: Altruistic persons who must use powers in purely positive ways Persons capable of both good and evil—perform negative acts against enemies	Extended family structure—usually includes relatives from both sides of family Elder members assume leadership roles	Most continue to speak their Indian language, as well as English Nonverbal communication	Time orientation—present Respect for age Going to hospital associated with illness or disease; therefore may not seek prenatal care, since pregnancy viewed as natural process

Continued.

‡This section was written by Mercedes Sandaval, PhD.

29

Cultural Characteristics Related to Health Care of Children and Families—cont'd

Cultural group	Health beliefs	Health practices	Family relationships	Communication	Comments
Native Americans (numerous tribes)—cont'd	Violation of a restriction or prohibition thought to cause illness Fear of witchcraft May carry objects believed to guard against witchcraft Theology and medicine strongly interwoven	Diviner-diagnosticians—diagnose but do not have powers or skill to implement medical treatment Specialists—use herbs and curative but nonsacred medical procedures Medicine persons—use herbs and ritual Singers—cure by the power of their song obtained from supernatural beings; effect cures by laying on of hands			Tend to take time to form an opinion of professionals Sexual matters not openly discussed with members of opposite sex

Multicultural Nursing Assessment

There must be an awareness of one's own ethnocultural heritage, both as a person and as a nurse. In addition, an awareness and sensitivity must be developed to the health beliefs and practices of a client's heritage. This awareness and sensitivity can be developed through careful assessment of a client's heritage and cultural beliefs. The factors that must be explored during a multicultural nursing assessment are as follows:

Cultural

What customs and values of the client may influence health behaviors and the provision of care?

Could the client's communication process or language affect the provision of care? How?

What health care beliefs and practices of the client may influence acceptance of and response to illness?

Could nutritional variables and preferences or restrictions affect the provision of care?

Sociological

Could the client's economic status affect the provision of care?

Could educational status affect the provision of care?

How does the client's social network affect the provision of care?

What family structural variables may influence the provision of care?

Are community support systems available, and do they help to fight against institutional racism?

Psychological

Could self-concept and identity factors affect the provision of care?

What are the client's defense mechanisms, and are they adaptive or maladaptive?

Could religious or cultural considerations affect the provision of care?

Biological and Physiological

Does the nurse need to take racial or anatomical characteristics or factors into account when providing care?

Do growth and development patterns influence physical assessment findings?

What variations in physical features and body systems are present?

Are there any culturally specific diseases to note? Are there any diseases to which the client has increased (decreased) resistance?

From Potter PA, Perry AG: *Basic nursing: a critical thinking approach*, ed 4, St. Louis, 1999, Mosby.

Cross-Cultural Examples of Cultural Phenomena That Affect Nursing Care

Nations of origin	Communication	Space	Time orientation	Social organization	Environmental control	Biological variations
Asian China Hawaii Philippines Korea Japan Southeast Asia (Laos, Cambodia, Vietnam)	National language preference Dialects, written characters Use of silence Nonverbal and contextual cuing	Noncontact people	Present	Family: hierarchical structure, loyalty Devotion to tradition Many religions, including Taoism, Buddhism, Islam, and Christianity Community social organizations	Traditional health and illness beliefs Use of traditional medicines Traditional practitioners: Chinese doctors and herbalists	Liver cancer Stomach cancer Coccidioidomycosis Hypertension Lactose intolerance
African West Coast (as slaves) Many African countries West Indian Islands Dominican Republic Haiti Jamaica	National languages Dialect: Pidgin, Creole, Spanish, and French	Close personal space	Present over future	Family: many female, single parent Large, extended family networks Strong church affiliation within community Community social organizations	Traditional health and illness beliefs Folk medicine tradition Traditional healer: root-worker	Sickle cell anemia Hypertension Cancer of the esophagus Stomach cancer Coccidioidomycosis Lactose intolerance

Ethnic/cultural group	Language	Space/touch	Time orientation	Social organization	Health care	Common diseases
Europe Germany England Italy Ireland Other European countries	National languages Many learn English immediately	Noncontact people Aloof Distant Southern countries: closer contact and touch	Future over present	Nuclear families Extended families Judeo-Christian religions Community social organizations	Primary reliance on modern health care system Traditional health and illness beliefs Some remaining folk medicine traditions	Breast cancer Heart disease Diabetes mellitus Thalassemia
Native American 170 Native American tribes Aleuts Eskimos	Tribal languages Use of silence and body language	Space very important and has no boundaries	Present	Extremely family oriented Biological and extended families Children taught to respect traditions Community social organizations	Traditional health and illness beliefs Folk medicine tradition Traditional healer: medicine man	Accidents Heart disease Cirrhosis of the liver Diabetes mellitus
Hispanic countries Spain Cuba Mexico Central and South America	Spanish or Portuguese primary language	Tactile relationships Touch Handshakes Embracing Value physical presence	Present	Nuclear family Extended families *Compadrazzo:* godparents Community social organizations	Traditional health and illness beliefs Folk medicine tradition Traditional healers: *Curandero* *Espiritista* *Partera, senora*	Diabetes mellitus Parasites Coccidioidomycosis Lactose intolerance

From Specter R: Culture, ethnicity, and nursing. In Potter PA, Perry AG, editors: *Fundamentals of nursing: concepts, process, and practice,* ed 3, St. Louis, 1993, Mosby.

33

Characteristic Food Patterns of Some Cultures

Ethnic group	Milk group	Protein group	Fruits and vegetables	Breads and cereals	Possible dietary problems
Native American (many tribal variations; many "Americanized")	Fresh milk Evaporated milk for cooking Ice cream Cream pies	Pork, beef, lamb, rabbit Fowl, fish, eggs Legumes Sunflower seeds Nuts: walnut, acorn, pine, peanut butter	Green beans, peas Beets, turnips, squash, peppers Leafy green and other vegetables	Refined bread Whole wheat Cornmeal Rice Dry cereals "Fry" bread Tortillas	Obesity, diabetes, alcoholism, nutritional deficiencies expressed in dental problems and iron deficiency anemia Inadequate amounts of all nutrients Excessive use of sugar
Middle Eastern* (Armenian, Greek, Syrian, Turkish)	Yogurt Little butter	Game meat Lamb Nuts Dried peas, beans, lentils Sesame seeds	Peppers, tomatoes, cabbage, grape leaves, cucumbers, squash Dried apricots, raisins, dates	Cracked wheat and dark bread	Many fried meats and vegetables Lack of fresh fruits Insufficient foods from milk group High consumption of sweeteners, lamb fat, and olive oil
African-American	Milk† Ice cream Cheese: longhorn, American	Pork: all cuts, plus organs, chitterlings Beef, lamb Chicken, giblets	Leafy vegetables Green and yellow vegetables Potatoes: white, sweet	Cornmeal and hominy grits Rice Biscuits, pancakes, white breads	Extensive use of frying, "smothering" in gravy, or simmering Fats: salt pork, bacon drippings, lard, gravies High consumption of sweets

Group	Milk products	Meat and protein	Fruits and vegetables	Bread and cereals	Nutritional considerations
Chinese (Cantonese most prevalent)	Milk: water buffalo	Eggs, Nuts, Legumes, Fish, game, Pork sausage‡, Eggs and pigeon eggs, Fish, Lamb, beef, goat, Fowl: chicken, duck, Nuts, Legumes, Soybean curd (tofu)	Stewed fruit, Bananas and other fresh fruit, Many vegetables, Radish leaves, Bean/bamboo sprouts	Rice/rice flour products, Cereals, noodles, Wheat, corn, millet seed	Insufficient citrus; Vegetables often boiled for long periods with pork fat and much salt; Limited amounts from milk group; †Tendency of some immigrants to use large amounts of grease in cooking; Limited use of milk and milk products; Often low in protein, calories, or both; May wash rice before cooking, removing vitamins added in fortification; Soy sauce (high sodium)
Polish	Milk, Sour cream, Cheese, Butter	Pork (preferred), Chicken	Vegetables, Cabbage, Roots, Fruits	Dark rye	Sodium in ham, sausages, pickles; High consumption of sweets; Tendency to overcook vegetables; Limited fruits (especially citrus), raw vegetables, and meats

Continued.

From Wong D, Perry S: *Maternal-child nursing care*, St. Louis, 1998, Mosby.

*Religious holidays may involve fasting, which is believed to increase the likelihood of preterm labor. Fasting requirement may be waived during pregnancy.

†Lactose intolerance relatively common in adults.

‡Lower in fat content than Western sausage.

Characteristic Food Patterns of Some Cultures—cont'd

Ethnic group	Milk group	Protein group	Fruits and vegetables	Breads and cereals	Possible dietary problems
Puerto Rican	Limited use of milk products Coffee with milk (*café con leche*)	Pork Poultry Eggs (Fridays) Beans (*habichuelas*)	Avocado, okra Eggplant Sweet yams Starchy vegetables and fruits (*viandas*)	Rice Cornmeal	Small amounts of pork and poultry Extensive use of fat, lard, salt pork, and olive oil Lack of milk products
Scandinavian: Danish, Finnish, Norwegian, Swedish	Cream Butter Cheeses	Wild game Reindeer Fish (fresh or dried) Eggs	Berries Dried fruit Vegetables: cole slaw, roots	Whole wheat, rye, barley, sweets (cookies, sweet breads)	Insufficient fresh fruits and vegetables High consumption of sweets, pickled, salted meats/fish Liberal use of fat
Southeast Asian: Vietnamese, Cambodian	Generally not taken Coffee with condensed cow's milk Plain yogurt Ice cream (rare) Soybean milk	Fish (daily): fresh, dried, salted Poultry/eggs: duck, chicken Pork Beef (seldom) Dry beans Tofu	Seasonal variety: fresh or preserved Green, leafy vegetables Yams Corn	Rice: grains, flour, noodles French bread "Cellophane" (bean starch) noodles	Fresh milk products generally not consumed Poultry/eggs may be limited Meat considered "unclean" is avoided Preference for diet high in salt/pepper and rice/pork High intake of MSG and soy sauce

	Milk	Meat	Vegetables/Fruits	Breads/Cereals	Comments
Jewish: Orthodox*	Milk§ Cheese§	Meat (bloodless; Kosher prepared): beef, lamb, goat, deer, poultry (all types), no pork Fish with fins and scales only No crustaceans	Wide variety	Wide variety	High intake of sodium in meat products
Filipino (Spanish-Chinese influence)	Flavored milk, milk in coffee Cheese: gouda, cheddar	Pork, beef, goat, deer, rabbit Chicken Fish Eggs, nuts, legumes	Many vegetables and fruits	Rice, cooked cereals Noodles: rice, wheat	Limited use of milk and milk products Tendency to prewash rice Tendency to have only small portions of protein foods
Italian	Cheese Some ice cream	Meat Eggs Dried beans	Leafy vegetables Potatoes Eggplant, tomatoes, peppers Fruits	Pasta White breads, some whole wheat Farina Cereals	Prefer expensive imported cheeses; reluctant to substitute less expensive domestic varieties Tendency to overcook vegetables Limited use of whole grains High consumption of sweets Extensive use of olive oil Insufficient servings from milk group

MSG, Monosodium L-glutamate.

*Religious holidays may involve fasting, which is believed to increase the likelihood of preterm labor. Fasting requirement may be waived during pregnancy.

§Milk and milk products not eaten with meat; milk may be taken before meal or 6 hours after meal; different sets of dishes and silverware are used to serve milk and meat products.

Continued.

37

Characteristic Food Patterns of Some Cultures—cont'd

Ethnic group	Milk group	Protein group	Fruits and vegetables	Breads and cereals	Possible dietary problems
Japanese (Isei, more Japanese influence; Nisei, more westernized)	Increasing amounts being used by younger generations	Pork, beef, chicken Fish Eggs Legumes: soya, red, lima beans Tofu Nuts	Many vegetables and fruits Seaweed	Rice, rice cakes Wheat noodles Refined bread, noodles	Excessive sodium: pickles, salty crisp seaweed, MSG, soy sauce Insufficient servings from milk group May use prewashed rice
Hispanic, Mexican-American	Milk Cheese Flan, ice cream	Beef, pork, lamb, chicken, tripe, hot sausage, beef intestines Fish Eggs Nuts Dry beans: pinto, chickpeas (often eaten more than once daily)	Spinach, wild greens, tomatoes, chilies, corn, cactus leaves, cabbage, avocado, potatoes Pumpkin, zapote, peaches, guava, papaya, citrus	Rice, cornmeal Sweet bread, pastries Tortilla: corn, flour Vermicelli (fideo)	Limited meats primarily because of cost Limited use of milk and milk products Large amounts of lard Abundant use of sugar Tendency to boil vegetables for long periods

MSG, Monosodium L-glutamate.

Cultural and Regional Foods

Name of food	Culture/region	Type of food	Description
Adobo	Filipino	Meat	Meat with soy sauce
Ajinomoto	Japanese	Grain	Wheat germ
Anadama	New England	Grain	Cornmeal-molasses yeast bread
Arroz blanco	Puerto Rican	Grain	Enriched white rice
Bacalao	Puerto Rican	Meat	Salted codfish
Bagels	Jewish	Grain	Bread dough, doughnut shaped, boiled in water and baked
Baklava	Greek	Dessert	Layered pastry made with honey
Bok choy	Oriental	Vegetable	Green leafy, stalklike vegetable
Brioche	French	Grain	Egg-rich cake bread, used as sweet roll or shell for entrees
Bulgur	Middle Eastern	Grain	Granular wheat product with nutlike flavor
Burrito	Mexican	Combination	Sandwich; tortilla filled with beef-bean mixture and fried or baked
Café con leche	Latin American	Beverage	Coffee with milk
Cape Cod turkey	New England	Meat	Codfish balls
Challah	Jewish	Grain	Sabbath or holiday twisted eggbread
Chayote	Mexican	Vegetable	Squashlike vegetable
Chitterlings	Southern U.S.	Meat	Intestine of young pigs, soaked, boiled, and fried
Chorizo	Mexican	Meat	Sausage
Cilantro	Mexican	Seasoning	Coriander; similar to parsley
Crackling	Southern U.S.	Snack	Crispy pieces of fried pork fat
Croissants	French	Grain	Buttery, flaky, crescent-shaped rolls
Crumpets	English	Grain	Muffinlike product cooked on griddle and then toasted
Cush	Montana	Grain	Cornbread mixed with butter and water and fried

Continued.

Modified from Burtis G, Davis J, Martin S: *Applied nutrition and diet therapy*, Philadelphia, 1988, Saunders.

Cultural and Regional Foods—cont'd

Name of food	Culture/region	Type of food	Description
Dandelion greens	Southern U.S.	Vegetable	Leaves from dandelion plant
Dolmathes	Greek	Combination	Grape leaves stuffed with beef
Enchiladas	Mexican	Combination	Tortilla filled with meat and cheese
Escargots	French	Meat	Snails
Falafel	Jewish	Meat	Mashed chick-peas mixed with spices and fried
Fatback	Southern U.S.	Fat	Fat from loin of pig
Feijoada	Brazilian	Meat	Black beans with meat
Feta	Greek	Milk	Soft, salty white cheese from sheep's or goat's milk
Finnan haddie	Scottish	Meat	Salted, smoked haddock
Frijoles fritos	Mexican	Meat	Refried pinto beans
Gazpacho	Spanish	Soup	Cold soup with chopped tomatoes, green peppers, and cucumbers
Gefilte fish	Jewish	Meat	Seasoned fish ground and shaped into balls
Goulash	Hungarian	Meat	Stew seasoned with paprika
Grits	Southern U.S.	Grain	Hulled and coarsely ground corn
Guava	Cuban	Fruit	Small, yellow or red sweet tropical fruit
Gumbo	Creole	Combination	Well-seasoned okra stew with meat or seafood
Hangtown fry	California	Meat	Fried oysters and eggs
Hoecake	Southeast U.S.	Grain	Thin corn cake
Hoppin' John	Southern U.S.	Combination	Blackeyed peas and rice
Hush puppies	Southern U.S.	Grain	Fried cornbread
Jalapeños	Latin American	Vegetable	Hot peppers
Jambalaya	Creole	Combination	Well-seasoned combination of seafoods, tomatoes, and rice
Kale	Southern U.S.	Vegetable	Dark green leafy vegetable, similar to spinach
Kasha	Jewish	Grain	Coarsely ground buckwheat, toasted before cooking in liquid

Kelp	Oriental	Vegetable	Seaweed
Kibbeh	Middle East	Meat	Fresh raw lamb, ground and seasoned, similar to meat loaf
Kielbasa	Polish	Meat	Sausage
Kimchi	Korean	Vegetable	Peppery fermented combination of pickled cabbage, turnips, radishes, and other vegetables
Kuchen	German	Dessert	Yeast cake
Lard	—	Fat	Shortening-like product from pork
Latkas	Jewish	Grain	Pancakes, sometimes from potatoes
Limpa	Swedish	Grain	Rye bread
Lox	Jewish	Meat	Smoked salmon
Matzoh	Jewish	Grain	Unleavened bread
Menudo	Mexican	Meat	Stew made with tripe (cow's stomach)
Minestrone	Italian	Soup	Vegetable soup
Miso	Oriental	Meat	Fermented soybean paste
Mog maw	Southern U.S.	Meat	Stomach of pig
Moussaka	Greek	Combination	Meat and eggplant casserole
Mush	Southwest U.S.	Grain	Cooked cereal, usually cornmeal
Pandowdy	New England	Dessert	Dumplings and fruit
Papaya	—	Fruit	Large, yellow, melonlike tropical fruit
Pasta	Italian	Grain	Macaroni, spaghetti, and noodles in various shapes made from wheat
Pepperoni	Italian	Meat	Hot sausage
Phyllo	Greek	Grain	Paper-thin pastry for making meat, vegetables, cheese and egg dishes, and sweet pastries
Pilaf	Middle Eastern	Grain	Rice enriched with fat and sometimes vegetables, bits of meat, and spices
Poi	Polynesian	Vegetable	Root vegetable, especially taro, cooked and pounded, mixed with water, and sometimes fermented

Continued.

Cultural and Regional Foods—cont'd

Name of food	Culture/region	Type of food	Description
Polenta	Italian	Grain	Cornmeal or cornmeal mush
Polk	Southern U.S.	Vegetable	Dark green leafy vegetable
Pot liquor (likker)	Southern U.S.	Vegetable	Liquid from cooking green vegetables or bones
Potato knishes	Jewish	Vegetable	Potato pancakes
Prickly pear	Native American	Fruit	Fruit of cactus
Prosciutto	Italian	Meat	Ready-to-eat, cured, smoked ham
Pumpernickel	—	Grain	Yeast bread with wheat, corn, rye, and potatoes
Ratatouille	French	Vegetable	Well-seasoned casserole of eggplant, zucchini, tomato, and green pepper
Redeye gravy	Southern U.S.	Gravy	Fried ham gravy
Sake	Oriental	Beverage	Rice wine
Salt pork	Southern U.S.	Fat	Salted pork fat from the belly
Sancocho	Puerto Rican	Combination	Soup with meat and viandas
Sashimi	Japanese	Meat	Raw fish
Sauerbraten	German	Meat	Pot roast in spicy, aromatic, sweet-and-sour marinade
Scones	English	Grain	Round, flat, unleavened sweetened bread

Scrapple	Pennsylvania Dutch	Combination	Solid mush from cornmeal and the by-products of hog butchering
Shoofly pie	Pennsylvania Dutch	Dessert	Molasses pie
Shoyu	Japanese	Seasoning	Soy sauce
Sofrito	Puerto Rican	Seasoning	Specially seasoned tomato sauce
Sopapillas	Mexican	Grain	Rich fried bread
Spatzle	German	Grain	Small dumplings
Spoonbread	Virginia	Grain	Baked dish with cornmeal
Spumoni	Italian	Dessert	Fruited ice cream
Stollen	German	Dessert	Christmas fruitcake
Stricle sheets	Pennsylvania Dutch	Dessert	Coffee cake
Strudel	German	Dessert	Light pastry filled with fruit or cheese
Tacos	Mexican	Combination	Fried tortillas filled with meat, vegetables, and hot sauce
Tamales	Mexican	Grain	Pancakelike leathery bread
Tempura	Japanese	Combination	Deep-fried seafood or vegetables
Teriyaki sauce	Hawaiian	Accessory	Sweetened soy sauce
Tofu	Oriental	Meat	Soybean curd
Trotters	Southern U.S.	Meat	Pig's feet
Viandas	Puerto Rican	Vegetable	Starchy tropical vegetables, including plantain, green bananas, and sweet potatoes

Cultural Behaviors Relevant to Health Assessment

Cultural group	Cultural variations (common belief/practice)	Nursing implications
African-Americans	Dialect and slang terms require careful communication to prevent error (e.g., "bad" may mean "good").	Question the client's meaning or intent.
Mexican-Americans	Eye behavior is important. An individual who looks at and admires a child without touching the child has given the child the "evil eye."	Always touch the child you are examining or admiring.
Native Americans	Eye contact is considered a sign of disrespect and is thus avoided.	Recognize that the client may be attentive and interested even though eye contact is avoided. Avoid excessive eye contact.
Appalachians	Eye contact is considered impolite or a sign of hostility. Verbal patter may be confusing.	Clarify statements.
American Eskimos	Body language is very important. The individual seldom disagrees publicly with others. Client may nod yes to be polite, even if not in agreement.	Monitor own body language closely, as well as client's, to detect meaning.

Jewish-Americans	Orthodox Jews consider excess touching, particularly from members of the opposite sex, offensive.	Establish whether client is an Orthodox Jew and avoid excessive touch.
Chinese-Americans	Individual may nod head to indicate yes or shake head to indicate no. Excessive eye contact indicates rudeness. Excessive touch is offensive.	Ask questions carefully and clarify responses. Avoid excessive eye contact and touch.
Filipino-Americans	Offending people is to be avoided at all costs. Nonverbal behavior is very important.	Monitor nonverbal behaviors of self and client, being sensitive to physical and emotional discomfort or concerns of the client. Use direct eye contact when communicating.
Haitian-Americans	Touch is used in conversation. Direct eye contact is used to gain attention and respect during communication. Women avoid eye contact as a sign of respect.	
East Indian Hindu-Americans	Avoidance of eye contact is a sign of respect.	Be aware that men may view eye contact by women as offensive. Avoid eye contact. Limit eye contact.
Vietnamese-Americans	The head is considered sacred; it is not polite to pat the head. An upturned palm is offensive in communication.	Touch the head only when mandated and explain clearly before proceeding to do so. Avoid hand gesturing.

From Kozier B et al.: *Techniques in clinical nursing*, ed 2, Menlo Park, Calif, 1993, Addison-Wesley.

Folk Healing Practices

Practice name	Ethnicity	Practice procedure	Purpose
Acupuncture	Asian (Chinese)	Needles in meridians (energy lines), herbs	Pain, sinus problems, injuries, stress, stroke, deafness, epilepsy, and so on
Cao Gio	Vietnamese, Cambodian	Coining produces ecchymosis, petechiae	Coughing, congestion, fever
Curanderismo	Hispanic	Bleeding, herbs, emetics, diuretics, prayers, penance, miracles	Physiological or psychological problems, social maladjustment
Folk practitioners	Haitian	Poultices, voodoo	Evil eye lifted
Hilot	Filipino	Faith healing through prayer, herbal medicine, massage, manipulation of bones and tissues	Most illnesses
Medicine men	Native American	Meditation, sweat lodges, herbal medicine, ritual	Any disease caused by an imbalance with nature
Moxa	Chinese	Burning of a plant on the skin	Mumps, convulsions, epistaxis
Root doctor	African-American	Herbs, laying on of hands	Any illness
Spiritual healer	White	Laying on of hands	Physiological, psychological, or social problems

Modified from Starn J: Family culture and chronic conditions. In Jackson PL, Vessey JA: *Primary care of the child with a chronic condition*, ed 2, St. Louis, 1996, Mosby.

Healers and Their Scope of Practice

Culture/folk practitioner	Preparation	Scope of practice
Hispanic Family member	Possesses knowledge of folk medicine.	Common illnesses of a mild nature that may or may not be recognized by modern medicine.
Curandero	May receive training in an apprenticeship. May receive a "gift from God" that enables her/him to cure. Knowledgeable in use of herbs, diet, massage, and rituals.	Treats almost all of the traditional illnesses. Some may not treat illness caused by witchcraft for fear of being accused of possessing evil powers. Usually admired by members of the community.
Espiritualista or spiritualist	Born with the special gifts of being able to analyze dreams and foretell future events. May serve apprenticeship with an older practitioner.	Emphasis on prevention of illness or bewitchment through use of medals, prayers, amulets. May also be sought for cure of existing illness.
Yerbero	No formal training. Knowledgeable in growing and prescribing herbs.	Consulted for preventive and curative use of herbs for both traditional and Western illnesses.
Sabador (may refer to a chiropractor by this title)	Knowledgeable in massage and manipulation of bones and muscles.*	Treats many traditional illnesses, particularly those affecting the musculoskeletal system. May also treat nontraditional illnesses.

Continued.

From Hautman MA: Folk health and illness beliefs, *Nurse Pract* 4(4):31, 1979.
*Preparation is for *sabador,* not chiropractor.

Healers and Their Scope of Practice—cont'd

Culture/folk practitioner	Preparation	Scope of practice
Blacks		
"Old lady"	Usually an older woman who has successfully raised her own family. Knowledgeable in child care and folk remedies.	Consulted about common ailments and for advice on child care. Found in rural and urban communities.
Spiritualist	Called by God to help others. No formal training. Usually associated with a fundamentalist Christian church.	Assists with problems that are financial, personal, spiritual, or physical. Predominantly found in urban communities.
Voodoo priest(ess) or *houngan*	May be trained by other priests(esses). In the United States the eldest son of a priest becomes a priest. A daughter of a priest(ess) becomes a priestess if she is born with a veil (amniotic sac) over her face.	Knowledgeable about properties of herbs; interpretation of signs and omens. Able to cure illness caused by voodoo. Uses communication techniques to establish a therapeutic milieu like psychiatrist. Treats Blacks, Mexican-Americans, and Native Americans.
Chinese		
Herbalist	Knowledgeable in diagnosis of illness and herbal remedies.	Both diagnostic and therapeutic. Diagnostic techniques include interviewing, inspection, auscultation, and assessment of pulses.

FAMILY ASSESSMENT

Family Coping Index

The family coping index was developed in 1964 as a tool for practice, as an approach to identifying the family need for nursing care and assessing the potential for behavioral changes, and as a method of determining in a more systematic way how the nurse can help the family to manage. This index continues to be used today as a relevant method of evaluating a family's ability to cope with life's daily challenges.

Scaling Cues

The following descriptive statements are "cues" to help you as you rate family coping. They are limited to three points: *1,* or no competence; *3,* moderate competence; and *5,* complete competence. You will find, however, that most families will fall somewhere in between these points. Mark the point you feel most nearly describes the level of competence they have. The descriptions are not complete but suggestive. In the long run it is your own professional judgment that will be needed to make a decision. When there is no problem or the area is not relevant, check the "no problem" column.

1. Physical independence

This category is concerned with ability to move about, for example, to get in and out of bed and to take care of daily grooming and walking. Note that it is the *family* competence that is measured—even though an individual is dependent, if the family is able to compensate for this the family may be independent. However, the quality as well as quantity of ability is important; hence, if the *focus* of care is poor—if a mother is giving care to a handicapped child that the child could give himself/herself, or if one person is giving care that should be shared with other members—the independence might be considered incomplete. The *causes* of dependence may vary—lack of physical independence in the family may be due to actual physical incapacity, to lack of "know-how," or to unwillingness or fear of doing the necessary tasks.

Developed jointly by the Richmond IVNA City Nursing Service and the Johns Hopkins School of Hygiene and Public Health, 1964. In Freeman R, Heinrich J: *Community health nursing practice*, ed 2, Philadelphia, 1981, Saunders.

1 = Family failing entirely to provide required personal care to one or more of its members. *Examples:* arthritic client unable to get out of bed alone, no one available to help; client "cannot" give his/her hypodermic medication because of fear.

3 = Family providing partially for needs of its members or providing care for some members but not for others. *Examples:* mother may be doing well with own and husband's care but failing to give daily care efficiently to newborn baby; daughter may be giving excellent physical care to aged mother but at cost of neglecting children somewhat, or with poor body mechanics that place undue strain upon herself.

5 = All family members, whether or not there is infirmity or disability in one or more members, are receiving the necessary care to maintain cleanliness, including skin care, are able to get about as far as possible within their physical abilities; are receiving assistance when needed without interruption or undue delay.

2. Therapeutic competence

This category includes all of the procedures or treatment prescribed for the care of illness, such as giving medications and using appliances (including crutches), dressings, exercises and relaxation, and special diets.

1 = Family either not carrying out procedures prescribed or doing it unsafely. For example, giving several medications without being able to distinguish one from the other, or taking them inappropriately, applying braces so they throw the limb out of line, measuring insulin incorrectly. Family resents, rejects, or refuses to give necessary care.

3 = Family carrying out some but not all of the treatments—for example, giving insulin but not adhering strictly to diet; carrying out procedures awkwardly, ineffectively, or with resentment or unnecessary anxiety. For example, crutch walking may be done, but with the helper using poor body mechanics or not giving the client enough security and confidence; client may give own hypodermic, but say, "I dread it every time." May be giving medications correctly, but not understanding purposes of the drug or symptoms to be observed.

5 = Family able to demonstrate that they can carry out the prescribed procedures safely and efficiently, with the understanding of the principles involved and with a confident and willing attitude.

3. Knowledge of health condition

This category is concerned with the particular health condition that is the occasion for care, for example, knowledge of the disease or disability, understanding of communicability of disease and modes of transmission, understanding of general pattern of development of a newborn baby and the basic needs of infants for physical care and tender loving care (TLC).

1 = Totally uninformed or misinformed about the condition. For example, believes tuberculosis is caused by sin, or syphilis cured when symptoms subside; believes stroke clients must be bedridden, and that it is cruel to make them do for themselves; that overweight in the school-age child is "healthy."

3 = Has some general knowledge of the disease or condition, but has not grasped the underlying principles, or is only partially informed. For instance, may recognize need for TLC but not relate this to placing the baby's crib near people when the baby is awake or holding the baby when feeding; may accept fact that client is dying but not see need to prepare family for this event; may understand dietary and insulin control of diabetes, but not needs such as special care of feet.

5 = Knows the salient facts about the disease well enough to take necessary action at the proper time, understands the rationale of care, able to observe and report significant symptoms.

4. Application of principles of personal and general hygiene

This is concerned with family action in relation to maintaining family nutrition, securing adequate rest and relaxation for family members, and carrying out accepted preventive measures such as immunizations, medical appraisal, and safe homemaking habits in relation to storing and preparing food.

1 = Family diet grossly inadequate or unbalanced, necessary immunizations not secured for children; house dirty, food handled in unsanitary way; members of family working beyond reasonable limits; children and adults getting too little sleep; family members unkempt, dirty, inadequately clothed in relation to weather.

3 = Failing to apply some general principles of hygiene—for instance, keeping house in excellent condition but expending too much energy and becoming overfatigued as a result; secured initial immunizations but not boosters, or some but not all available immunizations; general diet and homemaking skills good, but father carrying two full-time jobs.

5 = Household runs smoothly, family meals well selected; habits of sleep and rest adequate to needs.

5. Health care attitudes

This category is concerned with the way the family feels about health care in general, including preventive services, care of illness, and public health measures.

1 = Family resents and resists all health care; has no confidence in doctors, uses patent medicines and quack nostrums, feels illness is unavoidable and to be borne rather than treated; feels community health agencies should not interfere or bother the family members; practices folk medicine or superstitious rites in illness.

3 = Accepts health care in some degree, but with reservations. For example, may accept need for medical care for illness, but not general preventive measures; may have confidence in doctors generally, but not in the clinic or "free" doctors; may feel certain illnesses are hopeless (such as cancer), or care unnecessary—for instance, dental care for the young child.

5 = Understands and recognizes need for medical care in illness and for the usual preventive services, arranges for periodic physical appraisals and follows through with recommendations, accepts illness calmly and recognizes the limits it imposes while doing all possible to effect recovery and rehabilitation.

6. Emotional competence

This category has to do with the maturity and integrity with which the members of the family are able to meet the usual stresses and problems of life, and to plan for happy and fruitful living. This involves the degree to which individuals accept the necessary disciplines imposed by one's family and culture; the development and maintenance of individual responsibility and decision; and willingness to meet reasonable obligations, to accept adversity with fortitude, and to consider the needs of others as well as one's own.

1 = Family does not face realities—assumes moribund client will get well, that they can eventually pay a hospital bill far beyond their means, that an unwanted pregnancy is not so; one or more members lacking in any emotional control—uncontrollable rages, irresponsible sexual activities; one or more members alcoholic, family torn, suspicious of one another; evidences of great insecurity, guilt, or anxiety.

3 = Family members usually do fairly well, but one or more members evidence lack of security or maturity. For example, thumb sucking in late childhood; unusual concern with what the neighbors will think; failure to plan ahead for foreseeable emergencies; leaving children unattended, "fighting" in the family on occasion.

5 = All members of the family are able to maintain a reasonable degree of emotional calm, face up to illness realistically and hopefully; are able to discuss problems and differences with objectivity and reasonable emotional control; do not worry unduly about trivial matters, consider the needs and wishes of other family members, of neighbors, and of those with whom they work and live in making decisions or deciding upon action.

7. Family living patterns

This category is concerned largely with the interpersonal or group aspects of family life—how well the members of the family get along with one another, the ways in which they make decisions affecting the family as a whole, the degree to which they support one another and do things as a family, the degree of respect and affection they show for one another, the ways in which they manage the family budget, the kind of discipline that prevails.

1 = Family consists of a group of individuals indifferent or hostile to one another, or strongly dominated and controlled by a single family member; no control of children, or family members so totally dependent on one another that they are being stifled—for example, mother developing habits of dependence in sons so as to threaten future capacity for independence in own family life, no rational plan for managing available money; "battered" child.

3 = Family gets along but has habits or customs that interfere with their effectiveness or coherence as a family. For example, family members fond of one another, have many home activities, but dominated by a father in a kindly way; recreational habits separate family much of the time; children somewhat overprotected; expectations of the children unrealistic, for example, parents expecting children with low academic competence to enter professions.

5 = Family cohesive, does things together, each member acts with regard for the good of the family as a whole; children respect parents and vice versa; family tasks shared; evidence of planning.

8. Physical environment

This category is concerned with the home and community or work environment as it affects family health. This includes the conditions for housing, presence of accident hazards, screening, plumbing, facilities for cooking and for privacy; level of community (deteriorated or modern, presence of social hazards such as bars, street gangs, delinquency, pests such as rats), availability and condition of schools, and transportation.

1 = House in poor condition, unsafe, unscreened, poorly heated, neighborhood deteriorated, juvenile and adult delinquency among neighbors, no play space except streets.

3 = House requires some repair or painting but fundamentally sound; neighborhood poor but possible to protect children from social influence through school or other community activities; house crowded but adjustments to this fairly adequate.

5 = House in good repair, provides for privacy for members and is free of accidents and pest hazards; neighborhood respectable and provided with play space for children; free from undesirable social elements; opportunities for community activity.

9. Use of community facilities

This category has to do with the degree to which the family members know about and the wisdom with which they use available community resources for health, education, and welfare. This would include the ways in which they use services of private physicians, clinics, emergency rooms, hospitals, schools, welfare organizations, churches, and so forth. The *coping ability* does not indicate the level of the *need* for services, but rather the degree to which they can cope when they must seek such aid. Even though they have a severe housing problem, if they have used all appropriate facilities for enforcing landlord's compliance with sanitary regulations to secure public housing, their coping capacity in relation to *use* of community facilities is high, even though the underlying condition is not corrected.

1 = Family has obvious and serious social needs, but has not sought or found any help for them. For example, a family may be borrowing unreasonable sums of money for medical care, while not using available free hospitals or clinics; or leaving children without any supervision while the mother works; or failing to take steps to register for public housing when it is indicated. Using resources inappropriately, for example, calling ambulance or using emergency services for minor ills.

3 = Family knows about or uses some, but not all of the available community resources that are needed. For example, the family may be under welfare care, and know how to use the social worker responsible for their care, but have not recognized that the counselor in the school could help with educational planning, or that the church might provide recreational activities for the children as well as spiritual guidance.

5 = Family using the facilities they need appropriately and promptly. Know when to call for help and whom to call. Feel secure in their relationship with community workers such as social workers, teachers, and doctors.

Family coping estimate

Family _____   Nurse _____   Date _____

Initial _____   Periodic _____   Discharge _____

Coping area	Rating x-status 0-est. change Poor. . . . . . Excellent	Justification
Physical independence	1 2 3 4 5 Not applicable ☐	
Therapeutic independence	1 2 3 4 5 Not applicable ☐	
Knowledge of condition	1 2 3 4 5 Not applicable ☐	
Application of principles of hygiene	1 2 3 4 5 Not applicable ☐	
Attitude toward health care	1 2 3 4 5 Not applicable ☐	
Emotional competence	1 2 3 4 5 Not applicable ☐	
Family living patterns	1 2 3 4 5 Not applicable ☐	
Physical environment	1 2 3 4 5 Not applicable ☐	
Use of community resources	1 2 3 4 5 Not applicable ☐	

Comments

Sample Format for a Cross-Cultural Assessment of a Family With a Member With a Chronic Condition

Area of concern	Sample questions
Family demographics	Who lives in your family (i.e., members, ages, sexes)?
	What kind of work do members of the household do?
	What is your family's socioeconomic status?
	What kind of health insurance coverage do you have?
	Which family members are covered?
	What chronic conditions or symptoms do you have?
	How would you describe the problems that have brought you here today?
	Who is the primary caretaker in your family?
Orientation	Where were the members of the family born?
	What is the ethnic background of the family members?
	How many years have family members lived in the United States? (NOTE: Only ask if appropriate.)
	In your family is it important to be on time for an appointment or to get to an appointment when possible based on everyone's schedule for that day?
	Why do you think you have (the above-named) chronic condition (e.g., punishment for a parent's past behavior, such as conceiving a child out of wedlock; the result of a genetic problem; or a gift given because of the family's patience and love)?
Communication	What language(s) and dialect(s) are spoken at home?
	Who reads English in the family? If no one reads English, in what language would you prefer printed materials?
	Do parents and children look when spoken to or do they look down? To whom should questions be addressed?
	(NOTE: Avoid using a child as a translator, if at all possible, because of the strain this task imposes.)
Family relationships	Besides the immediate household, who else makes up the members of this family?
	Who makes the decisions in this family (e.g., mother-in-law, father, both partners, other family or friends, group decision)?

Modified from Starn J: Family culture and chronic conditions. In Jackson PL, Vessey JA: *Primary care of the child with a chronic condition*, ed 2, St. Louis, 1996, Mosby.

Sample Format for a Cross-Cultural Assessment of a Family With a Member With a Chronic Condition—cont'd

Area of concern	Sample questions
Family relationships—cont'd	Who cares for the client and the client's medical needs?
	What are the housing arrangements (e.g., space, number of rooms, members living in the home)?
	What is the family's usual daily routine like?
	To whom do you turn when you need help with, or have questions about, your condition?
Beliefs about health	What is the present health status of family members?
	What illnesses or conditions are present in the current family members?
	What illnesses or conditions were present in deceased family members?
	How often and for what reasons have family members used Western medicine in the past?
	What complementary therapies are used by your family routinely and specifically for the client (e.g., acupuncture, healers, prayer, massage)?
	What do you do when you are in pain?
	Is it important to keep the client at home or to use institutional placement?
	What do you think will help clear up the problem?
	Are there things that help you get better about which the health care providers should know?
	What problems has your illness caused your family?
Education	How much schooling have members of the family completed?
	What ways are the best for you to learn about your condition (e.g., pamphlets, videos, direct patient teaching, home visits, return demonstrations)?
	From whom are you most comfortable learning about your condition (e.g., doctor, nurse, social worker, home health aide, other family members)?
Religion	What religion(s) are practiced in your family?
	What religious things do you do to help yourself or your family (e.g., pray, meditate, attend a support group, practice the laying on of hands)?
	What things does your religion say you should *not* do (e.g., have blood transfusions, allow strangers or dangerous circumstances to affect you or your family)?
Nutrition	When are usual mealtimes for your family?
	With whom do you eat?
	What foods do you usually eat?
	What special foods do you eat when you are sick?
	What foods do you *not* eat and when?

Family APGAR Questionnaire

Part I

The following questions have been designed to help us better understand you and your family. You should feel free to ask questions about any item in the questionnaire.

The space for comments should be used when you wish to give additional information or if you wish to discuss the way the question is applied to your family. Please try to answer all questions.

Family is defined as the individual(s) with whom you usually live. If you live alone, your "family" consists of persons with whom you now have the strongest emotional ties.*

For each question, check only one box.

	Almost always	Some of the time	Hardly ever
I am satisfied that I can turn to my family for help when something is troubling me.	☐	☐	☐

Comments: _____

_____

| I am satisfied that my family talks over things with me and shares problems with me. | ☐ | ☐ | ☐ |

Comments: _____

| I am satisfied that my family accepts and supports my wishes to take on new activities or directions. | ☐ | ☐ | ☐ |

Comments: _____

| I am satisfied that my family expresses affection and responds to my emotions such as anger, sorrow, and love. | ☐ | ☐ | ☐ |

Comments: _____

_____

Modified from Smilkstein G et al.: Validity and reliability of the family by APGAR as a test of family function, *J Fam Prac* 15(2):303-311, 1982.

*According to which member of the family is being interviewed, the nurse may substitute for the word "family" either spouse, significant other, parents, or children.

Family APGAR Questionnaire—cont'd

	Almost always	Some of the time	Hardly ever
I am satisfied with the way my family and I share time together.	☐	☐	☐

Comments: _____

_____

Scoring. The client checks one of three choices, which is scored as follows: "Almost always" (2 points), "Some of the time" (1 point), or "Hardly ever" (0 points). The scores for each of the five questions are then totaled. A score of 7 to 10 suggests a highly functional family. A score of 4 to 6 suggests a moderately dysfunctional family. A score of 0 to 3 suggests a severely dysfunctional family.

Notes

Part II

Who lives in your home?* List the persons according to their relationship to you (for example, spouse, significant other,† child, or friend).

Check the column that best describes how you now get along with each member of the family listed.

Relationship	Age	Sex

Well	Fairly	Poorly

If you do not live with your own family, list the persons to whom you turn for help most frequently. List according to relationship (for example, family member, friend, associate at work, or neighbor).

Check the column that best describes how you now get along with each person listed.

Relationship	Age	Sex

Well	Fairly	Poorly

*If you have established your own family, consider your "home" as the place where you live with your spouse, children, or "significant other" (see next footnote for definition). Otherwise, consider home as your place of origin, for example, the place where your parents or those who raised you live.

†Significant other is the partner you live with in a physically and emotionally nurturing relationship but to whom you are not married.

CHILD ASSESSMENT

Pediatric Health History

The outline below provides a systematic procedure for completing a child health history. It is especially useful before completing a physical assessment to give the nurse essential background for health care planning.

Identifying information

1. Name
2. Address
3. Telephone number
4. Age and birth date
5. Birthplace
6. Race
7. Sex
8. Religion
9. Nationality
10. Date of interview
11. Informant

Additional information appropriate to older adolescent may include occupation, marital status, and temporary and permanent address.

Under informant include subjective impression of reliability, general attitude, willingness to communicate, overall accuracy of data, and any special circumstances such as use of an interpreter.

Informants should include parent and child, as well as others who may be primary caregivers, such as grandparent.

Chief complaint (CC)

To establish the major specific reason for the individual's seeking professional health attention.

Record in client's own words; include duration of symptoms.
If informant has difficulty isolating *one* problem, ask which problem or symptom led person to seek help *now*.
In case of routine physical examination, state CC as reason for visit.

Modified from Wong DL, Whaley LF: *Whaley and Wong's essentials of pediatric nursing,* ed 5, St. Louis, 1997, Mosby.

Present illness (PI)

To obtain all details related to the chief complaint.

In its broadest sense, *illness* denotes any problem of a physical, emotional, or psychosocial nature.

1. Onset
   a. Date of onset
   b. Manner of onset (gradual or sudden)
   c. Precipitating and predisposing factors related to onset (emotional disturbance, physical exertion, fatigue, bodily function, pregnancy, environment, injury, infection, toxins and allergens, or therapeutic agents)
2. Characteristics
   a. Character (quality, quantity, consistency, or other)
   b. Location and radiation (i.e., pain)
   c. Intensity or severity
   d. Timing (continuous or intermittent, duration of each, temporal relationship to other events)
   e. Aggravating and relieving factors
   f. Associated symptoms

Present information in chronological order; may be referenced according to one point in time, such as *prior to admission* (PTA).

3. Course since onset
   a. Incidence
      (1) Single acute attack
      (2) Recurrent acute attacks
      (3) Daily occurrences
      (4) Periodic occurrences
      (5) Continuous chronic episode
   b. Progress (better, worse, unchanged)
   c. Effect of therapy

Concentrate on reason for seeking help now, especially if problem has existed for some time.

Past history (PH)

To elicit a profile of the individual's previous illnesses, injuries, or operations.

1. Pregnancy (maternal)
   a. Number (gravida)
      (1) Dates of delivery

    b. Outcome (parity)
        (1) Gestation (full-term, premature, postmature)
        (2) Stillbirths, abortions
    c. Health during pregnancy
    d. Medications taken

Importance of perinatal history depends on child's age; the younger the child, the more important the perinatal history.

Explain relevance of obstetrical history in revealing important factors relating to the child's health.

Assess parents' emotional attitudes toward the pregnancy and birth.

  2. Labor and delivery
    a. Duration of labor
    b. Type of delivery
    c. Place of delivery
    d. Medications

Assess parent's feelings regarding delivery; investigate factors affecting bonding, such as if awake and able to hold infant or if asleep and separated from infant.

  3. Birth
    a. Weight and length
    b. Time of regaining birth weight
    c. Condition of health
    d. APGAR score
    e. Presence of congenital anomalies
    f. Date of discharge from nursery

If birth problems are reported, inquire about treatment, such as use of oxygen, phototherapy, or surgery, and parents' emotional response to the event.

  4. Previous illnesses, operations, or injuries
    a. Onset, symptoms, course, termination
    b. Occurrence of complications
    c. Incidence of disease in other family members or in community

Make positive statement about diphtheria, scarlet fever, measles, chicken pox, mumps, tonsillitis, pertussis, and common illnesses such as colds, earaches, or sore throats.

Elicit a description of disease to verify the diagnosis.

    d. Emotional response to previous hospitalization
    e. Circumstances and nature of injuries

Be alert to areas of injury prevention.

5. Allergies
    a. Hay fever, asthma, or eczema

Have parent describe the type of allergic reaction.

    b. Unusual reactions to foods, drugs, animals, plants, or household products

Note sensitivity to egg albumin and reactions to certain immunizations.

6. Current medications
    a. Name, dose, schedule, duration, and reason for administration

Assess parents' knowledge of correct dosage of common drugs such as acetaminophen; note underusage or overusage.

7. Immunizations
    a. Name, number of doses, ages when given
    b. Occurrence of reaction
    c. Administration of horse or other foreign serum, gamma globulin, or blood transfusion

May refer to immunization as "baby shots."
Whenever possible, confirm information by checking medical or school records.

8. Growth and development
    a. Weight at birth, 6 months, 1 year, and present
    b. Dentition
        (1) Age of eruption/shedding
        (2) Number
        (3) Problems with teething
    c. Age of head control, sitting unsupported, walking, first words
    d. Present grade in school, scholastic achievement
    e. Interaction with peers and adults
    f. Participation in organized activities such as scouts and sports

Compare parents' responses with own observations of child's achievement and results from objective tests such as Denver II or DASE.
School and social history can be more thoroughly explored under Family Assessment.

9. Habits
    a. Behavior patterns
        (1) Nail biting
        (2) Thumb sucking

(3) Pica
(4) Rituals such as "security blanket"
(5) Unusual movements (headbanging, rocking)
(6) Temper tantrums

Assess parents' attitudes toward habits and any remedies used to curtail them, such as punishment for bed-wetting.

b. Activities of daily living
  (1) Hour of sleep and arising
  (2) Duration of nocturnal sleep/naps
  (3) Age of toilet training
  (4) Pattern of stools and urination; occurrence of enuresis

Record child's usual terms for defecation and urination.

  (5) Type of exercise
c. Use/abuse of drugs, alcohol, coffee, or cigarettes

With adolescents, estimate the quantity of drugs used.

d. Usual disposition; response to frustration

Review of systems (ROS)

To elicit information concerning any potential health problem.

1. **General**—overall state of health, fatigue, recent or unexplained weight gain or loss, period of time for either, contributing factors (change of diet, illness, altered appetite), exercise tolerance, fevers (time of day), chills, night sweats (unrelated to climatic conditions), frequent infections, general ability to carry out activities of daily living

Explain relevance of questioning to parents (similar to pregnancy section) in comprising total health history of child.

Make positive statements about each system, for example, "Mother denies headaches, bumping into objects, squinting, or excessive rubbing of eyes."

Use terms parents are likely to understand, such as "bruises" for ecchymoses.

2. **Integument**—pruritus, pigment or other color changes, acne, eruptions, rashes (location), tendency for bruising, petechiae, excessive dryness, general texture, disorders or deformities of nails, hair growth or loss, hair color change (for adolescent, use of hair dyes or other potentially toxic substances such as hair straighteners)
3. **Head**—headaches, dizziness, injury (specific details)

4. **Eyes**—visual problems (ask about behaviors that indicate blurred vision, such as bumping into objects, clumsiness, sitting very close to television, holding a book close to the face, writing with head near desk, squinting, rubbing the eyes, bending the head in an awkward position), "cross-eye" (strabismus), eye infections, edema of lids, excessive tearing, use of glasses or contact lenses, date of last optic examination

5. **Nose**—nosebleeds (epistaxis), constant or frequent running or stuffy nose, nasal obstruction (difficulty in breathing), sense of smell

6. **Ears**—earaches, discharge, evidence of hearing loss (ask about behaviors such as need to repeat requests, loud speech, inattentive behavior), results of any previous auditory testing

7. **Mouth**—mouth breathing, gum bleeding, toothaches, toothbrushing, use of fluoride, difficulty with teething (symptoms), last visit to dentist (especially if temporary dentition is complete), response to dentist

8. **Throat**—sore throats, difficulty in swallowing, choking (especially when chewing food, which may be caused by poor chewing habits), hoarseness or other voice irregularities

9. **Neck**—pain, limitation of movement, stiffness, difficulty in holding head straight (torticollis), thyroid enlargement, enlarged nodes or other masses

10. **Chest**—breast enlargement, discharge, masses, enlarged axillary nodes (for adolescent female, ask about breast self-examination)

11. **Respiratory**—chronic cough, frequent colds (number per year), wheezing, shortness of breath at rest or on exertion, difficulty in breathing, sputum production, infections (pneumonia, tuberculosis), date of last chest x-ray examination; date of last tuberculin test and type of reaction, if any

12. **Cardiovascular**—cyanosis or fatigue on exertion, history of heart murmur or rheumatic fever, anemia, date of last blood count, blood type, recent transfusion

13. **Gastrointestinal**—(much of this in regard to appetite, food tolerance, and elimination habits has been asked elsewhere) concentrate on nausea, vomiting (if not associated with eating, it may indicate brain tumor or increased intracranial pressure), jaundice or yellowing skin or sclera, belching, flatulence, recent change in bowel habits (blood in stools, change of color, diarrhea, or constipation)

14. **Genitourinary**—pain on urination, frequency, hesitancy, urgency, hematuria, nocturia, polyuria, unpleasant odor of urine, direction and force of stream, discharge, change in size of scrotum,

date of last urinalysis (for adolescent, sexually transmitted disease, type of treatment; for adolescent male, ask about testicular self-examination)

15. **Gynecological**—menarche, date of last menstrual period, regularity or problems with menstruation, vaginal discharge, pruritus, date and result of last Pap test (include obstetrical history as discussed under birth history when applicable), if sexually active, type of contraception
16. **Musculoskeletal**—weakness, clumsiness, lack of coordination, unusual movements, back or joint stiffness, muscle pains or cramps, abnormal gait, deformity, fractures, serious sprains, activity level
17. **Neurological**—seizures, tremors, dizziness, loss of memory, general affect, fears, nightmares, speech problems, any unusual habits
18. **Endocrine**—intolerance to weather changes, excessive thirst, excessive sweating, salty taste to skin, signs of early puberty

Nutrition history
To elicit information about adequacy of child's dietary intake and eating patterns.

Family medical history
To identify the presence of genetic traits or diseases that have familial tendencies; to assess family habits and exposure to a communicable disease that may affect family members.

Choose terms wisely when asking about child's parentage, for example, inquire about paternal history by referring to the child's "father" rather than mother's husband; use term "partner" rather than spouse.

1. Family pedigree and guidelines for construction

A pedigree is a pictorial representation or diagram of a family tree to visualize patterns of disease transmission.

2. Familial diseases and congenital anomalies, such as heart disease, hypertension, cancer, diabetes mellitus, obesity, allergy, asthma, tuberculosis, sickle cell disease, mental retardation, convulsions, insanity or other emotional problems, syphilis, or rheumatic fever; indicate symptoms, treatment, and sequelae
3. Family habits such as smoking or chemical use
4. Geographical location such as recent travel or contact with foreign visitors

This is important for identification of endemic diseases.

Family personal/social history

To gain an understanding of the family's structure and function.

Sexual history

To elicit information concerning young person's concerns or activities and any pertinent data regarding adults' sexual activity that influences child.

1. Sexual concerns/activity of youngster
2. Sexual concerns/activity of adults if warranted

Sexual history is an essential component of preadolescents' and adolescents' health assessment.

Degree of investigation into parents' sexual history depends on its relevance to the child's health. It may be limited to family planning concerns, or it may be more detailed if overt sexual activity or abuse is suspected.

Investigate toward end of history when rapport is greatest.

Respect sensitive and complex nature of questioning.

Give parents and youngster option of discussing sexual matters alone with nurse.

Ensure confidentiality.

Clarify terms such as "sexually active" or "having sex."

Refer to sexual contacts as "partners," not "girlfriends" or "boyfriends," to avoid biasing discussion of homosexual activity.

Discussion may flow easily after review of genitourinary tract, such as asking female about menstruation or male about urinary problems.

Suggestions for beginning discussion include the following:

"Tell me about your social life."

"Who are your closest friends?"

"Is there one very special friend?"

"Some teenagers have decided to have sex. What do you think about that?"

Take detailed history of all contacts if sexually transmitted disease is suspected or diagnosed.

Client profile (C/P)

To summarize the interviewer's overall impression of the child's and family's physical, psychological, and socioeconomic background.

1. Health status
2. Psychological status
3. Socioeconomic status

A comprehensive summary often identifies nursing diagnoses based on subjective and objective feelings.

Physical Assessment and Examination of the Newborn

The following is a suggested guide for the physical examination of the newborn. In most instances this task is performed in the hospital, but there may be times when the nurse will want a copy of this assessment or need to perform such an assessment in the home.

Provide a normothermic and nonstimulating examination area.
Undress only body area examined to prevent heat loss.
Proceed in an orderly sequence (usually head to toe) with the following exceptions:
  Perform all procedures that require quiet first, such as auscultating the lungs, heart, and abdomen.
  Perform disturbing procedures, such as testing reflexes, last.
  Measure head, chest, and length at same time to compare results.
Proceed quickly to avoid stressing infant.
  Check that equipment and supplies are working properly and are accessible.
Comfort infant during and after examination; involve parent in the following:
  Talk softly.
  Hold infant's hands against chest.
  Swaddle and hold.
  Give pacifier or gloved finger to suck.

From Wong D: *Whaley and Wong's nursing care of infants and children,* ed 6, St. Louis, 1999, Mosby.

Summary of Physical Assessment of the Newborn

Usual findings	Common variations/minor abnormalities	Potential signs of distress/ major abnormalities
General measurements		
Head circumference—33-35 cm; about 2-3 cm larger than chest circumference	Molding after birth may decrease head circumference	Head circumference <10th or >90th percentile
Chest circumference—30.5-33 cm	Head and chest circumference may be equal for first 1-2 days after birth	
Crown-to-rump length—31-35 cm; approximately equal to head circumference		
Head-to-heel length—48-53 cm		
Birth weight—2700-4000 g	Loss of 10% of birth weight in first week; regained in 10-14 days	Birth weight <10th or >90th percentile
Vital signs		
Temperature		
Axillary—36.5°-37° C (97.9°-98° F)	Crying may increase body temperature slightly	Hypothermia
	Radiant warmer will falsely increase axillary temperature	Hyperthermia
Heart rate		
Apical—120-140 beats/min	Crying will increase heart rate; sleep will decrease heart rate	Bradycardia—Resting rate below 80-100 beats/min
	During first period of reactivity (6-8 hours), rate can reach 180 beats/min	Tachycardia—Rate above 160-180 beats/min
		Irregular rhythm

Respirations 30-60 breaths/min	Crying will increase respiratory rate; sleep will decrease respiratory rate During first period of reactivity (6-8 hours), rate can reach 80 breaths/min	Tachypnea—Rate above 60 breaths/min Apnea >15 seconds
Blood pressure Oscillometric—65/41 mm Hg in arm and calf	Crying and activity will increase BP Placing cuff on thigh may agitate infant; thigh blood pressure (BP) may be higher than arm or calf BP by 4-8 mm Hg	Oscillometric systolic pressure in calf 6-9 mm Hg less than in upper extremity (sign of coarctation of aorta)
General appearance *Posture*—Flexion of head and extremities, which rest on chest and abdomen	*Frank breech*—Extended legs, abducted and fully rotated thighs, flattened occiput, extended neck	Limp posture, extension of extremities
Skin At birth, bright red, puffy, smooth Second to third day, pink, flaky, dry Vernix caseosa Lanugo Edema around eyes, face, legs, dorsa of hands, feet, and scrotum or labia *Acrocyanosis*—Cyanosis of hands and feet	Neonatal jaundice after first 24 hours Ecchymoses or petechiae caused by birth trauma *Milia*—Distended sebaceous glands that appear as tiny white papules on cheeks, chin, and nose *Miliaria or sudamina*—Distended sweat (eccrine) glands that appear as minute vesicles, especially on face	Progressive jaundice, especially in first 24 hours Cracked or peeling skin Generalized cyanosis Pallor Mottling Grayness Plethora

Continued.

From Wong D, Perry S: *Maternal-child nursing care*, St. Louis, 1998, Mosby.

Summary of Physical Assessment of the Newborn—cont'd

Usual findings	Common variations/minor abnormalities	Potential signs of distress/ major abnormalities
Skin—cont'd		
Cutis marmorata—Transient mottling when infant is exposed to decreased temperature	*Erythema toxicum*—Pink papular rash with vesicles superimposed on thorax, back, buttocks, and abdomen: may appear in 24-48 hrs and resolve after several days	Hemorrhage, ecchymoses, or petechiae that persist
	Harlequin color change—Clearly outlined color changes as infant lies on side: lower half of body becomes pink, and upper half is pale	*Sclerema*—Hard and stiff skin
		Poor skin turgor
		Rashes, pustules, or blisters
	Mongolian spots—Irregular areas of deep blue pigmentation, usually in sacral and gluteal regions; seen predominantly in newborns of African, Native American, Asian, or Hispanic descent	*Café-au-lait spots*—Light brown spots
		Nevus flammeus—Port-wine stain
		Nevus vasculosis: Strawberry mark
	Telangiectatic nevi ("stork bites")—Flat, deep pink localized areas usually seen in back of neck	
Head		
Anterior fontanel—Diamond shaped, 2.5-4.0 cm	Molding after vaginal delivery	Fused sutures
Posterior fontanel—Triangular, 0.5-1 cm	Third sagittal (parietal) fontanel	Bulging or depressed fontanels when quiet
Fontanels should be flat, soft, and firm	Bulging fontanel because of crying or coughing	Widened sutures and fontanels

Widest part of fontanel measured from bone to bone, not suture to suture

Craniotabes—Snapping sensation along lambdoid suture that resembles indentation of ping-pong ball

Caput succedaneum—Edema of soft scalp tissue
Cephalhematoma (uncomplicated)—Hematoma between periosteum and skull bone

Eyes

Lids usually edematous
Color—Slate gray, dark blue, brown
Absence of tears
Presence of red reflex
Corneal reflex in response to touch
Pupillary reflex in response to light
Blink reflex in response to light or touch
Rudimentary fixation on objects and ability to follow to midline

Epicanthal folds in Asian infants
Searching nystagmus or strabismus
Subconjunctival (scleral) hemorrhages—Ruptured capillaries, usually at limbus

Pink color of iris
Purulent discharge
Upward slant in non-Asians
Hypertelorism (3 cm or greater)
Hypotelorism
Congenital cataracts
Constricted or dilated fixed pupil
Absence of red reflex
Absence of pupillary or corneal reflex
Inability to follow object or bright light to midline
Blue sclera
Yellow sclera

Ears

Position—Top of pinna on horizontal line with outer canthus of eye
Startle reflex elicited by a loud, sudden noise
Pinna flexible, cartilage present

Inability to visualize tympanic membrane because of filled aural canals
Pinna flat against head
Irregular shape or size
Pits or skin tags

Low placement of ears
Absence of startle reflex in response to loud noise
Minor abnormalities may be signs of various syndromes, especially renal

Continued.

Summary of Physical Assessment of the Newborn—cont'd

Usual findings	Common variations/minor abnormalities	Potential signs of distress/major abnormalities
Nose Nasal patency Nasal discharge—Thin white mucus Sneezing	Flattened and bruised	Nonpatent canals Thick, bloody nasal discharge Flaring of nares (alae nasi) Copious nasal secretions or stuffiness (may be minor)
Mouth and throat Intact, high-arched palate Uvula in midline Frenulum of tongue Frenum of upper lip Sucking reflex—Strong and coordinated Rooting reflex Gag reflex Extrusion reflex Absent or minimal salivation Vigorous cry	*Natal teeth*—Teeth present at birth; benign but may be associated with congenital defects *Epstein pearls*—Small, white epithelial cysts along midline of hard palate	Cleft lip Cleft palate Large, protruding tongue or posterior displacement of tongue Profuse salivation or drooling *Candidiasis (thrush)*—White, adherent patches on tongue, palate, and buccal surfaces Inability to pass nasogastric tube Hoarse, high-pitched, weak, absent, or other abnormal cry
Neck Short, thick, usually surrounded by skinfolds Tonic neck reflex	*Torticollis (wry neck)*—Head held to one side with chin pointing to opposite side	Excessive skinfolds Resistant to flexion Absence of tonic neck reflex Fractured clavicle

Chest		
Anteroposterior and lateral diameters equal	Funnel chest (*pectus excavatum*)	Depressed sternum
Slight sternal retractions evident during inspiration	Pigeon chest (*pectus carinatum*)	Marked retractions of chest and intercostal spaces during respiration
Xiphoid process evident	Supernumerary nipples	Asymmetric chest expansion
Breast enlargement	Secretion of milky substance from breasts ("witch's milk")	Redness and firmness around nipples
		Wide-spaced nipples
Lungs		
Respirations chiefly abdominal	Rate and depth of respirations may be irregular, periodic breathing	Inspiratory stridor
Cough reflex absent at birth, present by 1-2 days	Crackles shortly after birth	Expiratory grunt
Bilateral equal bronchial breath sounds		Retractions
		Persistent irregular breathing
		Periodic breathing with repeated apneic spells
		Seesaw respirations (paradoxical)
		Unequal breath sounds
		Persistent fine crackles
		Wheezing
		Diminished breath sounds
		Peristaltic sounds on one side, with diminished breath sounds on same side

Continued.

Summary of Physical Assessment of the Newborn—cont'd

Usual findings	Common variations/minor abnormalities	Potential signs of distress/major abnormalities
Heart		
Apex—Fourth to fifth intercostal space, lateral to left sternal border	*Sinus arrhythmia*—Heart rate increases with inspiration and decreases with expiration	*Dextrocardia*—Heart on right side
S_2 slightly sharper and higher in pitch than S_1	Transient cyanosis on crying or straining	Displacement of apex, muffled
		Cardiomegaly
		Abdominal shunts
		Murmurs
		Thrills
		Persistent cyanosis
		Hyperactive precordium
Abdomen		
Cylindric in shape	Umbilical hernia	Abdominal distention
Liver—Palpable 2-3 cm below right costal margin	*Diastasis recti*—Midline gap between recti muscles	Localized bulging
Spleen—Tip palpable at end of first week of age	*Wharton's jelly*—Unusually thick umbilical cord	Distended veins
Kidneys—Palpable 1-2 cm above umbilicus		Absent bowel sounds
Umbilical cord—Bluish white at birth with two arteries and one vein		Enlarged liver and spleen
Femoral pulses—Equal bilaterally		Ascites
		Visible peristaltic waves
		Scaphoid or concave abdomen
		Green umbilical cord
		Presence of only one artery in cord
		Urine or stool leaking from cord
		Palpable bladder distention following scanty voiding

Female genitalia

Labia and clitoris usually edematous

Urethral meatus behind clitoris

Vernix caseosa between labia

Urination within 24 hours

Pseudomenstruation—Blood-tinged or mucoid discharge

Hymenal tag

Enlarged clitoris with urethal meatus at tip

Fused labia

Absence of vaginal opening

Meconium from vaginal opening

No urination within 24 hours

Masses in labia

Ambiguous genitalia

Absent femoral pulses

Cord bleeding or hematoma

Male genitalia

Urethral opening at tip of glans penis

Testes palpable in scrotum

Scrotum usually large, edematous, pendulous, and covered with rugae; usually deeply pigmented in dark-skinned ethnic groups

Smegma

Urination within 24 hours

Urethral opening covered by prepuce

Inability to retract foreskin

Epithelial pearls—Small, firm, white lesions at tip of prepuce

Erection or priapism

Testes palpable in inguinal canal

Scrotum small

Hydrocele—Fluid in scrotum

Hypospadias—Urethral opening on ventral surface of penis

Epispadias—Urethral opening on dorsal surface of penis

Chordee—Ventral curvature of penis

Testes not palpable in scrotum or inguinal canal

No urination within 24 hours

Inguinal hernia

Hypoplastic scrotum

Masses in scrotum

Meconium from scrotum

Discoloration of testes

Ambiguous genitalia

Continued.

Summary of Physical Assessment of the Newborn—cont'd

Usual findings	Common variations/minor abnormalities	Potential signs of distress/major abnormalities
Back and rectum		
Spine intact, no openings, masses, or prominent curves	Green liquid stools in infant under phototherapy	Anal fissures or fistulas
Trunk incurvation reflex	Delayed passage of meconium in very-low-birth-weight neonates	Imperforate anus
Anal reflex		Absence of anal reflex
Patent anal opening		No meconium within 36 hours
Passage of meconium within 48 hours		Pilonidal cyst or sinus
		Tuft of hair along spine
		Spina bifida (any degree)
Extremities		
Ten fingers and toes	Partial syndactyly between second and third toes	*Polydactyly*—Extra digits
Full range of motion	Second toe overlapping into third toe	*Syndactyly*—Fused or webbed digits
Nail beds pink, with transient cyanosis immediately after birth	Wide gap between first (hallux) and second toes	*Phocomelia*—Hands or feet attached close to trunk
Creases on anterior two thirds of sole	Deep crease on plantar surface of foot between first and second toes	*Hemimelia*—Absence of distal part of extremity
Sole usually flat	Asymmetric length of toes	Hyperflexibility of joints
Symmetry of extremities	Dorsiflexion and shortness of hallux	Persistent cyanosis of nail beds
Equal muscle tone bilaterally, especially resistance to opposing flexion		Yellowing of nail beds
Equal bilateral brachial pulses		Sole covered with creases
		Transverse palmer (simian) crease
		Fractures
		Decreased or absent range of motion

Neuromuscular system		
Extremities usually maintain some degree of flexion	Quivering or momentary tremors	*Dislocated or subluxated hip*
Extension of an extremity followed by previous position of flexion		Limitation in hip abduction
Head lag while sitting, but momentary ability to hold head erect		Unequal gluteal or leg folds
Able to turn head from side to side when prone		Unequal knee height (Allis or Galeazz sign)
Able to hold head in horizontal line with back when held prone		Audible click on abduction (Ortolani sign)
		Asymmetry of extremities
		Unequal muscle tone or range of motion
		Hypotonia—Floppy, poor head control, extremities limp
		Hypertonia—Jittery, arms and hands tightly flexed, legs stiffly extended, startles easily
		Asymmetric posturing (except tonic neck reflex)
		Opisthotonic posturing—Arched back
		Signs of paralysis
		Tremors, twitches, and myoclonic jerks
		Marked head lag in all positions

Pediatric Physical Assessment

The following is a suggested guide for the physical examination of the child. The nurse may adapt the examination based on the child's age.

1. General
   a. Frequent colds, infections, or illnesses
   b. Frequent fevers, sweats
   c. Fatigue patterns
   d. Energetic or overactive patterns
2. Nutritional
   a. Recent weight gain or loss (describe)
   b. Appetite
   c. Twenty-four-hour recall, including types, amount of food eaten (formula, breast milk, meat, fruit, vegetables, cereals, juices, eggs, sweets, milk, snacks), and frequency (e.g., how many times a day or week)
   d. Child feeding self?
   e. Where does child eat?
   f. Whom does child eat with?
   g. Parent's perception of child's nutritional status (note problems)
   h. Vitamins?
   i. Junk food consumption (amount and kinds)
3. Integumentary
   a. Skin
      (1) Chronic rashes
      (2) Easy bruising or petechiae
      (3) Easy bleeding
      (4) Acne (treatment pattern)
      (5) Excessive sweating
      (6) Skin diseases, problems, or lesions
      (7) Itching
      (8) Pigmentation changes, discolorations, mottling
      (9) Excessive dryness
      (10) Skin growths or tumors
   b. Hair
      (1) Changes in amount, texture, characteristics
      (2) Infections, lice
      (3) Alopecia

Modified from Bowers AC, Thompson JM: *Clinical manual of health assessment,* ed 4, St. Louis, 1992, Mosby.

   c. Nails
      (1) Changes in appearance
      (2) Cyanosis
      (3) Texture

4. Head
   a. Headache (frequency, type, location, duration, care for)
   b. Past significant trauma
   c. Dizziness
   d. Syncope

5. Eyes
   a. Crossed eyes
   b. Strabismus
   c. Discharge
   d. Complaint of vision changes
   e. Reading difficulty
   f. Sitting close to television
   g. History of infections
   h. Pruritus
   i. Excessive tearing
   j. Pain in eyeball
   k. Swelling around eyes
   l. Cataracts
   m. Unusual sensations or twitching
   n. Excessive blinking
   o. Eye injury history
   p. Currently wears glasses
   q. Diplopia
   r. Blurring
   s. Gives history of inability to see distant images

6. Ears
   a. Multiple infections or earaches
   b. Myringotomy tubes in ears
   c. Discharge
   d. Cerumen
   e. Care habits
   f. Cracking or ringing
   g. Parent perceives problem in child's hearing

7. Nose, nasopharynx, and paranasal sinuses
   a. Discharge (character of)
   b. Epistaxis
   c. Allergies
   d. General olfactory ability
   e. Pain over sinuses

f. Postnasal drip
g. Sneezing
h. Nasal stuffiness

8. Mouth and throat
   a. Sore throats (frequent)
   b. Tonsils present
   c. Mouth sores
   d. Toothaches, caries
   e. Voice changes
   f. Hoarseness
   g. Mouth breathing
   h. Chewing difficulties
   i. Swallowing difficulties
   j. Teeth brushing pattern

9. Neck
   a. Swollen glands
   b. Tenderness
   c. Limitations of movement
   d. Stiffness

10. Breast: applicable only with teenagers; refer to adult database

11. Cardiovascular
    a. History of murmur
    b. History of heart problem
    c. Palpitations
    d. Hypertension
    e. Postural hypotension
    f. Cyanosis (what precipitates)
    g. Dyspnea on exertion
    h. Limitation of activities
    i. Frequent complaints of extremity coldness

12. Respiratory
    a. Breathing trouble
    b. Chronic cough
    c. Wheezing (precipitating factors)
    d. Croup history
    e. Noisy breathing
    f. Shortness of breath

13. Hematolymphatic
    a. Lymph node swelling (note frequency and location)
    b. Excessive bleeding or easy bruising
    c. Anemia
    d. Blood dyscrasias
    e. Lead exposures, deleading in past

14. Gastrointestinal
  a. Ulcer history
  b. Previously diagnosed problem
  c. Vomiting
  d. Diarrhea
  e. Constipation or stool-holding problems
  f. Rectal bleeding
  g. Stool color change
  h. Abdominal pains
  i. Pinworms by history
  j. Perianal pruritus
  k. Use of evacuation aids
  l. Toilet trained? If not, is it planned? Any problems?

15. Urinary
  a. Urinary tract infections during past year
  b. Previously diagnosed problems
  c. Characteristics of urine (cloudy, dark)
  d. Suprapubic pains
  e. Steadiness and force of urination stream
  f. Dysuria
  g. Nocturia
  h. Bed-wetting (Associated with emotional upsets? Family history of bed-wetting?)
  i. Urinary frequency
  j. Dribbling or incontinence
  k. Polyuria/oliguria
  l. Bubble bath used?

16. Genital
  a. Birth defects
  b. Discharges
  c. Odors
  d. Rashes, irritation
  e. Pruritus
  f. How is sexuality education handled in the home?
  g. Areas of concern
  h. If client is female and menstruating, refer to adult database for appropriate questioning

17. Musculoskeletal
  a. Muscles
    (1) Twitching
    (2) Cramping
    (3) Pain
    (4) Weakness
    (5) Pain with use

    b. Extremities
        (1) General complaints of pain, weakness, deformity
        (2) Night pains in legs
        (3) Gait ability—strength and coordination
    c. Bones and joints
        (1) Joint swelling
        (2) Joint pain
        (3) Redness, stiffness
        (4) Joint deformity
        (5) Fracture or dislocation history
    d. Back
        (1) History of back injury
        (2) Curvature of spine
        (3) Characteristics of problems and corrective measures
18. Central nervous system
    a. General
        (1) Unusual episodic behaviors
        (2) History of central nervous system diseases
        (3) Birth injury
    b. Seizure: febrile versus afebrile
    c. Speech
        (1) Stuttering
        (2) Speech misarticulations
        (3) Language delay
    d. Cognitive changes
        (1) Hallucinations
        (2) Passing out episodes
        (3) Staring spells
        (4) Learning difficulties
    e. Motor-gait
        (1) Coordination
        (2) Developmental clumsiness
        (3) Balance problems
        (4) Tic
        (5) Tremor, spasms
    f. Sensory
        (1) Pain pattern
        (2) Tingling sensations
19. Endocrine
    a. Diagnosis of disease states (e.g., thyroid, diabetes)
    b. Changes in skin texture (e.g., increased or decreased dryness or perspiration)

     c. Pigmentation
     d. Abnormal hair distribution
     e. Sudden or unexplained changes in height and weight
     f. Intolerance to heat or cold
     g. Exophthalmos
     h. Goiter
     i. Polydipsia (increased thirst)
     j. Polyphagia (increased food intake)
     k. Polyuria (increased urination)
     l. Anorexia (decreased appetite)
     m. Weakness
     n. Precocious puberty
20. Allergic and immunological
     a. Dermatitis (inflammation or irritation of the skin)
     b. Eczema
     c. Pruritus (itching)
     d. Urticaria (hives)
     e. Sneezing
     f. Vasomotor rhinitis (inflammation and swelling of mucous membrane of nose, nasal discharge)
     g. Conjunctivitis (inflammation of conjunctiva)
     h. Interference with activities of daily living
     i. Environmental and seasonal causes
     j. Treatment techniques

Performing a Pediatric Physical Examination

Perform examination in appropriate, nonthreatening area.
    Have room well lit and decorated with neutral colors.
    Have room temperature comfortably warm.
    Place all strange and potentially frightening equipment out of sight.
    Have some toys, dolls, stuffed animals, and games available for child.
    If possible, have rooms decorated and equipped for children of different ages.
    Provide privacy, especially for school-age children and adolescents.
Provide time for play and becoming acquainted.

From Wong D: *Whaley and Wong's nursing care of infants and children,* ed 6, St. Louis, 1999, Mosby.

Observe behaviors that signal child's readiness to cooperate:
  Talking to nurse
  Making eye contact
  Accepting offered equipment
  Allowing physical touching
  Choosing to sit on examining table rather than parent's lap
If signs of readiness are not observed, use the following techniques:
  Talk to parent while essentially "ignoring" child; gradually focus on
    child or a favorite object, such as a doll.
  Make complimentary remarks about child, such as appearance,
    dress, or a favorite object.
  Tell a funny story or play a simple magic trick.
  Have a nonthreatening "friend" available, such as a hand puppet to
    "talk" to child for the nurse.
If child refuses to cooperate, use the following techniques:
  Assess reason for uncooperative behavior; consider that a child who
    is unduly afraid may have had a previous traumatic experience.
  Try to involve child and parent in process.
  Avoid prolonged explanations about examining procedure.
  Use a firm, direct approach regarding expected behavior.
  Perform examination as quickly as possible.
  Have attendant gently restrain child.
  Minimize any disruptions or stimulation.
    Limit number of people in room.
    Use isolated room.
    Use quiet, calm, confident voice.
Begin examination in a nonthreatening manner for young children or
  children who are fearful:
  Use those activities that can be presented as games, such as test for
    cranial nerves or parts of developmental screening tests.
  Use approaches such as "Simon says" to encourage child to make a
    face, squeeze a hand, stand on one foot, and so on.
  Use "paper-doll" technique.
    Lay child supine on an examining table or floor that is covered
      with a large sheet of paper.
    Trace around child's body outline.
    Use body outline to demonstrate what will be examined, such as
      drawing a heart and listening with the stethoscope before per-
      forming the activity on child.
If several children in the family will be examined, begin with the most
  cooperative child to provide modeling of desired behavior.

Involve child in examination process:
    Provide choices such as sitting on table or in parent's lap.
    Allow child to handle or hold equipment.
    Encourage child to use equipment on a doll, family member, or examiner.
    Explain each step of the procedure in simple language.
Examine child in a comfortable and secure position:
    Sitting in parent's lap
    Sitting upright if in respiratory distress
Proceed to examine the body in an organized sequence (usually head to toe) with the following exceptions:
    Alter sequence to accommodate needs of children of different ages.
    Examine painful areas last.
    In emergency situation, examine vital functions (airway, breathing, and circulation) and injured area first.
Reassure child throughout examination, especially about bodily concerns that arise during puberty.
Discuss findings with family at end of examination.
Praise child for cooperation during examination; give reward such as a small toy or sticker.

Notes

Age-Specific Approaches to Physical Examination During Childhood

Position	Sequence	Preparation
Infant		
Before sits alone: supine or prone, preferably in parent's lap; before 4 to 6 months: can place on examining table	If quiet, auscultate heart, lungs, abdomen	Completely undress if room temperature permits
After sits alone: use sitting in parent's lap whenever possible	Record heart and respiratory rates	Leave diaper on male
If on table, place with parent in full view	Palpate and percuss same areas	Gain cooperation with distraction, bright objects, rattles, talking
	Proceed in usual head-to-toe direction	Have older infants hold a small block in each hand; until voluntary release develops toward end of the first year, infants will be unable to grasp other objects
	Perform traumatic procedures last (eyes, ears, mouth [while crying])	(e.g., stethoscope, otoscope)
	Elicit reflexes as body part examined	Smile at infant; use soft, gentle voice
	Elicit Moro reflex last	Pacify with bottle of sugar water or feeding
		Enlist parent's aid for restraining to examine ears, mouth
		Avoid abrupt, jerky movements
Toddler		
Sitting or standing on/by parent	Inspect body area through play: "count fingers," "tickle toes"	Have parent remove outer clothing
Prone or supine in parent's lap	Use minimal physical contact initially	Remove underwear as body part examined
	Introduce equipment slowly	Allow to inspect equipment; demonstrating use of equipment is usually ineffective

Auscultate, percuss, palpate whenever quiet

Perform traumatic procedures last (same as for infant)

Preschool child

Prefer standing or sitting

Usually cooperative prone/supine

Prefer parent's closeness

If cooperative, proceed in head-to-toe direction

If uncooperative, proceed as with toddler

If uncooperative, perform procedures quickly

Use restraint when appropriate; request parent's assistance

Talk about examination if cooperative; use short phrases

Praise for cooperative behavior

Request self-undressing

Allow to wear underpants if shy

Offer equipment for inspection; briefly demonstrate use

Make up "story" about procedure: "I'm seeing how strong your muscles are" (blood pressure)

Use paper-doll technique

Give choices when possible

Expect cooperation; use positive statement: "Open your mouth"

School-age child

Prefer sitting

Cooperative in most positions

Younger child prefers parent's presence

Older child may prefer privacy

Proceed in head-to-toe direction

May examine genitalia last in older child

Respect need for privacy

Request self-undressing

Allow to wear underpants

Give gown to wear

Explain purpose of equipment and significance of procedure, such as otoscope to see eardrum, which is necessary for hearing

Teach about body functioning and care

Continued.

From Wong DL: *Whaley and Wong's nursing care of infants and children,* ed 6, St. Louis, 1999, Mosby.

Age-Specific Approaches to Physical Examination During Childhood—cont'd

Position	Sequence	Preparation
Adolescent Same as for school-age child Offer option of parent's presence	Same as for older school-age child	Allow to undress in private Give gown Expose only area to be examined Respect need for privacy Explain findings during examination: "Your muscles are firm and strong" Matter-of-factly comment about sexual development: "Your breasts are developing as they should be" Emphasize normalcy of development Examine genitalia as any other body part; may leave to end

Environmental Assessment for Children

Pediatric Review of Children's Environmental Support and Stimulation (PROCESS)

I. Preparation of clinical observation
II. Clinical observation
III. Clinical observation guide
IV. Parent questionnaire
V. Toy checklist
VI. Scoring procedures
VII. PROCESS recording form

Preparation of the clinical observation

Not all visits to the health clinic or pediatric office provide the appropriate conditions for making the kinds of observations needed to score items on the Clinical Observation section of PROCESS. Generally, a 15- to 20-minute routine health maintenance visit is best suited for making the observation. The parent-child relationship is initially observed by the clinician while taking a medical history. During this portion of the visit, the child should be placed on the parent's lap. The child should remain on the parent's lap during the less intrusive parts of the physical examination. The child should be separated from the parent and placed on the examination table only for the more invasive aspects of the physical examination. This semi-structured format, which is typical for a health maintenance visit, allows observation of the parent-child relationship in increasingly stressful situations. However, it is not as constraining as a briefer clinic visit or a visit scheduled because of a child's illness. The 15 to 20 minutes used for such a visit provides an opportunity for a wide array of parenting behaviors to occur and, hopefully, provides the conditions for many parents to exhibit the kinds of behaviors typical of their behavior at home.

Prepared by Patrick Casey, MD, University of Arkansas for Medical Sciences and Robert Bradley, PhD, 1994, University of Arkansas at Little Rock.

Clinical observation

Child's name _____ Observation date _____

Child's age _____ Sex _____ Race _____ Height _____

Child's weight _____ Observer _____

_____ 1. Mother asks questions that are relevant and appropriate about the child.

      _____ irrelevant or no questions asked   _____ few questions asked are relevant

      _____ most questions asked are relevant   _____ all questions are relevant

_____ 2. Mother shows interest in baby's behavior.

      _____ little or no interest   _____ only somewhat interested

      _____ moderately interested   _____ very interested

_____ 3. Mother reports how smart or how good baby is.

      _____ never   _____ once

      _____ 2 or 3 times   _____ many times

_____ 4. Mother talks, sings, or otherwise vocalizes to baby.

      _____ never   _____ once

      _____ 2 or 3 times   _____ many times

_____ 5. Mother is comfortable in caring for baby.

      _____ very uncomfortable/ awkward   _____ somewhat uncomfortable

      _____ comfortable   _____ very comfortable

_____ 6. Mother responds to child's social initiations with social response, for example, smile, eye contact, or laugh.

      _____ never   _____ once

      _____ 2 or 3 times   _____ many times

_____ 7. Mother initiates verbal interchanges with observer, for example, asks questions or makes spontaneous comments.

      _____ never   _____ once

      _____ 2 or 3 times   _____ many times

_____ 8. Mother expresses ideas freely and easily; uses statements of appropriate length for conversation (more than brief answers).

      _____ very poor expressive skills: one or two word answers   _____ poor expressive skills

      _____ appropriate expressive skills   _____ very expressive

_____ **9.** Mother is eager to pat or pick up crying baby to quiet or comfort.

_____ ignores child, needs prompting

_____ adequate response

_____ slow responding

_____ monitors child during distress and eager to respond

_____ **10.** Mother attends to baby's responses during the examination.

_____ never

_____ usually

_____ once

_____ almost all the time

_____ **11.** Mother is detached and/or inwardly absorbed.

_____ not interested in visit or communication, may be hostile

_____ shows moderate interest and communication

_____ not interested but neutral in emotion and communication

_____ extremely interested and involved

_____ **12.** Mother has eye-to-eye contact with the baby.

_____ never

_____ 2 or 3 times

_____ once

_____ many times

_____ **13.** Mother stays within reach of the child.

_____ never

_____ most of the time

_____ only in distress

_____ always physically available

_____ **14.** Mother responds to child's vocalization with verbal responses.

_____ never

_____ 2 or 3 times

_____ once

_____ many times

_____ **15.** Mother demonstrates negative responses or feelings toward child.

_____ many times

_____ once

_____ 2 or 3 times

_____ never

_____ **16.** Mother caresses or strokes baby gently.

_____ never

_____ 2 or 3 times

_____ once

_____ many times

_____ **17.** Mother looks at baby with warmth and tenderness.

_____ never

_____ 2 or 3 times

_____ once

_____ many times

_____ **18.** Mother shows positive emotional response to praise of child offered by examiner.

_____ no response

_____ some response

_____ little or poor response

_____ very positive response

_____ **19.** Mother smiles at baby.

_____ never

_____ 2 or 3 times

_____ once

_____ many times

_____ **20.** Baby is clean. (Not every item necessary to score on a given level.)

_____ smells bad, diaper area not clean, fingernails dirty, hair oily and matted, scalp dirty and crusty looking

_____ body and hair clean

_____ diaper area not clean, fingernails dirty, body dirty, hair dirty

_____ hair is fixed and clean, smells of recent bath, powdered and "perfumed"

Observation total: _____

Clinical observation guide

Note: Throughout the Clinical Observation Guide, the items have been stated for the mother, but this may be any person who is the prime caregiver, for example, foster mother, grandmother, or father.

1. Mother asks questions that are relevant and appropriate about the child or situation.

   The key word is *relevant*. Credit is given for the quality of questions asked, not the quantity. "Most questions asked are relevant" means that most of the questions themselves were relevant in nature, not that there were many in number. If only one question is asked, but it is relevant, then credit is given for "most questions asked are relevant."

2. Mother shows interest in baby's behavior.

   Mother shows interest by close observation and may talk to the child in response to behavior. She may sit forward in the chair or stand to observe the exam more closely.

3. Mother reports how smart or how good baby is.

   The mother will make a *spontaneous* comment about the "good things" the baby does. It will be more than a flat response to "what has he/she learned" or other questions.

4. Mother talks, sings, or otherwise vocalizes to baby.

   Credit for this will include the soft humming, comforting sounds, as well as the more audible vocalizations that may occur.

5. Mother is comfortable in caring for baby.

   The mother seems at ease and relaxed with the child and her ability to meet the child's needs. She appears to *enjoy* the child and what he/she is doing. Discomfort can be awkwardness in handling the child (holding, diapering) or difficulty organizing self and the baby.

6. Mother responds to child's social initiations with social response.

   This is a response to an action initiated by the child. If the child makes no overtures to the parent, the answer will be "never." The mother must respond to the baby's attention-getting actions (look, vocalization, touch, or gesture) by responding directly to the child.

7. Mother initiates verbal interchanges with observer.

   The mother converses with the examiner besides responding to questions. For example, she talks about the child's progress, problems, behavior, or concerns.

8. Mother expresses ideas freely and easily; uses statements of appropriate length for conversation.

   "Very expressive" indicates good language use, expressing thoughts or concerns spontaneously; appropriate language and ease of manner. "Appropriate expressive" indicates more a simpler speech pattern with shorter sentences, but the speaker is generally fluent. Poor ability involves hesitancy in conversing, short answers, little or no spontaneous communication, sometimes saying things such as "I don't know how to say it." "Very poor expressive skills" indicates much difficulty conversing. Responses consist of one-word answers, or prompting and/or assistance is needed. There is no spontaneous speech.

9. Mother is eager to pat or pick up crying baby to quiet or comfort.

   The mother who monitors during the exam stands close to the child, has some reaching or touching, speaks to the child to comfort, and picks up child immediately upon conclusion of the exam. She may appear anxious during the child's distress. "Adequate response" involves more passivity or remaining seated, but watching attentively and picking up the child when certain the exam is completed. A slow response involves a mother who remains seated or at a distance, waits to respond after the exam, and moves to the child slowly. The mother who ignores or needs prompting must be told to get the child or have the child handed to her upon completion of the exam.

10. Mother attends to baby's responses during the examination.

    The mother who *attends* monitors the child carefully and with interest throughout the exam. She is aware of the child's responses and may discuss them with the examiner. "Usually" involves attending during most of the exam and observing whether standing by the child or not. "Some" indicates attending only when the child is easily visible. The mother remains seated and makes no special effort to monitor child. "Never" indicates the mother pays little or no attention to the exam, seems preoccupied, looks around, or does something else.

11. Mother is detached and/or inwardly absorbed.

    This mother is noncommunicative, shows little interest or no interest, and may be hostile. The mother who is not interested but neutral shows little interest or involvement but is not hostile. A moderately interested mother may stand back or look away, but is communicative. The extremely interested and involved mother is "present" both physically and mentally during the exam, is verbal and attentive to the child's behavior, and stays nearby.

12. Mother has eye-to-eye contact with baby.

The eye contact involves the child's looking at mother and the mother's returning the gaze. If the child does not look at the mother, record this as "never" even though the mother looks at the child.

13. Mother stays within reach of the child.

Mother stays nearby and within reach of the child. The mother is easily accessible to the child unless a physician removes the child for some reason, for example, to observe walking or other motor skill.

14. Mother responds to vocalization with verbal responses.

The mother makes some vocalization (words or sounds) in response to sounds made by the child. These may be imitative of the child's sound or verbal interpretations of what the child "says." May hold a "conversation" with the child. Credit is also given for verbal responses by the mother to the child's crying.

15. Mother demonstrates negative responses or feelings toward child.

"Negative" means angry looks, frowning or scowling at the child; sharp verbal reprimands or commands; abrupt and/or rough handling (i.e., jerky or rough picking up or moving of the child); pulling or pushing roughly, thumping, pinching, or grabbing. May also include giving the child to someone else to care for, especially if the child is being difficult to manage.

16. Mother caresses or strokes baby gently.

This includes gentle hugs, pats, petting strokes, and any other soft touch.

17. Mother looks at baby with warmth and tenderness.

This is more than "just watching" to be sure the child is safe. It includes a genuine show of interest and pleasure, often accomplished by a soft smile and/or lingering look.

18. Mother shows positive emotional response to praise.

"Very positive response" involves a positive comment, proud smile, and a further expansion of praised action, a "thank you" with enthusiasm. "Some response" indicates a brief general comment of a "thank you" with little enthusiasm. "Little or poor response" on the part of the mother may include only a nod, "yes," "uh-uh," or some other generalized reaction, usually flat and expressionless in tone. "No response" is completely ignoring the praise.

19. Mother smiles at baby.

Mother smiles at the child's actions, seemingly showing approval of behavior or appearance. It is not in response to the child's social contact.

20. Baby is clean.

Very clean babies are really "fixed up." The hair is "done up," the child smells good, obviously has been bathed recently, and is powdered and "perfumed." The clean baby has been bathed and is not dirty, but is not especially "fixed up." The dirty baby in general has marginally clean hair and/or scalp, evidence of not having been bathed recently, diaper area *not* clean, or dirty fingernails. The really dirty baby in general smells bad, the diaper area is not clean, the body is dirty, hair matted and oily, scalp dirty and/or crusty looking. There is evidence of not having been bathed and smell of old urine.

Parent questionnaire

CHILD'S NAME _____ TODAY'S DATE _____

BIRTH DATE _____ SEX _____ RACE _____ AGE _____

CAREGIVER'S NAME _____

RELATIONSHIP TO CHILD:

Mother	_____	Grandmother	_____
Foster mother	_____	Other	_____

PARENT'S AGE:

Mother	_____	Father	_____

PARENT'S EDUCATION:

Mother	_____	Father	_____

PARENT'S OCCUPATION:

Mother	_____	Income	_____
Father	_____	Income	_____

NUMBER OF CHILDREN: _____

BIRTH ORDER OF THIS CHILD: _____

CHILD LIVES WITH (list everyone who lives in household): _____

_____

HOME ADDRESS: _____

_____

TELEPHONE:

Home: _____   Work: _____

PARENT QUESTIONNAIRE INSTRUCTIONS— PLEASE READ

1. Please **answer ALL questions.** Your answers will remain confidential.
2. Be **HONEST**—there are no right or wrong answers.
3. Mark the answer that is **MOST** appropriate for your situation when two answers seem to be correct. If the question **DOES NOT** seem to fit your child, for example, because of his/her age, mark the answer that is closest to what you would do in the situation given.
4. If you need help or have questions about any part of the questionnaire, **PLEASE ASK.**

THANK YOU FOR YOUR TIME AND ASSISTANCE.

_____ 1. How long do you spend talking with your child each day?
    _____ 10 to 20 minutes   _____ 20 to 60 minutes
    _____ 1 to 2 hours   _____ more than 2 hours a day

_____ 2. How often do you ask your friends or family for their suggestions on how to raise your baby?
    _____ hardly ever   _____ occasionally
    _____ about once a month   _____ about once a week or more

_____ 3. How often do you read the articles from newspapers, magazines, or books on how to raise a baby?
    _____ very rarely   _____ only occasionally
    _____ about once a month   _____ about once a week

_____ 4. How often does your child's father or other adult male do some caregiving for your child (dress, feed, bathe, put to bed, baby-sit while you are away)?
    _____ not very often   _____ once a week
    _____ about three to four times a week   _____ nearly every day

_____ 5. What do you do when your baby starts to cry?
    _____ try to ignore the crying until he/she stops   _____ go to the baby only if the crying keeps on for a while
    _____ see if there is anything wrong, and if he/she is OK, let him/her cry   _____ pick him/her up and hold or play with him/her for a while

_____ **6.** Where does your baby usually sleep at nap time?

_____ wherever he/she falls asleep

_____ in whatever room I am in

_____ in a room alone while I go on with my household activity

_____ in a room alone, and I keep the rest of the house quiet

_____ **7.** How would you describe your child?

_____ often fussy and hard to care for

_____ sometimes fussy, but can be comforted without too much trouble

_____ usually happy and easy to care for

_____ always happy and easy to care for

_____ **8.** How much is the TV or radio on while your child is awake?

_____ nearly all the time

_____ about 3 to 5 hours

_____ about 1 to 2 hours

_____ never

_____ **9.** How often do you feel uncomfortable caring for your baby?

_____ frequently

_____ some of the time

_____ hardly ever

_____ never

_____ **10.** Where does your child sleep at night?

_____ in bed with parents

_____ in bed with his/her brother or sister

_____ in his/her own bed

_____ in his/her own room

_____ in his/her bed— sharing a room

_____ **11.** What do you usually do when your child keeps on acting bad or misbehaving?

_____ shake or spank him/her

_____ scold him/her

_____ leave him/her alone

_____ try to get him/her interested in something else

_____ **12.** How regular is your child's sleeping schedule?

_____ at different times most every day

_____ at the same time only 2 or 3 days a week

_____ at the same time 5 or 6 days a week

_____ at about the same time every day

_____ **13.** Where does your child spend his/her awake or play time?

_____ in a playpen so I know where he/she is

_____ in his/her room

_____ my child can go where he/she wants as long as he/she does not get hurt

_____ I keep my child within sight and check on him/her often

_____ **14.** In how many places have you and your child lived in the past 2 years?

    _____ four or more   _____ three

    _____ two   _____ only one

_____ **15.** How often do you change decorations or objects in your child's room?

    _____ do not change them   _____ seldom change them

    _____ occasionally change   _____ change them often
         them

_____ **16.** How many people live in the same house with you and your baby?

    _____ more than six   _____ four to six others

    _____ two or three others   _____ one other

_____ **17.** About how much time do you spend helping your child learn new things (crawling, walking, talking, using a spoon, holding/playing with a toy)?

    _____ hardly any   _____ 10 to 15 minutes a

    _____ 15 to 30 minutes   couple of times a week
         a day   _____ an hour or more a day

_____ **18.** How do you think young babies learn new things?

    _____ Babies usually will   _____ Babies need some help
         learn new things as   when they are learning
         they grow up.   a few things like
    _____ Babies need help   feeding or dressing
         when they are *first*   themselves and using
         learning to do some-   the potty.
         thing, just to show   _____ Babies need help all
         them how, then   the time when they are
         they will learn by   learning to do things.
         themselves.

_____ **19.** How often do you play with your baby using toys that will help him/her learn a new skill?

    _____ once or twice a   _____ several times a
         month   week
    _____ almost every day   _____ several times every day

_____ **20.** What do you do when you get a new toy for your child?

_____ I buy only toys I know he/she can play with without help.

_____ I let him/her figure out how to use it by him/herself.

_____ I show him/her once or twice what to do, then let him/her play with it and figure it out.

_____ I play with him/her and the toy until he/she can use it easily.

_____ **21.** When your child is fussy, what do you do? (This is at times other than when he/she is tired or hungry.)

_____ scold or spank him/her

_____ try to get him/her interested in a toy or something

_____ let him/her fuss

_____ play with or hold him/her

IF YOUR CHILD IS **YOUNGER THAN 8 MONTHS OF AGE,** PLEASE ANSWER THE QUESTIONS 22a–24a. THEN COMPLETE THE **TOY CHECKLIST** on p. 103.

_____ **22a.** Who feeds your baby?

_____ I usually let the baby feed him/herself or prop the bottle

_____ me or one other person (this _must_ be the same "other person" each time)

_____ whoever is available to help

_____ I usually feed the baby myself

_____ **23a.** How often do you have to get someone else to hold or play with your baby when he/she is fussy so you can finish your work?

_____ several times every day

_____ only once or twice a week

_____ every day

_____ hardly ever/never

_____ **24a.** On what kind of feeding schedule is your baby?

_____ a very set schedule

_____ a regular schedule about 3 or 4 days a week

_____ no set schedule— whenever he/she cries

_____ a regular schedule, but it will change to meet his/her needs if necessary

IF YOUR CHILD IS **8 MONTHS OF AGE OR OLDER,** ANSWER THE QUESTIONS 22b–24b, THEN COMPLETE THE **TOY CHECKLIST** on p 103.

_____ **22b.** How are family meals handled?

_____ unplanned, every-one gets his/her own

_____ unplanned, food is fixed whenever someone is hungry

_____ planned, with foods cooked but not always served at regular times

_____ planned, with foods cooked and served at regular times every day

_____ **23b.** How often does your child have at least one meal with you and his/her father or other adult male figures? (The other adult male must be the same adult male each time, for example, grandfather or uncle.)

_____ less than once a week

_____ about once a week

_____ three or four times a week

_____ every day

_____ **24b.** When does your child usually eat?

_____ whenever he/she is hungry, seems like all the time

_____ whenever he/she is hungry, usually about four or five times a day

_____ two or three times a day, but not on a regular basis

_____ three meals a day on a regular schedule, with one or two snacks during the day

TOY CHECKLIST

We are interested in finding out what kinds of toys children have in their homes. The items below are for children of different ages.

Please check any of the following that you have in your home and that your child is allowed to play with. Do not check the ones you do not have now or that are broken.

_____ doll	_____ homemade toys (for example, doll)
_____ stroller	
_____ toy telephone	_____ boxes or plastic containers to fill
_____ children's books	
_____ crib gym	_____ pots and pans he/she can play with
_____ squeeze toys	
_____ car, truck, or train	_____ jump seat or door swing
_____ teething ring	
_____ stacking rings	_____ record player
_____ surprise box	_____ toy dishes
_____ plastic keys on a ring	_____ busy bath
_____ children's records	_____ toy animals
_____ measuring cups	_____ walker
_____ stuffed animal	_____ ball
_____ push or pull toy	_____ building toys
_____ mobile	_____ blocks
_____ plastic snap together beads	_____ swing
	_____ pounding toy
_____ shape sorting ball or box	_____ mirror
	_____ bathtub toys
_____ musical toy or music box	_____ bucket or pail
	_____ rattles
_____ shovel or other digging toy	_____ busy box
	_____ pacifier

Thank you for your responses and time.

Scoring procedures

PROCESS consists of three major sections:

1. Clinical observation (20 items, each with four choices)
2. Parent questionnaire (24 items, each with four choices)
3. Toy checklist (40 items)

All items in the Clinical Observation and Parent Questionnaire sections are arranged in the following way:

Description of item:

_____ response A   _____ response B
_____ response C   _____ response D

Scoring for each item is as follows:

response A = 1 point   response B = 2 points
response C = 3 points   response D = 4 points

PROCESS recording form

On the PROCESS recording form are places to record scores for each section of PROCESS. Complete this form as follows:

1. **Enter** the score for each Clinical Observation item in the appropriate numbered space.

    Then **add** the points for each item in the columns to obtain an **Observation Total.**

2. **Enter** the score for each Parent Questionnaire item in the appropriate numbered space.

    Then **add** the points for items in the column labeled *Developmental Stimulation* to get the **DS Total.**

    Then **add** the points for items in the column labeled *Organization* to get the **Org Total.**

    Then **add** the **DS Total** and the **Org Total** to get the **Parent Quest. Total.**

3. **Compute** the **Toy Score** using the *Toys Table.*

    Then **compute** the **Weighted Toys Total** as presented on the Process Recording Form.

4. **Enter** the **Total** for each section in the **Summary Table** of the Process Recording Form.

    Then **add** the three **Total** scores to obtain the **PROCESS Total.**

Child's Name _____

Date _____

Date of Birth _____

PROCESS Recording Form

Parent questionnaire	
Developmental Stimulation	**Org**anization
Item 1:	Item 2:
Item 3:	Item 4:
Item 5:	Item 6:
Item 7:	Item 8:
Item 9:	Item 10:
Item 11:	Item 12:
Item 13:	Item 14:
Item 15:	Item 16:
Item 17:	
Item 18:	
Item 19:	
Item 20:	
Item 21:	Item 22:
Item 23:	Item 24:
DS Total =	**Org** Total =
PARENT QUEST. TOTAL =	

Summary table
Parent quest. total =
Weighted toys total =
Observation total =
PROCESS TOTAL =

Clinical observation	
Item 1:	Item 11:
Item 2:	Item 12:
Item 3:	Item 13:
Item 4:	Item 14:
Item 5:	Item 15:
Item 6:	Item 16:
Item 7:	Item 17:
Item 8:	Item 18:
Item 9:	Item 19:
Item 10:	Item 20:
OBSERVATION TOTAL =	

Toys Table	
# of Toys:	**Toy Score =**
0	0
1-5	1
6-10	2
11-15	3
16-20	4
21-25	5
26-30	6
31-35	7
36-40	8
Toy Score _____ × 6 = _____	
WEIGHED TOYS TOTAL	

ADULT ASSESSMENT

Adult Health History

The outline below suggests a systematic procedure for completing an adult health history. It is especially useful before a physical assessment to give the nurse background data for health care planning.

1. Biographical data
2. Reason for visit (chief complaint)
3. Present health status (general summary and symptom analysis; also known as history of present illness—HOPI)
4. Current health data
5. Past health status
6. Family history
7. Review of physiological systems
8. Psychosocial history

Biographical data
Name
Age
Race
Culture
Address and telephone number
Marital status
Children and family in home (if not family, significant others)
Occupation
Means of transportation to health care facility if pertinent
Description of home and size and type of community

Reason for visit
One statement that describes the reason for the client's visit or the chief complaint, stated in the client's own words.

Present health status
Summary of client's current major health concerns
If illness is present, record symptom analysis
  1. When client was last well
  2. Date of problem onset

From Bowers A, Thompson J: *Clinical manual of health assessment,* ed 4, St. Louis, 1992, Mosby.

3. Character of complaint
4. Nature of problem onset
5. Course of problem
6. Client's hunch of precipitating factors
7. Location of problem
8. Relation to other body symptoms, body positions, and activity
9. Patterns of problem
10. Efforts of client to treat
11. Coping ability

Current health data

Current medications
1. Type (prescription, over-the-counter drugs, vitamins, etc.)
2. Prescribed by whom
3. When first prescribed
4. Amount per day
5. Problems

Allergies (description of agent and reactions)
1. Drugs
2. Foods
3. Contact substances
4. Environmental factors

Last examinations (physician/clinic, findings, advice, instructions)
1. Physical
2. Dental
3. Vision
4. Hearing
5. EKG
6. Chest radiograph
7. Pap smear (females)
8. Interdermal tuberculin test

Immunization status (dates or year of last immunization)
1. Tetanus, diphtheria, pertussis
2. Mumps
3. Rubella, rubeola
4. Polio
5. Influenza
6. Hepatitis B
7. Chicken pox
8. Lyme disease

Past health status

Although each of the following is asked separately, the examiner must summarize and record the data *chronologically:*

Childhood illnesses: rubeola, rubella, mumps, pertussis, scarlet fever, chicken pox, strep throat

Serious or chronic illnesses: scarlet fever, diabetes, kidney problems, hypertension, sickle cell anemia, seizure disorders, blood infections

Serious accidents or injuries: head injuries, fractures, burns, other trauma

Hospitalizations: description of, including reason for, location, primary care providers, duration

Operations: what, where, when, why, by whom

Emotional health: past problems, help sought, support persons

Obstetrical history

1. Complete pregnancies: number, pregnancy course, postpartum course, and condition, weight, and sex of each child
2. Incomplete pregnancies: duration, termination, circumstances (including abortions and stillbirths)
3. Summary of complications

Family history

Family members include the client's blood relatives, spouse, and children. Specifically the interviewer should inquire about the client's maternal and paternal grandparents, parents, aunts, uncles, spouse, and children, as well as about the general health, stress factors, and illnesses of other family members. Questions should include a survey of the following:

Alzheimer's disease	Mental illnesses
Cancer	Developmental delay
Diabetes	Alcoholism
Heart disease	Endocrine diseases
Hypertension	Sickle cell anemia
Epilepsy (or seizure disorder)	Kidney disease
	Unusual limitations
Emotional stresses	Other chronic problems

The most concise method to record these data is by a family tree. Figure 1 is an example.

Review of physiological systems

The purpose of this component of the database is to collect information about the body regions or systems and their function.

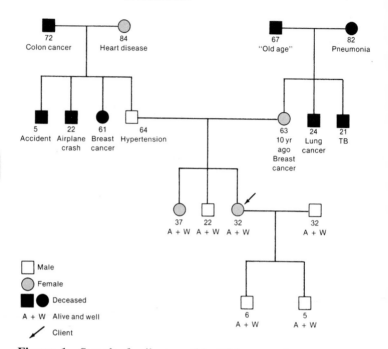

Figure 1 Sample family tree (identifying grandparents, parents, aunts and uncles, siblings, spouse, and children).

General—reflect from client's previous description of current health status

1. Fatigue patterns
2. Exercise and exercise tolerance
3. History of weakness episodes, if any
4. History of fever, sweats, if any
5. Frequency of colds, infections, or illnesses
6. Ability to carry out activities of daily living

Nutritional

1. Client's average, maximum, and minimum weights during past month; 1 year; 5 years
2. History of weight gains or losses (time element); specific efforts to change weight
3. Twenty-four-hour diet recall (helpful to mail the client a chart to fill in before visit)
4. Cultural or religious practices regarding intake
5. Current appetite
6. Extreme deviations in physical activity that would affect appetite (e.g., athletic or immobilization influences)

7. Person(s) who buys and prepares food
8. Person(s) client normally eats with
9. Availability of money to buy preferred food
10. Status of ability to chew; condition of teeth or dentures
11. Client's self-evaluation of nutritional status

Integumentary
1. Skin
   a. Skin disease, problems, lesions (wounds, sores, ulcers)
   b. Skin growths, tumors, masses
   c. Excessive dryness, sweating, odors
   d. Pigmentation changes or discolorations
   e. Pruritus (itching)
   f. Texture changes
   g. Temperature changes
2. Hair
   a. Changes in amount, texture, character
   b. Alopecia (loss of hair)
   c. Use of dyes
3. Nails
   a. Changes in appearance, texture

Head
1. Headache (characteristics, including frequency, type, location, duration, care for)
2. Past significant trauma
3. Dizziness
4. Syncope

Eyes
1. Discharge (characteristics)
2. History of infections, frequency, treatment
3. Pruritus
4. Lacrimation (excessive tearing)
5. Pain in eyeball
6. Spots (floaters)
7. Swelling around eyes
8. Cataracts, glaucoma
9. Unusual sensations or twitching
10. Vision changes (generalized or vision field)
11. Use of corrective or prosthetic devices
12. Diplopia (double vision)
13. Blurring
14. Photophobia
15. Difficulty reading
16. Interference with activities of daily living

Ears
1. Pain (characteristics)
2. Cerumen (wax)
3. Infection
4. Hearing changes (describe)
5. Use of prosthetic devices
6. Increased sensitivity to environmental noise
7. Vertigo
8. Ringing and cracking
9. Care habits
10. Interference with activities of daily living

Nose, nasopharynx, and paranasal sinuses
1. Discharge (characteristics)
2. Epistaxis
3. Allergies
4. Pain over sinuses
5. Postnasal drip
6. Sneezing
7. General olfactory ability

Mouth and throat
1. Sore throats (characteristics)
2. Tongue or mouth lesion (abscess, sore, ulcer)
3. Bleeding gums
4. Hoarseness
5. Voice changes
6. Use of prosthetic devices (dentures, bridges)
7. Altered taste
8. Chewing difficulty
9. Swallowing difficulty
10. Pattern of dental hygiene

Neck
1. Node enlargement
2. Swellings, masses
3. Tenderness
4. Limitation of movement
5. Stiffness

Breasts
1. Pain or tenderness
2. Swelling
3. Nipple discharge
4. Changes in nipples
5. Lumps, dimples
6. Unusual characteristics

   7. Date of mammogram

   8. Breast examination (pattern, frequency)

Cardiovascular

   1. Cardiovascular

      a. Palpitations

      b. Heart murmur

      c. History of heart disease

      d. Hypertension

      e. Chest pain (character and frequency)

      f. Shortness of breath

      g. Orthopnea

      h. Paroxysmal nocturnal dyspnea

   2. Peripheral vascular

      a. Coldness, numbness

      b. Discoloration

      c. Peripheral edema

      d. Varicose veins

      e. Intermittent claudication

Respiratory

   1. History of asthma

   2. Other breathing problems (when, precipitating factors)

   3. Sputum production

   4. Hemoptysis

   5. Chronic cough (characteristics)

   6. Shortness of breath (precipitating factors)

   7. Night sweats

   8. Wheezing or noise with breathing

Hematolymphatic

   1. Lymph node swelling

   2. Excessive bleeding or easy bruising

   3. Petechiae, ecchymoses

   4. Anemia

   5. Blood transfusions

   6. Excessive fatigue

   7. Radiation exposure

Gastrointestinal

   1. Food idiosyncrasies

   2. Change in taste

   3. Aphagopraxia or dysphagia (inability to swallow or difficulty in swallowing)

   4. Indigestion or pain (associated with eating?)

   5. Pyrosis (burning sensation in esophagus and stomach with sour eructation)

6. Ulcer history
7. Nausea/vomiting (time, degree, precipitating or associated factors)
8. Hematemesis
9. Jaundice
10. Ascites
11. Bowel habits (diarrhea/constipation)
12. Stool characteristics
13. Change in bowel habits
14. Hemorrhoids (pain, bleeding, amount)
15. Dyschezia (constipation resulting from habitual neglect in responding to stimulus to defecate)
16. Use of digestive or evacuation aids (what, how often)

Urinary
1. Characteristics of urine
2. History of renal stones
3. Hesitancy
4. Urinary frequency (in 24-hour period)
5. Change in stream of urination
6. Nocturia (excessive urination at night)
7. History of urinary tract infection, dysuria (painful urination), urgency, flank pain
8. Suprapubic pain
9. Dribbling or incontinence
10. Stress incontinence
11. Polyuria (excessive excretion of urine)
12. Oliguria (decrease in urinary output)
13. Pyuria

Genital
1. General
   a. Lesions
   b. Discharges
   c. Odors
   d. Pain, burning, pruritus
   e. Venereal disease history
   f. Satisfaction with sexual activity
   g. Birth control methods practiced
   h. Sterility
2. Men
   a. Prostate problems
   b. Penis and scrotum self-examination practices
3. Women
   a. Menstrual history (age of onset, last menstrual period [LMP], duration and amount of flow, problems)

    b. Amenorrhea (absence of menses)
    c. Menorrhagia (excessive menstruation)
    d. Dysmenorrhea (painful menses), treatment method
    e. Metrorrhagia (uterine bleeding at times other than during menses)
    f. Dyspareunia (pain with intercourse)
    g. Date of last Pap test

Musculoskeletal
  1. Muscles
    a. Twitching
    b. Cramping
    c. Pain
    d. Weakness
  2. Extremities
    a. Deformity
    b. Gait or coordination difficulties
    c. Interference with activities of daily living
    d. Walking (amount per day)
  3. Bones and joints
    a. Joint swelling
    b. Joint pain
    c. Redness
    d. Stiffness (time-of-day related)
    e. Joint deformity
    f. Crepitus (noise with joint movement)
    g. Limitations of movement
    h. Interference with ADLs (activities of daily living)
  4. Back
    a. History of back injury (characteristics of problems, corrective measures)
    b. Interference with ADLs

Central nervous system
  1. History of central nervous system disease
  2. Fainting episodes
  3. Seizures
    a. Characteristics
    b. Medications
  4. Cognitive changes
    a. Inability to remember (recent versus distant)
    b. Disorientation
    c. Phobias
    d. Hallucinations
    e. Interference with ADLs

   5. Motor-gait
      a. Coordinated movement
      b. Ataxia, balance problems
      c. Paralysis (partial versus complete)
      d. Tic, tremor, spasm
      e. Interference with ADLs
   6. Sensory
      a. Paresthesia (patterns)
      b. Tingling sensations
      c. Other changes
Endocrine
   1. Diagnosis of disease states (e.g., thyroid, diabetes)
   2. Changes in skin pigmentation or texture
   3. Changes in or abnormal hair distribution
   4. Sudden or unexplained changes in height and weight
   5. Intolerance of heat or cold
   6. Exophthalmos
   7. Goiter
   8. Hormone therapy
   9. Polydipsia (increased thirst)
   10. Polyphagia (increased food intake)
   11. Polyuria
   12. Anorexia (decreased appetite)
   13. Weakness
Allergic and immunological (optional; use if client indicates allergy history; note precipitating factors in each case)
   1. Dermatitis (inflammation or irritation of skin)
   2. Eczema
   3. Pruritus
   4. Urticaria (hives)
   5. Sneezing
   6. Vasomotor rhinitis (inflammation and swelling of mucous membrane of nose, nasal discharge)
   7. Conjunctivitis (inflammation of conjunctiva)
   8. Interference with ADLs
   9. Environmental and seasonal correlation
   10. Treatment techniques
Any other physiological problems or disease states not specifically discussed. (If present, explore in detail [e.g., fatigue, insomnia, nervousness]).

Psychosocial history

General statement of client's feelings about self

Feelings of satisfaction or frustration in interpersonal relationships

  1. Home, occupants
  2. Client's position in home relationships
  3. Most significant relationship (in and out of home)
  4. Community activities
  5. Work or school relationships
  6. Family cohesiveness patterns

Activities of daily living

  1. General description of work, leisure, and rest distribution
  2. Significant hobbies or methods of relaxation
  3. Family demands
  4. Community activities and involvement
  5. Ability to accomplish all that is desired during period of day/week

General statement about client's ability to cope with ADLs

Occupational history

  1. Jobs held in past
  2. Current employer
  3. Educational preparation
  4. Satisfaction with present and past employment
  5. Time spent at work versus time spent at play

Recent changes or stresses in client's lifestyle (e.g., divorce, moving, new job, family illness, new baby, financial stresses)

Patterns in which client copes with situations of stress

Response to illness

  1. Client's ability to cope during own or others' illness
  2. Client's family's and friends' response during periods of illness

History of psychiatric care or counseling

Feelings of anxiety or nervousness (characteristics and coping mechanisms)

Feelings of depression (such symptoms as insomnia, crying, fearfulness, marked irritability, or anger)

Changes in personality, behavior, or mood

Use of medications or other techniques during times of anxiety, stress, or depression

Habits

  1. Alcohol
     a. Kinds (beer, wine, mixed drinks)
     b. Frequency per week
     c. Pattern over past 5 years; 1 year

    d. Drinking companions

    e. Alcohol consumption variances (increase) when anxious or stressed

2. Smoking

    a. Kind (pipe, cigarette, cigar)

    b. Amount per week; day

    c. Pattern over past 5 years; 1 year

    d. Enclosed with others who smoke

    e. Smoking amount variances (increase) when anxious or stressed

    f. Desire to quit smoking (methods, attempts)

3. Coffee and tea

    a. Amount per day

    b. Pattern over past 5 years; 1 year

    c. Consumption variances (increase) when anxious or stressed

    d. Physiological effects

4. Other

    a. Overeating or sporadic eating (e.g., always in refrigerator, soft drink abuse, cookie jar syndrome)

    b. Nail biting

    c. "Street drug" usage

    d. Nervous noneating

    e. Seat belt use

Financial status

    1. Sources

    2. Adequacy

    3. Recent changes in resources and expenditures

Notes

Functional Health Patterns Assessment: Adult

Health perception–health management pattern

1. History
   a. How has general health been?
   b. Any colds in past year? If appropriate: Absences from work?
   c. Most important things you do to keep healthy? Think these things make a difference to health? (Include family folk remedies if appropriate.) Use of cigarettes, alcohol, drugs? Breast self-examination?
   d. Accidents (home, work, driving)?
   e. In past, been easy to find ways to follow things doctors or nurses suggest?
   f. If appropriate: What do you think caused this illness? Actions taken when symptoms perceived? Results of action?
   g. If appropriate: Things important to you in your health care? How can we be most helpful?
2. Examination
   a. General health appearance.

Nutritional-metabolic pattern

1. History
   a. Typical daily food intake. (Describe.) Supplements (vitamins, type of snacks)?
   b. Typical daily fluid intake. (Describe.)
   c. Weight loss/gain? (Amount.) Height loss/gain? (Amount.)
   d. Appetite?
   e. Food or eating: Discomfort? Swallowing? Diet restrictions?
   f. Heal well or poorly?
   g. Skin problems: Lesions, dryness?
   h. Dental problems?
2. Examination
   a. Skin: Bony prominences? Lesions? Color changes? Moistness?
   b. Oral mucous membranes: Color, moistness, lesions?
   c. Teeth: General appearance and alignment. Dentures? Cavities? Missing teeth?
   d. Actual weight, height.
   e. Temperature.
   f. Intravenous feeding/parenteral feeding (specify)?

Data from Gordon M: *Nursing diagnosis: process and application,* ed 3, St. Louis, 1994, Mosby; Gordon M: *Manual of nursing diagnosis: 1995–1996,* St. Louis, 1995, Mosby. In Mandle CL, Castle JE: Health promotion and the individual. In Edelman CL, Mandle CL: *Health promotion throughout the lifespan,* ed 4, St. Louis, 1998, Mosby.

Elimination pattern

1. History
   a. Bowel elimination pattern. (Describe.) Frequency? Character? Discomfort? Problem in control? Laxatives and so on?
   b. Urinary elimination pattern. (Describe.) Frequency? Problem in control?
   c. Excessive perspiration? Odor problems?
   d. Body cavity drainage, suction, and so on (specify)?
2. Examination
   a. If indicated: Examine excreta or drainage color and consistency.

Activity-exercise pattern

1. History
   a. Sufficient energy for desired/required activities?
   b. Exercise pattern? Type? Regularity?
   c. Spare-time (leisure) activities? Child: Play activities?
   d. Perceived ability (code for level) for:

Feeding _____	Dressing _____	Cooking _____
Bathing _____	Grooming _____	Shopping _____
Toileting _____	General mobility _____	
Bed mobility_____	Home maintenance_____	

   Functional Level Codes:
   Level 0:   Full self-care
   Level I: Requires use of equipment or device
   Level II: Requires assistance or supervision from another person
   Level III: Requires assistance or supervision from another person and equipment or device
   Level IV: Is dependent and does not participate
2. Examination
   a. Demonstrated ability (code listed above) for:

Feeding _____	Dressing _____	Cooking _____
Bathing _____	Grooming _____	Shopping _____
Toileting _____	General mobility _____	
Bed mobility_____	Home maintenance_____	

   b. Gait _____ Posture _____ Absent body part? (Specify) _____
   c. Range of motion (joints) _____ Muscle firmness _____
   d. Hand grip _____ Can pick up a pencil? _____
   e. Pulse (rate) _____ (rhythm) _____ Breath sounds _____
   f. Respirations (rate) _____ (rhythm) _____ Breath sounds _____
   g. Blood pressure _____
   h. General appearance (grooming, hygiene, energy level)

Sleep-rest pattern

1. History
   a. Generally rested and ready for daily activities after sleep?
   b. Sleep onset problems? Aids? Dreams (nightmares)? Early awakening?
   c. Rest-relaxation periods?
2. Examination
   a. If appropriate: Observe sleep pattern.

Cognitive-perceptual pattern

1. History
   a. Hearing difficulty? Hearing aid?
   b. Vision? Wear glasses? Last checked? When last changed?
   c. Any change in memory lately?
   d. Important decision easy/difficult to make?
   e. Easiest way for you to learn things? Any difficulty?
   f. Any discomfort? Pain? If appropriate: How do you manage it?
2. Examination
   a. Orientation.
   b. Hears whisper?
   c. Reads newsprint?
   d. Grasps ideas and questions (abstract, concrete)?
   e. Language spoken.
   f. Vocabulary level. Attention span.

Self-perception–self-concept pattern

1. History
   a. How describe self? Most of the time, feel good (not so good) about self?
   b. Changes in body or things you can do? Problem to you?
   c. Changes in way you feel about self or body (since illness started)?
   d. Things frequently make you angry? Annoyed? Fearful? Anxious?
   e. Ever feel you lose hope?
2. Examination
   a. Eye contact. Attention span (distraction).
   b. Voice and speech pattern. Body posture.
   c. Nervous (5) or relaxed (1); rate from 1 to 5.
   d. Assertive (5) or passive (1): rate from 1 to 5.

Roles-relationships pattern

1. History
   a. Live alone? Family? Family structure (diagram)?
   b. Any family problems you have difficulty handling (nuclear/extended)?
   c. Family or others depend on you for things? How managing?
   d. If appropriate: How family/others feel about illness/hospitalization?
   e. If appropriate: Problems with children? Difficulty handling?
   f. Belong to social groups? Close friends? Feel lonely (frequency)?
   g. Things generally go well at work? (School?)
   h. If appropriate: Income sufficient for needs?
   i. Feel part of (or isolated in) neighborhood where living?
2. Examination
   a. Interaction with family member(s) or others (if present).

Sexuality-reproductive pattern

1. History
   a. If appropriate to age and situation: Sexual relationships satisfying? Changes? Problems?
   b. If appropriate: Use of contraceptives? Problems?
   c. Female: When menstruation started? Last menstrual period? Menstrual problems? Para? Gravida?
2. Examination
   a. None unless problem identified or pelvic examination is part of full physical assessment.

Coping–stress tolerance pattern

1. History
   a. Any big changes in your life in the last year or two? Crisis?
   b. Who is most helpful in talking things over? Available to you now?
   c. Tense or relaxed most of the time? When tense, what helps?
   d. Use any medicines, drugs, alcohol?
   e. When (if) have big problems (any problems) in your life, how do you handle them?
   f. Most of the time, is this (are these) way(s) successful?
2. Examination: None.

Values-beliefs pattern

1. History
   a. Generally get things you want from life? Important plans for the future?
   b. Religion important in life? If appropriate: Does this help when difficulties arise?

   c. If appropriate: Will being here interfere with any religious practices?
2. Examination: None.
3. Other concerns
   a. Any other things we have not talked about that you would like to mention?
   b. Any questions?

Adult Physical Examination

There is no one right way to put together the parts of the physical examination so that the end product is an easily flowing process that minimizes the number of times the client has to change position and that conserves energy. The following is a suggested approach. In reality, this or any other approach may require adaptation to a particular setting, client condition, or client disability.

General inspection

Begin the inspection as you greet the client on entering the room, and look for signs of distress or disease. You can perform parts of your physical examination at any time as long as the client is within your view. There are no blank moments when you are with the client. On your first greeting, you can judge the alacrity with which you are met; the moistness of the palm when you shake hands; the gait as you walk back to the room; and the eyes, their luster, and their expression of emotion. All of this contributes to your examination, along with assessments of the following:

1. Skin color
2. Facial expression
3. Mobility
   a. Use of assistive devices
   b. Gait
   c. Sitting, rising from chair
   d. Taking off coat
4. Dress and posture
5. Speech pattern, disorders, foreign language
6. Difficulty hearing, assistive devices
7. Stature and build

Modified from Seidel H et al.: *Mosby's guide to physical examination,* ed 4, St. Louis, 1999, Mosby.

8. Musculoskeletal deformities
9. Vision problems, assistive devices
10. Eye contact with examiner
11. Orientation, mental alertness
12. Nutritional state
13. Respiratory problems
14. Significant others accompanying client

Client instructions

Instruct the client to empty bladder, remove clothing, and put on gown. Then begin the examination. A suggested sequence follows.

Measurement

1. Measure height.
2. Measure weight.
3. Assess distance vision: Snellen chart.
4. Document vital signs: temperature, pulse, respiration, and blood pressure in both arms.

Client seated, wearing gown

Client is seated on examining table; examiner stands in front of client.

Head and face

1. Inspect skin characteristics.
2. Inspect symmetry and external characteristics of eyes and ears.
3. Inspect configuration of skull.
4. Inspect and palpate scalp and hair for texture, distribution, and quantity of hair.
5. Palpate facial bones.
6. Palpate temporomandibular joint while client opens and closes mouth.
7. Palpate sinus regions; if tender, transilluminate.
8. Inspect ability to clench teeth, squeeze eyes tightly shut, wrinkle forehead, smile, stick out tongue, puff out cheeks (CN V, VII).
9. Test light sensation of forehead, cheeks, chin (CN V).

Eyes

1. External examination
   a. Inspect eyelids, eyelashes, palpebral folds.
   b. Determine alignment of eyebrows.
   c. Inspect sclera, conjunctiva, iris.
   d. Palpate lacrimal apparatus.
2. Near vision screening: Rosenbaum chart (CN II)

3. Eye function
  a. Test pupillary response to light and accommodation.
  b. Perform cover-uncover test and light reflex.
  c. Test extraocular eye movements (CN III, IV, VI).
  d. Assess visual fields (CN II).
  e. Test corneal reflex (CN V).
4. Ophthalmoscopic examination
  a. Test red reflex.
  b. Inspect lens.
  c. Inspect disc, cup margins, vessels, retinal surface, vitreous humor.

Ears

1. Inspect alignment.
2. Inspect surface characteristics.
3. Palpate auricle.
4. Assess hearing with whisper test or ticking watch (CN VIII).
5. Perform otoscopic examination.
  a. Inspect canals.
  b. Inspect tympanic membranes for landmarks, deformities, inflammation.
6. Perform Rinne and Weber tests.

Nose

1. Note structure, position of septum.
2. Determine patency of each nostril.
3. Inspect mucosa, septum, and turbinates with nasal speculum.
4. Assess olfactory function: test sense of smell (CN I).

Mouth and pharynx

1. Inspect lips, buccal mucosa, gums, hard and soft palates, floor of mouth for color and surface characteristics.
2. Inspect oropharynx: note anteroposterior pillars, uvula, tonsils, posterior pharynx, mouth odor.
3. Inspect teeth for color, number, surface characteristics.
4. Inspect tongue for color, characteristics, symmetry, movement (CN XII).
5. Test gag reflex and "ah" reflex (CN IX, X).
6. Perform taste test (CN VII).

Neck

1. Inspect for symmetry and smoothness of neck and thyroid.
2. Inspect for jugular venous distention.
3. Inspect and palpate range of motion; test resistance against examiner's hand.

4. Test shoulder shrug (CN IX).
5. Palpate carotid pulses.
6. Palpate tracheal position.
7. Palpate thyroid.
8. Palpate lymph nodes: preauricular and postauricular, occipital, tonsillar, submaxillary, submental, superficial cervical chain, posterior cervical, deep cervical, supraclavicular.
9. Auscultate carotid arteries and thyroid for bruits.

Upper extremities
1. Observe and palpate hands, arms, and shoulders.
   a. Skin and nail characteristics
   b. Muscle mass
   c. Musculoskeletal deformities
   d. Joint range of motion: fingers, wrists, elbows, shoulders
2. Assess pulses: radial, brachial.
3. Palpate epitrochlear nodes.
4. Perform Allen test.

Client seated, back exposed
Client is still seated on examining table. Gown is pulled down to the waist for males so the entire chest and back are exposed; back is exposed, but breasts are covered for females. Examiner stands behind the client.

Back and posterior chest
1. Inspect skin and thoracic configuration.
2. Inspect symmetry of shoulders, musculoskeletal development.
3. Inspect and palpate scapula and spine.
4. Palpate and percuss costovertebral angle.

Lungs
1. Inspect respiration: excursion, depth, rhythm, pattern.
2. Palpate for expansion and tactile fremitus.
3. Palpate scapular and subscapular nodes.
4. Percuss posterior chest and lateral walls systematically for resonance.
5. Percuss for diaphragmatic excursion.
6. Auscultate systematically for breath sounds: note characteristics and adventitious sounds.

Client seated, chest exposed
Examiner moves around to front of the client. The gown is lowered in females to expose anterior chest.

Anterior chest, lungs, and heart

1. Inspect skin, musculoskeletal development, symmetry.
2. Inspect respirations: client posture, respiratory effort.
3. Inspect for pulsations or heaving.
4. Palpate chest wall for stability, crepitation, tenderness.
5. Palpate precordium for thrills, heaves, pulsations.
6. Palpate left chest to locate apical impulse.
7. Palpate for tactile fremitus.
8. Palpate nodes: infraclavicular, axillary.
9. Percuss systematically for resonance.
10. Auscultate systematically for breath sounds.
11. Auscultate systematically for heart sounds: aortic area, pulmonic area, second pulmonic area, apical area.

Female breasts

1. Inspect in the following positions: client's arms extended over head, pushing hands on hips, hands pushed together in front of chest, client leaning forward.
2. Palpate breasts in all four quadrants, tail of Spence, over areolae; if breasts are large, perform bimanual palpation.
3. Palpate nipple; compress breasts to observe for discharge.

Male breasts

1. Inspect breasts and nipples for symmetry, enlargement, surface characteristics.
2. Palpate breast tissue.

Client reclining 45 degrees

Assist the client to a reclining position at a 45-degree angle. Examiner stands to the right side of the client.

1. Inspect chest in recumbent position.
2. Inspect jugular venous pulsations and measure jugular venous pressure.

Client supine, chest exposed

Assist the client into a supine position. If the client cannot tolerate lying flat, maintain head elevation at 30-degree angle. Uncover the chest while keeping abdomen and lower extremities draped.

Female breasts

1. Inspect in recumbent position.
2. Palpate systematically with client's arm over head and arm at side.

Heart
1. Palpate chest wall for thrills, heaves, pulsations.
2. Auscultate systematically; you can turn client slightly to left side and repeat auscultation.

Client supine, abdomen exposed
Client remains supine. Cover the chest with the client's gown. Arrange draping to expose the abdomen from pubis to epigastrium.

Abdomen
1. Inspect skin characteristics, contour, pulsations, movement.
2. Auscultate all quadrants for bowel sounds.
3. Auscultate aorta, renal arteries, femoral arteries for bruits, venous hums.
4. Percuss all quadrants for tone.
5. Percuss liver borders and estimate span.
6. Percuss left midaxillary line for splenic dullness.
7. Lightly palpate all quadrants.
8. Deeply palpate all quadrants.
9. Palpate right costal margin for liver border.
10. Palpate left costal margin for spleen.
11. Palpate for right and left kidneys.
12. Palpate midline for aortic pulsation.
13. Test abdominal reflexes.
14. Have client raise head as you inspect abdominal muscles.

Inguinal area
Palpate for lymph nodes, pulses, hernias.

External genitalia, males
1. Inspect penis, urethral meatus, scrotum, pubic hair.
2. Palpate scrotal contents.

Client supine, legs exposed
Client remains supine. Arrange drapes to cover abdomen and pubis and to expose lower extremities.

Feet and legs
1. Inspect for skin characteristics, hair distribution, muscle mass, musculoskeletal configuration.
2. Palpate for temperature, texture, edema, pulses (dorsal pedis, posterior tibial, popliteal).
3. Test range of motion and strength of toes, feet, ankles, knees.
4. Check for postural color changes.

Hips
1. Palpate hips for stability.
2. Test range of motion and strength of hips.

Client sitting, lap draped

Assist the client to a sitting position. Client should have gown on with drape across lap.

Musculoskeletal
1. Observe client moving from lying to sitting position.
2. Note coordination, use of muscles, ease of movement.

Neurological
1. Test sensory function: dull and sharp sensation of forehead, paranasal sinus area, lower arms, hands, lower legs, feet.
2. Test vibratory sensation of wrists, ankles.
3. Test two-point discrimination of palms, thighs, back.
4. Test stereognosis, graphesthesia.
5. Test fine motor function, coordination, and position sense of upper extremities.
   a. Touch nose with alternating index fingers.
   b. Rapidly alternate fingers to thumb.
   c. Rapidly move index finger between own nose and examiner's finger.
6. Test fine motor function, coordination, and position sense of lower extremities.
   a. Run heel down tibia of opposite leg.
   b. Alternately and rapidly cross leg over knee.
7. Test deep tendon reflexes and compare bilaterally: biceps, triceps, brachioradial, patellar, Achilles.
8. Test Babinski reflex bilaterally.

Client standing

Assist client to a standing position. Examiner stands next to client.

Spine
1. Inspect and palpate spine as client bends over at waist.
2. Test range of motion: hyperextension, lateral bending, rotation of upper trunk.

Neurological
1. Observe gait.
2. Test proprioception and cerebellar function.

a. Assess Romberg test.
b. Ask the client to walk heel to toe.
c. Ask the client to stand on one foot then the other with eyes closed.
d. Ask the client to hop in place on one foot then the other.
e. Ask the client to do deep knee bends.

Abdominal/genital
Test for inguinal and femoral hernias.

Female client, lithotomy position
Assist female clients into lithotomy position and drape appropriately. Examiner is seated.

External genitalia
1. Inspect pubic hair, labia, clitoris, urethral opening, vaginal opening, perineal and perianal area, anus.
2. Palpate labia and Bartholin's glands; milk Skene's glands.

Internal genitalia
1. Perform speculum examination.
   a. Inspect vagina and cervix.
   b. Collect Pap smear and other necessary specimens.
2. Perform bimanual palpation to assess for characteristics of vagina, cervix, uterus, adnexae.
3. Perform rectovaginal examination to assess rectovaginal septum, broad ligaments.
4. Perform rectal examination.
   a. Assess anal sphincter tone and surface characteristics.
   b. Obtain rectal culture if needed.
   c. Note characteristics of stool when gloved finger is removed.

Male client, bending forward
Assist male clients in leaning over examining table or into knee-chest position. Examiner is behind client.

1. Inspect sacrococcygeal and perianal areas.
2. Perform rectal examination.
   a. Palpate sphincter tone and surface characteristics.
   b. Obtain rectal culture if needed.
   c. Palpate prostate gland and seminal vesicles.
   d. Note characteristics of stool when gloved finger is removed.

Assessment Tests

Name of test	How to perform	Interpretation
Adson's test	Have client sit with arms pronated, chin raised high and pointed toward side being examined. Have client inspire and hold his or her breath. Check radial pulse to see if it is still present. If present, is it diminished?	If radial pulse is absent or diminished, test is positive—indicates subclavian compression or scalenus anticus syndrome.
Allen's test	Have client sit with arms supinated. Occlude both radial arteries with your fingers and have client pump his or her hands 3 times. Have client open his or her hands with radial artery still compressed. Observe color of client's palm. Repeat test, occluding ulnar arteries.	If palms are not a normal pink color but are white or very pale pink, this indicates that either radial or ulnar artery is occluded.
Anvil test	Raise limb of supine client from table with knee in extension; strike calcaneus with fist, using a moderate blow in direction of hip.	This maneuver causes pain in early hip joint disease.
Babinski's reflex	Using a blunt object, stroke along lateral side of foot from heel to ball, and across ball of foot to medial side.	Dorsiflexion of big toe with extension fanning of other toes is a positive reflex. This reflex is normal in infants and abnormal in children and adults—indicates pyramidal tract disease.

From Dunn S: *Mosby's primary care consultant,* St. Louis, 1998, Mosby.

Continued.

Assessment Tests—cont'd

Name of test	How to perform	Interpretation
Bárány's test (caloric test)	Alternately irrigate ears with warm water or air and cold water or air. Warm irrigation produces rotary nystagmus toward irrigated side, and cold irrigation produces rotary nystagmus away from irrigated side.	If ear is diseased, less nystagmus is produced.
Barre's pyramidal sign	With client in recumbent position, watch lateral or vertical movement of one leg.	If opposite leg makes a similar movement, this sign is positive, indicating a prefrontal brain lesion.
Brodie-Trendelenburg test	With client supine, elevate leg vertically until veins are empty. Client then stands, and examiner observes filling of veins.	If valves are incompetent, veins fill from above. If valves are normal, veins fill from bottom. Incompetent valves are seen in varicose veins.
Brudzinski's sign	With client supine, passively flex neck to chin while holding down thorax.	Involuntary hip flexion occurs with nuchal rigidity.
CAGE questionnaire*	C Feels need to *cut down* on drinking A Is *annoyed* by criticism G Feels *guilty* E Has an *eye-opener*	Any positive answer indicates that alcoholism is possible.
Chaddock's reflex	Firmly stroke ulnar surface of forearm.	Flexion of wrist and extension of fingers in a fanlike position is a positive reflex. This reflex is abnormal and is seen in hemiplegia.
Chadwick's sign	Perform internal examination of female genitalia.	If cervix is bluish purple, this sign is positive; Chadwick's sign is a presumptive sign of pregnancy.

Charcot's triad	Assess for intention tremors, nystagmus, and scanning speech. Presence of Charcot's triad is a sign of brainstem involvement in multiple sclerosis.
Chvostek's sign	Tap facial nerve against bone just anterior to ear. Ipsilateral contraction of facial muscle is a positive sign of tetany, as in parathyroid deficit; may indicate calcium or magnesium deficit.
Costovertebral tenderness	Strike with heel of palm between spine and twelfth rib. Tenderness indicates inflammation of kidney.
Cranial nerves	I—olfactory Test smell.
	II—optic Test vision (fundoscopic examination).
	III—oculomotor Test eye movement (pupillary reflex and size, shape, and equality of pupils).
	IV—trochlear Test eye movement (ability to follow moving objects).
	V—trigeminal Test head and face movement and sensation to pain, touch, and temperature.
	VI—abducens Test lateral rectus muscle.
	VII—facial Test muscles of face, scalp, and auricula.
	VIII—acoustic Test hearing and for nystagmus.
	IX—glossopharyngeal Test with vagus nerve.
	X—vagus Test uvula elevation, gag reflex, and swallow reflex.
	XI—accessory Test resistance of trapezii; turn head against resistance.
	XII—hypoglossal Test tongue muscle strength.
Crossed-leg raise	Have client with low-back pain lie supine and raise unaffected leg with knee extended. Pain in affected leg and sciatic pain in unaffected leg indicate herniated disc.

Continued.

*From Ewing JA: CAGE questionnaire, *JAMA* 252:1908, 1984.

Assessment Tests—cont'd

Name of test	How to perform	Interpretation
Drawer's sign	With client supine, have client flex affected knee at right angle. Sit on client's foot. With both hands grasp upper part of legs with fingers in popliteal fossa and pull head of tibia toward you.	Movement more than 1 cm is positive sign—indicates rupture of anterior cruciate ligament.
Finger-to-nose test	With arms extended and eyes open, ask client to quickly bring his or her finger in a wide arc to nose.	In cerebellar disease, this motion is accompanied by an action tremor.
Goodell's sign	Assess during bimanual female examination.	Softening of cervix is a probable sign of pregnancy.
Graenslen's test	With client supine, have him or her hold knee of affected side with both hands, flexing knee and hip to fix lumbar spine to table; hyperextend other thigh by pushing it over end of table.	An affected sacroiliac joint will emit pain.
Hegar's sign	Assess during bimanual female examination.	Softening of lower uterine segment is a probable sign of pregnancy.
Homans' sign	Assess dorsiflexion of foot.	Pain produced in calf of same leg indicates thrombophlebitis or thrombosis.
Hoover's sign	Have client in supine position. Stand at foot and take each heel in one of your palms, and rest your hands on table. Have client attempt to raise affected limb.	This test is used to differentiate hysterical paralysis from organic paralysis. In organic disease, the movement causes unaffected heel to press downward. In hysteria, it does not.

Kernig's sign	With client supine, passively flex hip, with knee flexed at 90 degrees. Keep hip flexed and attempt to straighten knee.	This reliable sign of meningeal irritation can occur with herniated disc or tumor of cauda equina. Resistance to knee extension is a positive sign.
McBurney's sign	Palpate McBurney's point, which is a point in right lower quadrant of abdomen. It is about 2 inches from right anterosuperior iliac spine, in a line between spine and umbilicus.	Severe pain and tenderness are found in appendicitis.
McMurray's test	Have client supine or standing on affected side. Place one hand on foot and one on knee. Flex knee until heel nearly touches buttocks. Rotate foot laterally and extend knee to 90 degrees.	Click indicates torn medial meniscus.
Murphy's sign	Palpate subhepatic area deeply.	Inspiratory arrest secondary to extreme tenderness indicates cholecystitis.
Naffziger's sign	Compress external jugular vein.	If maneuver produces nerve root irritation, it is diagnostic for sciatica or herniated nucleus pulposus.
Ortolani's sign	Place infant on his or her back on examining table, flex hips and knees at right angles, and abduct until lateral aspect of knees touch table. Examiner's hands should be around infant's thighs and knees. Attempt internal and external rotation.	Click or popping sound indicates joint instability.
Patrick's test	With client supine, flex knee and place foot on opposite patella. Pull flexed knee lateralward as far as possible.	No pain means test is negative and excludes hip joint disease.

Continued.

Assessment Tests—cont'd

Name of test	How to perform	Interpretation
Phalen's maneuver	Flex both wrists to 90 degrees with dorsal surfaces in opposition for 60 seconds.	Tingling, pain, or numbness indicates carpal tunnel syndrome. Extension brings relief.
Pulse deficit	Two examiners are needed. One counts radial pulse, and other counts apical pulse.	If radial pulse is less than apical pulse, there is a lack of peripheral perfusion.
Rebound tenderness	In region of abdomen remote to suspect area, push deeply and then withdraw abruptly.	Pain experienced in affected area is sign of peritoneal irritation (e.g., peritonitis or appendicitis).
Rinne test	Hold vibrating tuning fork on mastoid process; when sound is no longer heard, hold fork in air next to ear.	AC > BC is positive test (normal); BC > AC is negative test.
Romberg's test	Have client standing with legs together and arms at sides, first with eyes open and then with eyes closed.	Loss of balance is positive test—indicates cerebellar ataxia or vestibular dysfunction.
Simmonds' test	With client prone and with feet off table, squeeze calf muscle transversely.	Plantar flexion indicates normal or incomplete rupture of Achilles tendon. There is no motion with complete rupture.
Straight-leg raises (SLRs)	With client supine, elevate each leg passively with knee extended.	Radicular pain at 30 to 60 degrees is positive test.
Tinel's sign	Light percussion on radial side of palmaris longus tendon.	Tingling sensation indicates carpal tunnel syndrome.
Trendelenburg's sign	Have client stand on one foot unsupported.	In normal hip, buttock rises and falls; in dislocation of hip, there is weakness of gluteal muscle or paralysis.

Trousseau's sign	Occlude brachial artery for 3 minutes with a BP cuff.	No response is normal. Carpal spasm indicates latent tetany, as seen in hypocalcemia or hypomagnesemia.
2-minute orthopedic examination[†]	Stand facing examiner.	Assess acromioclavicular joints and general habitus.
	Look at ceiling, floor, over both shoulders; touch ears to shoulders.	Assess cervical spine motion.
	Shrug shoulders (examiner resists).	Assess trapezius strength.
	Abduct shoulders 90 degrees (examiner resists at 90 degrees).	Assess deltoid strength.
	Perform full external rotation of arms.	Assess shoulder motion.
	Flex and extend elbows.	Assess elbow motion.
	With arms at sides and elbows 90 degrees flexed, pronate and supinate wrists.	Assess elbow and wrist motion.
	Spread fingers; make fist.	Assess hand or finger motion and deformities.
	Tighten quadriceps; relax quadriceps.	Assess symmetry and knee effusion, as well as ankle effusion.
	Duck walk 4 steps (away from examiner with buttocks on heels).	Assess hip, knee, and ankle motion.
	Turn back to examiner.	Assess for symmetry. Back is asymmetric in scoliosis.
	Rise up on toes, raise heels.	Assess for calf symmetry and leg strength.
	With knees straight, touch toes.	Assess for scoliosis, hip motion, and hamstring tightness.
Weber test	Place vibrating tuning fork in midline of skull.	In normal hearing, sound is heard the same in both ears. In conductive loss, sound lateralizes to bad ear. In sensorineural loss, sound lateralizes to good ear.

From Dunn S: *Mosby's primary care consultant,* St. Louis, 1998, Mosby.

ELDERLY ASSESSMENT

Important Aspects of the History in the Elderly

Social history
Living arrangements
Relationships with family and friends
Economic status
Abilities to perform activities of daily living
Social activities and hobbies
Mode of transportation

Past medical history
Previous surgical procedures
Major illnesses and hospitalizations
Immunization status
    Influenza, pneumococcal, tetanus
Tuberculosis history and testing
Medications (use the "brown bag" technique)
    Previous allergies
    Knowledge of current medication regimen
    Compliance
Perceived beneficial or adverse drug effects

Systems review
Ask questions about general symptoms that may indicate treatable underlying disease such as fatigue, anorexia, weight loss, and insomnia. Attempt to elicit key symptoms in each organ system, including:

System	Key symptoms
Respiratory	Increasing dyspnea
	Persistent cough
Cardiovascular	Orthopnea
	Edema
	Angina
	Claudication
	Palpitations
	Dizziness
	Syncope

From Kane R, Ouslander J, Abrass I: *Essentials of clinical geriatrics,* ed 3, New York, 1994, McGraw-Hill.

System	Key symptoms
Gastrointestinal	Difficulty chewing
	Dysphagia
	Abdominal pain
	Change in bowel habit
Genitourinary	Frequency
	Urgency
	Nocturia
	Hesitancy, intermittent stream, straining to void
	Incontinence
	Hematuria
	Vaginal bleeding
Musculoskeletal	Focal or diffuse pain
	Focal or diffuse weakness
Neurological	Visual disturbances (transient or progressive)
	Progressive hearing loss
	Unsteadiness or falls
	Transient focal symptoms
Psychological	Depression
	Anxiety or agitation
	Paranoia
	Forgetfulness or confusion

Normal Physical Assessment Findings for Elderly Clients

Cardiovascular changes

Cardiac output	Heart loses elasticity; therefore decreased heart contractility in response to increased demands
Arterial circulation	Decreased vessel compliance with increased peripheral resistance to blood flow resulting from general or localized arteriosclerosis
Venous circulation	Does not exhibit change with aging in the absence of disease
Blood pressure	Significant increase in the systolic, slight increase in the diastolic, increase in peripheral resistance and pulse pressure
Heart	Dislocation of the apex because of kyphoscoliosis; therefore diagnostic significance of location is lost
	Increased premature beats, rarely clinically important

From Ebersole P, Hess P: *Toward healthy aging,* ed 5, St. Louis, 1998, Mosby.

Normal Physical Assessment Findings for Elderly Clients—cont'd

Cardiovascular changes—cont'd

Murmurs	Diastolic murmurs in over half the aged; the most common heard at the base of the heart because of sclerotic changes on the aortic valves
Peripheral pulses	Easily palpated because of increased arterial wall narrowing and loss of connective tissue; feeling of tortuous and rigid vessels
	Possibility that pedal pulses may be weaker as a result of arteriosclerotic changes; colder lower extremities, especially at night; possibility of cold feet and hands with mottled color
Heart rate	No changes with age at normal rest

Respiratory changes

Pulmonary blood flow and diffusion	Decreased blood flow to the pulmonary circulation; decreased diffusion
Anatomic structure	Increased anterior-posterior diameter
Respiratory accessory muscles	Degeneration and decreased strength; increased rigidity of chest wall
	Muscle atrophy of pharynx and larynx
Internal pulmonic structure	Decreased pulmonary elasticity creates senile emphysema
	Shorter breaths taken with decreased maximum breathing capacity, vital capacity, residual volume, and functional capacity
	Airway resistance increases; less ventilation at the base of the lung and more at the apex

Integumentary changes

Texture	Skin loses elasticity; wrinkles, folding, sagging, dryness
Color	Spotty pigmentation in areas exposed to sun; face paler, even in the absence of anemia
Temperature	Extremities cooler; decreased perspiration
Fat distribution	Less on extremities; more on trunk
Hair color	Dull gray, white, yellow, or yellow-green
Hair distribution	Thins on scalp, axilla, pubic area, upper and lower extremities; decreased facial hair in men, women may develop chin and upper lip hair
Nails	Decreased growth rate

Genitourinary and reproductive changes

Renal blood flow	Because of decreased cardiac output, reduced filtration rate and renal efficiency; possibility of subsequent loss of protein from kidneys
Micturition	In men possibility of increased frequency as a result of prostatic enlargement
	In women decreased perineal muscle tone; therefore urgency and stress incontinence
	Increased nocturia for both men and women
	Possibility that polyuria may be diabetes related
	Decreased volume of urine may relate to decrease in intake but evaluation needed
Incontinence	Increased occurrence with age, specifically in those with dementia
Male reproduction	
Testosterone production	Decreases; phases of intercourse slower, lengthened refractory time
Frequency of intercourse	No changes in libido and sexual satisfaction; decreased frequency to one or two times weekly
Testes	Decreased size; decreased sperm count; diminished viscosity of seminal fluid
Female reproduction	
Estrogen	Decreased production with menopause
Breasts	Diminished breast tissue
Uterus	Decreased size; mucous secretions cease; possibility that uterine prolapse may occur as a result of muscle weakness
Vagina	Epithelial lining atrophies; narrow and shortened canal
Vaginal secretions	Become more alkaline as glycogen content increases and acidity declines

Gastrointestinal changes

Mastication	Impaired because of partial or total loss of teeth, malocclusive bite, and ill-fitting dentures
Swallowing and carbohydrate digestion	Swallowing more difficult as salivary secretions less diminish
Esophagus	Decreased esophageal peristalsis
	Increased incidence of hiatus hernia with accompanying gaseous distention
Digestive enzymes	Decreased production of hydrochloric acid, pepsin, and pancreatic enzymes
Fat absorption	Delayed, affecting the absorption rate of fat-soluble vitamins A, D, E, and K
Intestinal peristalsis	Reduced gastrointestinal motility
	Constipation because of decreased motility and roughage

Continued.

Normal Physical Assessment Findings for Elderly Clients—cont'd

Musculoskeletal changes

Muscle strength and function	Decrease with loss of muscle mass; bony prominences normal in aged, since muscle mass decreased
Bone structure	Normal demineralization, more porous
	Shortening of the trunk as a result of intervertebral space narrowing
Joints	Become less mobile; tightening and fixation occur
	Activity may maintain function longer
	Normal posture changes; some kyphosis
	Range of motion limited
Anatomic size and height	Total decrease in size as loss of body protein and body water occurs in proportion to decrease in basal metabolic rate
	Increased body fat; diminished in arms and legs, increased in trunk
	Decreased height from 2.5 to 10 cm from young adulthood

Nervous system changes

Response to stimuli	All voluntary or automatic reflexes slower
	Decreased ability to respond to multiple stimuli
Sleep patterns	Stage IV sleep reduced in comparison to younger adulthood; increased frequency of spontaneous awakening
	Stay in bed longer but get less sleep; insomnia a problem which should be evaluated
Reflexes	Deep tendon reflexes responsive in the healthy aged
Ambulation	Kinesthetic sense less efficient; may demonstrate an extrapyramidal Parkinson-like gait
	Basal ganglions of the nervous system influenced by the vascular changes and decreased oxygen supply
Voice	Decreased range, duration, and intensity of voice; may become higher pitched and monotonous

Sensory changes

Vision	
Peripheral vision	Decreases
Lens accommodation	Decreases, requires corrective lenses
Ciliary body	Atrophy around disc
Iris	Development of arcus senilis
Choroid	Atrophy around disc
Lens	May develop opacity, cataract formation; more light necessary to see
Color	Fades or disappears

Sensory changes—cont'd

Macula	Degenerates
Conjunctiva	Thins and looks yellow
Tearing	Decreases; increased irritation and infection
Pupil	May differ in size
Cornea	Presence of arcus senilis
Retina	Observable vascular changes
Stimuli threshold	Increased threshold for light touch and pain
	Ischemic paresthesias common in the extremities
Hearing	Less perceptible high-frequency tones; hence greatly impaired language understanding; promotes confusion and seems to create increased rigidity in thought processes
Gustatory	Decreased acuity as taste buds atrophy; may increase the amount of seasoning on food

SITUATIONAL ASSESSMENT

The nurse encounters a variety of situational interruptions when caring for clients. Assessment of selected and common events will assist the nurse to develop an appropriate plan of care. The following tools are examples to help the nurse working with clients in the community.

ACTIVITIES OF DAILY LIVING

The assessment of the client's ability to perform the activities of daily living provides the nurse with data to indicate the client's self-care ability. The following tools may be used to plan the assistance given to the client to regain a maximum level of independence, and to plan for support services. Basic activities of daily living and instrumental activities of daily living are both given.

Index of Independence in Basic Activities of Daily Living

The Index of Independence in Basic Activities of Daily Living is based on an evaluation of the functional independence or dependence of clients in bathing, dressing, going to toilet, transferring, continence, and feeding. Specific definitions of functional independence and dependence appear below the index.

A—Independent in feeding, continence, transferring, going to toilet, dressing, and bathing.

B—Independent in all but one of these functions.

C—Independent in all but bathing and one additional function.

D—Independent in all but bathing, dressing, and one additional function.

E—Independent in all but bathing, dressing, going to toilet, and one additional function.

F—Independent in all but bathing, dressing, going to toilet, transferring, and one additional function.

G—Dependent in all six functions.

Other—Dependent in at least two functions but not classifiable as C, D, E, or F.

Independence means without supervision, direction, or active personal assistance, except as specifically noted. This is based on actual status and not on ability. A client who refuses to perform a function is considered as not performing the function, even though the client is deemed able.

Bathing (sponge, shower, or tub)

Independent: assistance only in bathing a single part (as back or disabled extremity) or bathes self completely

Dependent: assistance in bathing more than one part of body; assistance in getting in or out of tub or does not bathe self

Dressing

Independent: gets clothes from closets and drawers; puts on clothes, outer garments, braces; manages fasteners; act of tying shoes is excluded

Dependent: does not dress self or remains partly undressed

Going to toilet

Independent: gets to toilet; gets on and off toilet; arranges clothes; cleans organs of excretion (may manage own bedpan used at night only and may or may not be using mechanical supports)

Dependent: uses bedpan or commode or receives assistance in getting to and using toilet

Transfer

Independent: moves in and out of bed independently and moves in and out of chair independently (may or may not be using mechanical supports)

Dependent: assistance in moving in or out of bed or chair; does not perform one or more transfers

Continence

Independent: urination and defecation entirely self-controlled

Dependent: partial or total incontinence in urination or defecation; partial or total control by enemas, catheters, or regulated use of urinals or bedpans

Feeding

Independent: gets food from plate or its equivalent into mouth (precutting of meat and preparation of food, as buttering bread, are excluded from evaluation)

Dependent: assistance in act of feeding (see above); does not eat at all or parenteral feeding

Evaluation form

Name _____   Date of evaluation _____

For each area of functioning listed below, check description that applies.
  (The word "assistance" means supervision, direction of personal assistance.)

Bathing—either sponge bath, tub bath, or shower

☐	☐	☐
Receives no assistance (gets in and out of tub by self if tub is usual means of bathing)	Receives assistance in bathing only one part of the body (such as back or a leg)	Receives assistance in bathing more than one part of the body (or not bathed)

Dressing—gets clothes from closets and drawers—including underclothes, outer garments, and using fasteners (including braces if worn)

☐	☐	☐
Gets clothes and gets completely dressed without assistance	Gets clothes and gets dressed without assistance except for assistance in tying shoes	Receives assistance in getting clothes or in getting dressed, or stays partly or completely undressed

Toileting—going to the "toilet room" for bowel and urine elimination; cleaning self after elimination, and arranging clothes

☐	☐	☐
Goes to "toilet room," cleans self, and arranges clothes without assistance (may use object for support such as cane, walker, or wheelchair and may manage night bedpan or commode, emptying same in morning)	Receives assistance in going to "toilet room," in cleansing self, or in arranging clothes after elimination or in use of night bedpan or commode	Does not go to room termed "toilet" for the elimination process

Transfer—

☐	☐	☐
Moves in and out of bed as well as in and out of chair without assistance (may be using object for support such as cane or walker)	Moves in or out of bed or chair with assistance	Does not get out of bed

Continence—

☐
Controls urination and bowel movement completely by self

☐
Has occasional "accidents"

☐
Supervision helps keep urine or bowel control; catheter is used, or is incontinent

Feeding—

☐
Feeds self without assistance

☐
Feeds self except for getting assistance in cutting meat or buttering bread

☐
Receives assistance in feeding or is fed partly or completely by using tubes or intravenous fluids

Instrumental Activities of Daily Living

Evaluation of autonomy of the older adult helps in making decisions with family and clients about client care. This scale can be an effective therapeutic tool in planning care and in identifying strengths and limitations of the older adult.

Instructions

The instrumental activities of daily living (IADL) has eight categories of activities that help the nurse determine the client's level of functioning beyond simple physical tasks of self-care. The highest possible score for both males and females is *eight.* For males, the possible score for each item in a category appears in the first column at the right of the category items. For females, the possible score for each item in a category appears in the second column at the right of the category items. The highest possible score for a category is one and the lowest possible score is zero.

Give a score for each category, choosing the category item that best reflects the client's level of functioning. For example, A: Ability to use telephone = **1.** Item chosen: #2—Dials a few well-known numbers.

Modified from Lawton M, Brody E: Assessment of older people: self-maintaining and instrumental activities of daily living, *The Gerontologist* 9:179-186, 1969. Copyright © The Gerontological Society of America.

Sum the score.

A score of 7-8 = high level independence

5-6 = moderate level independence

3-4 = moderate level dependence

1-2 = dependence

Although a summed score will give an overall picture of the level of independence in IADL, each category should be considered separately to determine the rehabilitative needs of clients.

Category	Male score	Female score
A. Ability to use telephone		
1. Operates telephone on own initiative—looks up and dials numbers, etc.	1	1
2. Dials a few well-known numbers.	1	1
3. Answers telephone but does not dial.	1	1
4. Does not use telephone at all.	0	0
B. Shopping		
1. Takes care of all shopping needs independently.	1	1
2. Shops independently for small purchases.	0	0
3. Needs to be accompanied on any shopping trip.	0	0
4. Completely unable to shop.	0	0
C. Food preparation	(if applicable)	
1. Plans, prepares, and serves adequate meals independently.	1	1
2. Prepares adequate meals if supplied with ingredients.	0	0
3. Heats and serves prepared meals, or prepares meals but does not maintain adequate diet.	0	0
4. Needs to have meals prepared and served.	0	0
D. Housekeeping	(if applicable)	
1. Maintains house alone or with occasional assistance (e.g., "heavy work–domestic help").	1	1
2. Performs light daily tasks such as dish washing, bed making.	1	1
3. Performs light daily tasks but cannot maintain acceptable level of cleanliness.	1	1
4. Needs help with all home maintenance tasks.	1	1
5. Does not participate in any housekeeping tasks.	0	0
E. Laundry	(if applicable)	
1. Does personal laundry completely.	1	1
2. Launders small items—rinses socks, stockings, etc.	1	1
3. All laundry must be done by others.	0	0

Category	Male score	Female score
F. Mode of transportation		
1. Travels independently on public transportation or drives own car.	1	1
2. Arranges own travel via taxi, but does not otherwise use public transportation.	1	1
3. Travels on public transportation when assisted or accompanied by another.	0	1
4. Travel limited to taxi or automobile with assistance of another.	0	0
5. Does not travel at all.	0	0
G. Responsibility for own medications		
1. Is responsible for taking medication in correct dosages at correct time.	1	1
2. Takes responsibility if medication is prepared in advance in separate dosages.	0	0
3. Is not capable of dispensing own medication.	0	0
H. Ability to handle finances		
1. Manages financial matters, independently budgets, writes checks, pays rent, bills, goes to bank, collects and keeps track of income.	1	1
2. Manages own finances with assistance for banking.	1	1
3. Is not capable of managing finances.	0	0

Dementia Assessment

Dementia involves loss of intellectual functioning and memory over time, which results in dysfunction in daily living. It is important for the nurse to compute the results of an assessment of dementia to provide anticipatory guidance needed for education and support of clients and family.

A. History

1. Active medical conditions

_____

_____

_____

From Kane R, Ouslander J, Abrass I: *Essentials of clinical geriatrics,* New York, 1994, McGraw-Hill.

2. Medications

_____

_____

_____

3. History of (describe):

_____ Hypertension

_____ Stroke

_____ Transient ischemic attack

_____ Depression

_____ Other psychiatric disorder

4. Current symptoms (complaints of client or family)

_____ Memory loss

_____ Forgets recent events

_____ Forgets things just said

_____ Forgets names of people

_____ Forgets words

_____ Gets lost

_____ Asks questions or tells stories repeatedly

_____ Confused about date or place

_____ Cannot do simple calculations

_____ Cannot understand what is read or said

_____ Impairment of other cognitive functions

_____ Anxiety/agitation

_____ Paranoia

_____ Delusions/hallucinations

_____ Wandering

_____ Disruptive behavior

_____ Incontinence

5. Onset of symptoms

_____ Recent (days to few weeks)

_____ Longer duration (months)

_____ Uncertain

6. Progression of symptoms

_____ Rapid

_____ Gradual

_____ Stepwise (irregular, stuttering deteriorations)

_____ Uncertain

7. Activities of daily living (ADL)

Does the impairment of cognitive function interfere with instrumental ADL?

_____ Yes   _____ No

If yes, which ones? _____

Basic ADL? _____ Yes _____ No

If yes, which ones? _____

B. Physical examination

1. General appearance
   _____ Normal
   _____ Abnormal (Describe: _____)

2. Blood pressure
   Right arm _____ / _____
   Left arm _____ /_____

3. Hearing

	Normal	Abnormal
Normal voice	_____	_____
1024-Hz tuning fork	_____	_____

4. Orientation

	No	Yes
Person	_____	_____
Place	_____	_____
Time	_____	_____
Situation	_____	_____

5. Memory function

	Normal	Impaired
Remote	_____	_____
Recent (object recall after 5 minutes)	_____	_____
Immediate (digit repetition)	_____	_____

6. Short Portable Status Questionnaire
   (Many other standardized tests are also available.)

Right	Wrong	
_____	_____	What is the date today (month/day/year)?
_____	_____	What day of the week is it?
_____	_____	What is the name of this place?
_____	_____	What is your telephone number? (If no telephone, what is your street address?)
_____	_____	How old are you?
_____	_____	When were you born (month/day/year)?
_____	_____	Who is the current president of the United States?
_____	_____	Who was the president just before him?
_____	_____	What was your mother's maiden name?
_____	_____	Subtract 3 from 20 and keep subtracting 3 from each new number you get, all the way down.

   Number of errors _____
   0-2 errors—intact
   3-4 errors—mild intellectual impairment
   5-6 errors—moderate intellectual impairment
   8-10 errors—severe intellectual impairment

7. Other cognitive functions

	Normal	Impaired
Remote	————	————
General fund of knowledge	————	————
Simple calculations	————	————
Ability to write name	————	————
Ability to copy diagrams	————	————
Interpretations of proverbs	————	————
Naming common objects	————	————
Insight	————	————
Judgment	————	————
Ability to follow simple written commands (e.g., "Close your eyes")	————	————
Ability to follow simple verbal commands (e.g., "Touch your left ear with your right hand")	————	————

8. Thought content
   _____ Normal
   _____ Delusions
   _____ Paranoid ideation
   _____ Other (Describe: _____)

9. Mood/affect
   _____ Appropriate _____ Depressed _____ Labile _____ Agitated
   _____ Other (Describe: _____)

10. Behavior during examinations

	Yes	No
Good attention and concentration	————	————
Good effort to answer questions and perform tasks	————	————
Many "don't know" answers	————	————

11. Remainder of neurological examination
    _____ Focal neurological signs (Describe: _____)
    _____
    _____ Signs of parkinsonism (Describe: _____)
    _____
    Pathological reflexes:
    _____ Babinski
    _____ Hoffman
    _____ Grasp
    _____ Palmomental
    Gait:
    _____ Normal
    _____ Abnormal (Describe: _____)
    _____ Other abnormality (Describe: _____)

Sensory examination:
_____ Normal
_____ Abnormal (Describe _____)

12. Hachinski ischemia score

Characteristic	Point score
Abrupt onset	2
Stepwise deterioration	1
Somatic complaints	1
Emotional incontinence	1
History or presence of hypertension	1
History of strokes	2
Focal neurological symptoms	2
Focal neurological signs	2

Total score: _____
(Score of 4 or more suggests multiinfarct dementia.)

C. Diagnostic studies

	Normal	Abnormal
Blood:		
CBC	_____	_____
Sedimentation rate	_____	_____
Glucose	_____	_____
BUN	_____	_____
Electrolytes	_____	_____
Calcium	_____	_____
Liver function tests	_____	_____
Free thyroxine index	_____	_____
TSH	_____	_____
VDRL	_____	_____
Vitamin B_{12}	_____	_____
Folate	_____	_____
Radiographic:		
Chest film	_____	_____
CT scan	_____	_____
Other:		
Urinalysis	_____	_____
EKG	_____	_____
EEG	_____	_____
Lumbar puncture	_____	_____
Audiology	_____	_____

D. Diagnosis

_____ Probable primary degenerative dementia (Alzheimer's type)
_____ Multiinfarct dementia
_____ Mixed
_____ Other (describe)
_____ Depression
_____ Other potentially reversible cause of dementia (describe)

Focused Assessment for Clients With Cognitive Impairment

Assessment	Clinical example
Orientation	
Is the client oriented to time?	Perceives time passing rapidly; confused about whether it is spring or summer; perceives date as 10 years earlier.
Is the client oriented to place?	Believes that he is living in a resort and not a nursing home; goes to nurse's station asking for his bill because he wants to check the room-service charges.
Is the client oriented to person?	Does not recognize her children.
Does the client become more disoriented late in the day or at night? Does the client exhibit symptoms of sundown syndrome?	Becomes agitated, yelling at people as twilight approaches.
Thought processes	
Is there evidence of forgetfulness that is creating problems or indicating potentially serious problems? Has the forgetfulness increased recently?	Puts pot of soup on to boil and forgets, resulting in burning pot and its contents; constantly misplacing things; goes to bed in clothes worn during the day and does not change into night clothes; increasing forgetfulness.
Is there evidence that the immediate, recent, or remote memory is impaired?	When shown how to put right arm in sleeve is unable to duplicate the action with left arm; shortly after meeting someone, asks who person is; appears to enjoy talking about childhood experiences with other clients.
Is the client able to follow verbal/written directions?	Begins asking where home is located; becomes more distractible; shortening attention span.
Is there evidence of "substitution behavior"?	When asked to get coat in preparation for a trip out to a mall, goes to the kitchen and begins cleaning the sink.

Continued.

From Haber J et al.: *Comprehensive psychiatric nursing*, ed 5, St. Louis, 1997, Mosby.

Focused Assessment for Clients With Cognitive Impairment—cont'd

Assessment	Clinical example
Is the client able to describe a situation (current/past) in a logical and coherent way?	Attempts to describe visit and dinner with family. Description is interspersed with incidents that occurred during a previous vacation; activities of ordering food, eating, and trip back to nursing home not presented in a logical time frame or exposition of ideas.
Is client able to engage in problem solving?	Inability to think about information logically impairs steps in problem-solving process.
Does the client exhibit symptoms that reflect dementia or pseudodementia?	Deficits in self-care hygiene; unable to button shirt until specific directions are provided; tells spouse lunch was delicious, but 1 hour later cannot recall having eaten or what was eaten at the meal.
Does the client exhibit deficits in calculating, using a fund of information, or learning new tasks?	When playing a simple game, client is told to pick up six chips and give three to partner; unable to count required chips.
Does the client exhibit language impairments? Is speech more impoverished than it has been in the past?	Cannot ask for eating utensils when they are missing; asks for a shovel and pitchfork instead of fork and spoon.
Does the client fail to recognize familiar objects?	Does not recognize a toothbrush or recall what it is used for.
When the client is asked a question, does the response reflect confabulation?	When asked to explain the reason he put all his clothing in a bag outside his room, he tells the nurse that he is packing for a vacation and that a bus will be picking him up and driving to Florida for the winter.

Affect and mood
Is there evidence of emotional lability or inappropriate affect, blunting, shallowness, unresponsiveness, euphoria, irrational anger, or sadness?

Little or no facial expression, affect flat; unresponsive toward family members when they visit; outbursts of tearfulness or exaggerated laughing in the absence of stimuli; cannot provide reason for emotional outburst.

Is there evidence that the client is/was involved in a grieving process?

Currently withdrawn, tearful, disheveled appearance; makes statements: "Why did this happen to me?" "I've lost myself" and "Where is my home?"

What is client's emotional response to the disease process: unlike or like responses to past crises?

Response has been characterized by irritability and hostility toward others, reflective of past behavioral responses to crises.

Sensory perception
Does the client exhibit delusional thinking or report illusions or hallucinations?

Complains often of people watching him, spying on him, and coming into his room at night and reorganizing it; misperceives spouse entering room at night as her daughter; tells nurse she hears angel voices talking to her.

Motor activity
Does the client exhibit motor impairments?

Unsteady gait, unable to use cane effectively, safer ambulation with walker; hyperactivity has been replaced with increasing retardation of motor activity.

Biological rhythms
Have there been changes in eating, sleeping, or other patterns recently? In the past year?

Nocturnal wandering has occurred recently. Now needs help feeding self. Asks for food in the early morning hours and after bedtime; needs to be encouraged to eat at mealtime even though there are complaints of not feeling hungry.

Continued.

Focused Assessment for Clients With Cognitive Impairment—cont'd

Assessment	Clinical example
Self-care	
Is self-care deteriorating?	Does not bathe unless supervised; disheveled appearance.
Behavior and personality	
What changes in behavior have occurred during the past few months? past year?	Behavior had been very ritualistic last year; currently is disorganized.
Has there been evidence of social disinhibition?	Has begun undressing in public places.
What behavioral changes have occurred?	Initially very ritualistic; has become increasingly disorganized and agitated; wanders.
Is there evidence of personality changes that have been observed over time or described in behavioral terms by significant others?	Wife states that her husband had been an open, friendly, and trusting man but has become chronically suspicious.
Is the client's judgment becoming unreliable or dangerous to self or others?	Withdrew large sums of money from the bank, asked for small bills, closed out his accounts, took money home, and hid it in his refrigerator and stove.
Have there been changes in the way the client managed interpersonal relationships?	Instigates fights with others; is intrusive; lacks respect for other clients' space and possessions; overbearing and demanding.
How would you describe the client's sociability?	Sociability is decreasing.
Are there changes in the client's behavior that violate social conventions and have potential for causing embarrassment or being labeled deviant?	Was observed voiding by a tree in the front yard.
What coping mechanisms is the client using to defend against awareness of the deficits?	Denies being lost and blames it on wife's moving to a strange town when environment becomes unfamiliar.

Behavior and personality—cont'd

Is the client becoming isolated and withdrawing from social contact with others?

Chooses to sit alone in dining room; does not participate in group therapy; walks away when clients and staff attempt to talk with him.

Does the client exhibit impaired functioning in particular situations? What types of behavior occur? What types of situations elicit the dysfunctional behavior?

Becomes agitated and hostile when family members visit; is relatively calm at home alone with wife; appears disorganized by the noise and presence of others.

Does the client avoid situations that would expose the loss of memory or intellectual functioning?

Walked out of admission interview and refused to join other clients in group and recreational activities.

Do the client's deficits contribute to behavior that is a danger to others?

When rules are enforced, such as smoking in a designated area, he becomes combative.

Do the client's deficits require protection from self-injury?

Unable to use electric razor to shave; wife caught him attempting to rinse it under running water while it was plugged in.

Incontinence Assessment

The control of urine is said to be a requirement for social acceptability. There are a number of underlying causes of incontinence. Assessment of incontinence is essential for referral and establishment of appropriate physiological management.

I. Assessment of acute incontinence

If incontinence is of recent onset (within a few days) or associated with an acute illness, check for any of the following:

_____ Acute urinary tract infection

_____ Fecal impaction

_____ Acute confusion (delirium)*

_____ Immobility*

_____ Drug effects (e.g., excessive sedation, polyuria caused by diuretics, urinary retention, other autonomic effects)

_____ Metabolic abnormality with polyuria (e.g., hyperglycemia, hypercalcemia)

---

*Such that ability to get to a toilet (or toilet substitute) is impaired. If incontinence persists despite management of any of these conditions or resolution of an acute illness, further assessment (as shown in Part II) should be pursued.

II. Assessment of persistent incontinence

A. History

1. Do you ever leak urine when you do not want to?

   _____ No, never   _____ Yes

2. Do you ever have trouble getting to the toilet on time or have accidents getting your clothes or bed wet?

   _____ No, never   _____ Yes

3. How long have you had a problem with urinary leakage?

   _____ Less than 1 week

   _____ 1 to 4 weeks

   _____ 1 to 3 months

   _____ 4 to 12 months

   _____ 1 to 5 years

   _____ Longer than 5 years

From Kane R, Ouslander J, Abrass I: *Essentials of clinical geriatrics,* New York, 1994, McGraw-Hill.

4. How often do you leak urine?

_____ Less than once per week

_____ More than once per week, but less than once per day

_____ About once per day

_____ More than once per day

_____ Continual leakage

_____ Variable

5. When does the leakage occur?

_____ Mainly during the day

_____ Mainly at night

_____ Both night and day

6. When you leak urine, how much leaks?

_____ Just a few drops

_____ More than a few drops, but less than a cupful

_____ More than a cupful (enough to wet clothes or bed linens)

_____ Variable

_____ Unknown

7. Do any of the following cause you to leak urine?

_____ Coughing

_____ Laughing

_____ Exercise or other forms of straining

_____ Inability to get to the toilet in time

8. How often do you normally urinate?

_____ Every 6 to 8 hours or less often

_____ About every 3 to 5 hours

_____ About every 1 or 2 hours

_____ At least every hour or more often

_____ Frequency varies

_____ Unknown

9. Do you wake up at night to urinate?

_____ Never or rarely

_____ Yes, usually between one and three times

_____ Yes, four or more times per night

_____ Yes, but frequency varies

10. Once your bladder feels full, how long can you hold your urine?

_____ As long as you want (several minutes at least)

_____ Just a few minutes

_____ Less than a minute or two

_____ Not at all

_____ Cannot tell when bladder is full

11. Do you have any of the following when you urinate?
    _____ Difficulty in getting the urine started
    _____ Very slow stream or dribbling
    _____ Straining to finish
    _____ Discomfort or pain
    _____ Burning
    _____ Blood in the urine

12. Are you using any of the following to help with the urinary leakage?
    _____ Bed or furniture pads
    _____ Sanitary napkins
    _____ Other types of pads in your underwear
    _____ Special undergarments
    _____ Medication
    _____ Bedside commode
    _____ Urinal
    _____ Other (Describe: _____)

13. Is the urinary leakage enough of a problem that you would like further evaluation and treatment?
    _____ Yes _____ No

14. Do you ever have uncontrolled loss of stool?
    _____ No, never _____ Yes

15. Relevant medical history
    _____ Stroke
    _____ Dementia
    _____ Parkinson's disease
    _____ Prior CNS trauma/surgery
    _____ Other neurological disorder
    _____ Diabetes
    _____ Congestive heart failure
    _____ Other (Specify: _____)

16. Prior genitourinary history
    _____ Multiple vaginal deliveries
    _____ Cesarean section(s)
    _____ Abdominal hysterectomy
    _____ Vaginal hysterectomy
    _____ Bladder suspension
    _____ TURP (transurethral prostate resection)
    _____ Suprapubic prostatectomy
    _____ Urethral stricture/dilatation
    _____ Bladder tumor
    _____ Pelvic irradiation
    _____ Recurrent urinary tract infections

17. Medications
    Diuretic   _____

_____

    Antihypertensive   _____

_____

    Other drugs that   _____
    affect the autonomic   _____
    nervous system   _____

B. Physical examination

1. Mental status
    _____ Normal
    _____ Mild/moderate cognitive impairment
    _____ Severe cognitive impairment (unaware of toileting needs)

2. Mobility
    _____ Ambulates independently, with adequate speed
    _____ Ambulates independently, but slowly (so that ability to get to a toilet is impaired)
    _____ Not independently ambulatory, but able to use urinal, bedpan, or bedside commode independently
    _____ Chair- or bed-bound, but able to use urinal or bedpan independently
    _____ Dependent on others for toileting

3. Abdominal examination
    _____ Bladder enlarged and palpable
    _____ Bladder not palpable

4. Neurological examination of lower extremities
    _____ Normal
    _____ Evidence of upper motor neuron lesion
    _____ Evidence of lower motor neuron lesion
    _____ Peripheral neuropathy

5. Rectal examination
    _____ Decreased rectal sphincter tone
    _____ Decreased perianal sensation
    _____ Absent bulbocavernosus reflex
    _____ Prostate enlarged
    _____ Prostate cancer suspected

6. External genitalia
    _____ Skin irritation
    _____ Diminished sensation
    _____ Abnormal (Describe: _____)

7. Vaginal examination
   _____ Atrophic vaginitis
   _____ Mild prolapse
   _____ Moderate/severe prolapse
   _____ Rectocele
   _____ Adnexal or uterine mass

C. Diagnostic studies
1. Pad test with full bladder
   _____ No leakage
   _____ Leakage, small amount
   _____ Leakage, large amount
   _____ Delayed leakage
2. Voided volume
   _____ Unable   _____ ml
3. Post void residual
   _____ ml (or volume in bladder _____ ml)
4. Bladder filling (if done)
   Capacity: _____ ml
   _____ Stable
   _____ Involuntary contraction (at _____ ml)
   Amount lost: _____ ml
5. Stress maneuvers
   Volume in bladder: _____ ml

Supine	Standing	
_____	_____	No leakage
_____	_____	Leak small amount
_____	_____	Leak large amount
_____	_____	Delayed leakage

6. Voided volume
   _____ ml
7. Calculated residual
   _____ ml
8. Urinalysis
   _____ Normal
   _____ Hematuria (>2 RBC per high-power field)
   _____ Pyuria (>5 WBC per high-power field)
   _____ Bacteriuria (>1+)
9. Urine culture
   _____ Sterile
   _____ Insignificant growth ($<10^5$ colonies/ml)
   _____ Significant growth ($>10^5$ colonies/ml)

Organism(s)_____

Sensitive to _____

_____

D. Disposition

_____ Treat reversible factors (describe)

_____ Treat for urge incontinence

_____ Treat for stress incontinence

_____ Treat for mixed incontinence

_____ Refer for further evaluation

Reason: _____

List specific treatment program

_____

_____

URO-Log Voiding Diary

Using the following formula, the nurse can predict some episodes of incontinence.

$$\frac{D}{T_2} > T_1 = \text{Incontinence}$$

where

T_1 = Time between onset and desire of micturition and uncontrolled micturition

T_2 = Rate at which individual can walk

D/T_2 = Distance individual must walk to reach toilet

An absolute last resort in dealing with incontinence is the use of urinary appliances.

To be completed by your next visit.

Name _____

Date _____

Time of day	Type and amount of fluid intake	Type and amount of food eaten	Amount voided (in ounces)	Amount of leakage (small, medium, large)	Activity engaged in when leakage occurred	Was urge present?

From NAFC, Spartanburg, SC.

Hospice Psychosocial/Spiritual Assessment

Patient: Spiritual Psychosocial Assessment:

Source of Information: ☐ Pt. ☐ Family ☐ Chart ☐ Other ___
Describe/Comment: _____
_____
_____

☐ Anxious/
☐ Fearful
☐ Angry
☐ Guilty
☐ Depressed

Who is Primary Support: _____

☐ Confused
☐ Accepting
Death

Method of coping: ☐ Faith ☐ Family/Friends ☐ Denial
☐ Avoidance ☐ Stoicism ☐ Alcohol/drugs
☐ Other

Describe: _____
_____

Plan: _____
_____

Patient: Life Interests:

Occupation: _____
_____
Hobbies/Recreation: _____
Comments: _____
_____

Patient: Religious Info:

Religious Affiliation: _____ Importance in Life: _____
Church/Synagogue/Other: _____
Help requested in processing spiritual/religious issues?   ☐ Yes   ☐ No
Primary Spiritual Caregiver: _____ Phone #: _____
Plan: _____

Family/Caregiver: Assessment:

Primary Contact/Caregiver: _____
Relationship: _____
Address: _____
Phone #: _____
Family's Primary Support: _____
Name: _____ Relationship: _____
Phone #: _____
Comments: _____
_____
_____

☐ Health Problems

☐ Drug/alcohol Abuse
_____

☐ Transportation Difficulty
_____

☐ Fatigued

☐ Other Losses (list)

Plan: Bereavement Program Discussed
☐ Yes   ☐ No
Grief Packet Given
☐ Yes   ☐ No
Comments: _____
_____
_____
_____
_____

Completed By: _____ Date: _____ Time: _____

Bereavement Discharge Summary:

A. Name of Deceased _____ Date of Death _____
Name of Bereaved _____ Relationship _____
Date of Discharge From Bereavement
Follow-Up/Counseling _____
Month   Day   Year

B. Bereavement Follow-Up Completed:
☐ Sympathy Card   ☐ Volunteer Contact
☐ Information Packet   ☐ 6-month Letter   Summary: ___
☐ Contact by Bereavement Counselor ☐ 12-month Letter
_____
_____

Recorded By _____
Signature and Title   Date

Courtesy Northwest Hospital, Seattle, Wash.

JAREL Spiritual Well-Being Scale

Directions: Please circle the choice that *best* describes how much you agree with each statement. Circle only *one* answer for each statement. There is no right or wrong answer.

	Strongly agree	Moderately agree	Agree	Disagree	Moderately disagree	Strongly disagree
1. Prayer is an important part of my life.	SA	MA	A	D	MD	SD
2. I believe I have spiritual well-being.	SA	MA	A	D	MD	SD
3. As I grow older, I find myself more tolerant of other's beliefs.	SA	MA	A	D	MD	SD
4. I find meaning and purpose in my life.	SA	MA	A	D	MD	SD
5. I feel there is a close relationship between my spiritual beliefs and what I do.	SA	MA	A	D	MD	SD
6. I believe in an afterlife.	SA	MA	A	D	MD	SD
7. When I am sick I have less spiritual well-being.	SA	MA	A	D	MD	SD
8. I believe in a supreme power.	SA	MA	A	D	MD	SD
9. I am able to receive and give love to others.	SA	MA	A	D	MD	SD
10. I am satisfied with my life.	SA	MA	A	D	MD	SD

	SA	MA	A	D	MD	SD
11. I set goals for myself.	SA	MA	A	D	MD	SD
12. God has little meaning in my life.	SA	MA	A	D	MD	SD
13. I am satisfied with the way I am using my abilities.	SA	MA	A	D	MD	SD
14. Prayer does not help me in making decisions.	SA	MA	A	D	MD	SD
15. I am able to appreciate differences in others.	SA	MA	A	D	MD	SD
16. I am pretty well put together.	SA	MA	A	D	MD	SD
17. I prefer that others make decisions for me.	SA	MA	A	D	MD	SD
18. I find it hard to forgive others.	SA	MA	A	D	MD	SD
19. I accept my life situations.	SA	MA	A	D	MD	SD
20. Belief in a supreme being has no part in my life.	SA	MA	A	D	MD	SD
21. I cannot accept change in my life.	SA	MA	A	D	MD	SD

Developed by Hungelmann J, Kenkel-Rossi E, Klassen L, Stollenwerk R: Marquette University College of Nursing, Milwaukee, Wis. In Hungelmann J et al.: Focus on spiritual well-being: harmonious interconnectedness of mind-body-spirit—use of the JAREL spiritual well-being scale, *Geriatric Nurs* 17(6):262, 1996.

The JAREL Spiritual Well-Being Scale was developed by nurse researchers to provide nurses and other health care professionals with a simple tool for assessing a client's spiritual well-being. The tool was developed for clients from Christian, non-Christian, and atheist belief systems. Items on the tool comprise three key dimensions: the faith/belief dimension, life/self-responsibility, and life satisfaction/self-actualization. The tool is simple to use, requiring clients to rate their level of agreement with each item along a five-point scale (strongly agree to strongly disagree). For clients with visual or literacy problems, the nurse can read the items and record the client's response. If the client's score on any item, group of items, or a particular dimension is low, it may indicate an area to explore further.

The tool helps the nurse explore with a client any perceptions or concerns he or she might have. For example, if a client disagrees about accepting life situations, the nurse needs to spend time understanding how illness is being accepted and managed by the client. Whether a nurse uses a tool like the JAREL scale or directs an assessment with questions that are based on principles of spirituality, it is important not to impose personal value systems on the client. This is particularly true when the client's values and beliefs are similar to those of the nurse, as it can then become very easy to make false assumptions.

Barthel Index

The Barthel Index is of value in obtaining baseline functional data and in monitoring improvement in mobility and self-care over time. It measures performance ability in personal care activities of daily living and mobility. The client's ability to perform independently or with help is appraised and scored according to performance in 10 categories of function. The authors of this instrument devised a weighted scoring system that ranges from 0 to 100. A total score of 100 indicates complete independence, independent performance in all 10 domains. To be considered "independent," the client must not require assistance at any time, either before, during, or after the performance of the task.

	With help	Independent
1. Feeding (if food must be in cup, score as "with help")	5	10
2. Moving from wheelchair to bed and return (includes sitting up in bed)	5-10	15
3. Personal toilet (wash face, comb hair, shave, clean teeth)	0	5
4. Getting on and off toilet (handling clothes, wipe, flush)	5	10
5. Bathing self	0	5
6. Walking on level surface	10	15
If unable to walk, propelling wheelchair (score only if unable to walk)	0	5
7. Ascending and descending stairs	5	10
8. Dressing (includes tying shoes, fastening fasteners)	5	10
9. Controlling bowels	5	10
10. Controlling bladder	5	10

From Mahoney FI, Barthel DW: Functional evaluation: the Barthel index, *Md State Med J* 14:2, 1965.

Assessment Data for Persons Experiencing a Loss

Name _____

Date _____

Age _____

1. Nature of the lost object (or person)
2. Meaning the lost object (or person) had for the mourner
3. Mourner's typical coping patterns
4. Mourner's social and cultural milieu
5. Mourner's attitude toward death (if applicable)
6. Special resources (support systems) the mourner possesses for coping with the loss

From Detherage KS, Mandle CL: Stress management and crisis intervention. In Edelman CL, Mandle CL, editors: *Health promotion throughout the lifespan*, ed 4, St. Louis, 1998, Mosby.

7. Factors that influence the mourning process:
   Importance of the lost object (or person) as a source of support
   Degree of ambivalence toward the lost object (or person)
   Age of the deceased (if applicable)
   Quantity and quality of other relationships
   Degree of preparation for the loss, which was
       Sudden _____
       Gradual _____
   Mourner's physical, psychological, social, and spiritual health

CHILDBEARING ASSESSMENT

PREGNANCY

Postnatal care following pregnancy is a mainstay in the practice of nursing. The nurse assists the woman during this critical time by teaching, observing, and supporting her and her family through this usually normal process. A significant contribution of the nurse is early identification of risk. The following tools will help achieve this goal.

Notes

Signs of Pregnancy

Time of occurrence (gestational age)	Sign	Other possible cause
Presumptive signs		
3-4 weeks	Breast changes	Premenstrual changes, oral contraceptives
4 weeks	Amenorrhea	Stress, vigorous exercise, early menopause, endocrine problems, malnutrition
4-14 weeks	Nausea, vomiting	Gastrointestinal virus, food poisoning
6-12 weeks	Urinary frequency	Infection, pelvic tumors
12 weeks	Fatigue	Stress, illness
16-20 weeks	Quickening	Gas, peristalsis
Probable signs		
5 weeks	Goodell's sign	Pelvic congestion
6-8 weeks	Chadwick's sign	Pelvic congestion
6-12 weeks	Hegar's sign	Pelvic congestion
4-12 weeks	Positive pregnancy test (serum)	Hydatidiform mole, choriocarcinoma
6-12 weeks	Positive result to pregnancy test (urine)	False positive results may be because of pelvic infection, tumors
16 weeks	Braxton Hicks contractions	Myomas, other tumors
16-28 weeks	Ballottement	Tumors, cervical polyps
Positive signs		
5-6 weeks	Visualization of fetus by ultrasound examination	No other causes
16 weeks	Visualization of fetus by x-ray study	
6 weeks	Fetal heart tones detected by ultrasound examination	
10-17 weeks	Fetal heart tones detected by Doppler ultrasound, stethoscope	
17-19 weeks	Fetal heart tones detected by fetal stethoscope	
19-22 weeks	Fetal movements palpated	
Late pregnancy	Fetal movements visible	

From Lowdermilk DL, Perry SE, Bobak IM: *Maternity and women's health care,* ed 6, St. Louis, 1997, Mosby.

Categories of High Risk Factors

Biophysical factors

1. *Genetic considerations.* Genetic factors may interfere with normal fetal or neonatal development, result in congenital anomalies, or create difficulties for the mother. These factors include defective genes, transmissible inherited disorders and chromosome anomalies, multiple pregnancy, large fetal size, and ABO incompatibility.

2. *Nutritional status.* Adequate nutrition, without which fetal growth and development cannot proceed normally, is one of the most important determinants of pregnancy outcome. Conditions that influence nutritional status include the following: young age; three pregnancies in the previous 2 years; tobacco, alcohol, or drug use; inadequate dietary intake because of chronic illness or food fads; inadequate or excessive weight gain; and hematocrit value less than 33%.

3. *Medical and obstetrical disorders.* Complications of current and past pregnancies, obstetrical-related illnesses, and pregnancy losses put the client at risk.

Psychosocial factors

1. *Smoking.* A strong, consistent, causal relationship has been established between maternal smoking and reduced birth weight. Risks include low–birth-weight infants, higher neonatal mortality rates, increased spontaneous abortions, and increased incidence of premature rupture of membranes. These risks are aggravated by low socioeconomic status, poor nutritional status, and concurrent use of alcohol.

2. *Caffeine.* Birth defects in humans have not been related to caffeine consumption. High intake (three or more cups of coffee per day) has been related to a slight decrease in birth weight.

3. *Alcohol.* Although its exact effects in pregnancy have not been quantified and its mode of action is largely unexplained, alcohol exerts adverse effects on the fetus, resulting in fetal alcohol syndrome, fetal alcohol effects, learning disabilities, and hyperactivity.

4. *Drugs.* The developing fetus may be adversely affected by drugs through several mechanisms. They can be teratogenic, cause metabolic disturbances, produce chemical effects, or cause

From Lowdermilk DL, Perry SE, Bobak IM: *Maternity and women's health care,* ed 6, St. Louis, 1997, Mosby.

depression or alteration of central nervous system function. This category includes medications prescribed by a health care provider or bought over-the-counter, as well as commonly abused drugs such as heroin, cocaine, and marijuana.

5. *Psychological status.* Childbearing triggers profound and complex physiological, psychological, and social changes, with evidence to suggest a relationship between emotional distress and birth complications. This risk factor includes conditions such as specific intrapsychic disturbances and addictive lifestyles; a history of child or spouse abuse; inadequate support systems; family disruption or dissolution; maternal role changes or conflicts; noncompliance with cultural norms; unsafe cultural, ethnic, or religious practices; and situational crises.

Sociodemographic factors

1. *Low income.* Poverty underlies many other risk factors and leads to inadequate financial resources for food and prenatal care, poor general health, increased risk of medical complications of pregnancy, and greater prevalence of adverse environmental influences.

2. *Lack of prenatal care.* Failure to diagnose and treat complications early is a major risk factor arising from financial barriers or lack of access to care; depersonalization of the system resulting in long waits, routine visits, variability in health care personnel, and unpleasant physical surroundings; lack of understanding of the need for early and continued care or cultural beliefs that do not support the need; and fear of the health care system and its providers.

3. *Age.* Women at both ends of the childbearing age spectrum have a higher incidence of poor outcomes; however, age may not be a risk factor in all cases. Both physiological and psychological risks should be evaluated.

   Adolescents—More complications are seen in young mothers (less than 15 years old), who have a 60% higher mortality rate than those over age 20, and in pregnancies occurring less than 3 years after menarche. Complications include anemia, pregnancy-induced hypertension (PIH), prolonged labor, and contracted pelvis and cephalopelvic disproportion. Long-term social implications of early motherhood are lower educational status, lower income, increased dependence on government support programs, higher divorce rates, and higher parity.

   Mature mothers—The risks to older mothers are not from age alone but from other considerations such as number and spacing of previous pregnancies; genetic disposition of the parents; and medical history, lifestyle, nutrition, and prenatal care. The increased likelihood of chronic diseases and complications that arises from more invasive medical management of a pregnancy and labor combined with demographic characteristics put an older woman at risk. Medical conditions more likely to be experienced by mature women include hypertension and PIH, diabetes, extended labor, cesarean birth, placenta previa, abruptio placentae, and mortality. Her fetus is at greater risk for low birth weight and macrosomia, chromosomal abnormalities, congenital malformations, and neonatal mortality.

4. *Parity.* The number of previous pregnancies is a risk factor that is associated with age and includes all first pregnancies, especially a first pregnancy at either end of the childbearing age continuum. The incidence of PIH and dystocia is higher with a first birth.

5. *Marital status.* The increased mortality and morbidity rates for nonmarried women, including a greater risk for PIH, are often related to inadequate prenatal care and a younger childbearing age.

6. *Residence.* The availability and quality of prenatal care varies widely with geographical residence. Women in metropolitan areas have more prenatal visits than those in rural areas, who have fewer opportunities for specialized care and consequently a higher incidence of maternal mortality. Health care in the inner city, where residents are usually poorer and begin childbearing earlier and continue for longer, may be of lower quality than in a more affluent neighborhood.

7. *Ethnicity.* Although ethnicity by itself is not a major risk, race is an indicator of other sociodemographic risk factors. Nonwhite women are more than 3 times as likely as white women to die of pregnancy-related causes. African-American babies have the highest rates of prematurity and low birth weight, with the infant mortality rate among African-Americans being more than double that for whites.

Environmental factors

Various environmental substances can affect fertility and fetal development, the chance of a live birth, and the child's subsequent mental and physical development. Environmental influences include infections, radiation, chemicals such as pesticides, therapeutic drugs, illicit drugs, industrial pollutants, cigarette smoke, stress, and diet. Paternal exposure to mutagenic agents in the workplace has been associated with an increased risk of spontaneous abortion.

Specific Pregnancy Problems and Related Risk Factors

Preterm labor
Age less than 16 or more than 35 years
Low socioeconomic status
Maternal weight below 50 kg (110 lb)
Poor nutrition
Previous preterm birth
Incompetent cervix
Uterine anomalies
Smoking
Drug addiction and alcohol abuse
Pyelonephritis, pneumonia
Multiple gestation
Anemia
Abnormal fetal presentation
Preterm rupture of membranes
Placental abnormalities
Infection

Polyhydramnios
Diabetes mellitus
Multiple gestation
Fetal congenital anomalies
Isoimmunization (Rh or ABO)
Nonimmune hydrops
Abnormal fetal presentation

Intrauterine growth restriction (IUGR)
Multiple gestation
Poor nutrition
Maternal cyanotic heart disease
Chronic hypertension
Pregnancy-induced hypertension
Recurrent antepartum hemorrhage
Smoking

From DeCherney AH, Pernoll ML, editors: *Current obstetric and gynecologic diagnosis and treatment,* ed 8, Norwalk, Conn, 1994, Appleton & Lange.

Maternal diabetes with vascular problems
Fetal infections
Fetal cardiovascular anomalies
Drug addiction and alcohol abuse
Fetal congenital anomalies
Hemoglobinopathies

Oligohydramnios
Renal agenesis (Potter's syndrome)
Prolonged rupture of membranes
IUGR
Intrauterine fetal death

Postterm pregnancy
Anencephaly
Placental sulfatase deficiency
Perinatal hypoxia, acidosis
Placental insufficiency

Chromosomal abnormalities
Maternal age 35 years or more
Balanced translocation (maternal and paternal)

Prenatal Assessment Guide

Aspects of adaptation
Age
Initial response to pregnancy
Planned or unplanned pregnancy
Feelings about pregnancy
Desired family size
Perception of pregnancy affecting present activities and responsibilities
Perception of parenthood affecting future activities and plans
Current developmental task of pregnancy: coping mechanisms, fantasies about pregnancy, changes in mood and effect on others
Sexual functioning during pregnancy: changes, feelings, problems
Nature of verbal interest expressed about self and fetus

From Becker C: *JOGN Nursing,* Nov/Dec 1982, 375-378.

Preparations for prenatal classes (type, when completed), place of delivery, other children in mother's absence, and new sibling

Menstrual history: problems, last normal menstrual period, expected date of confinement

Height and prepregnancy weight

Past obstetrical history: dates, course, outcomes

Present obstetrical status: course, abdominal assessment, quickening, fetal heart sound, blood pressure, urinalysis, weight and pattern of gain, signs of any major complications of pregnancy

Past medical history: illness, date, treatment, outcome, surgery, childhood diseases, current immunization status, allergies, venereal disease, emotional problems

Family medical history: illnesses, emotional problems, genetic defects (both sides of family)

Loss of significant other in past year

Food intolerances (lactose, nausea and vomiting), food cravings, and pica

Iron-vitamin-mineral dietary supplements used

Elimination patterns: changes, problems with remedies used

Pattern of rest, sleep: difficulties, remedies used

Aspects of personal belief system and lifestyle

Date first sought prenatal care this pregnancy and in prior pregnancies

Reasons for seeking and receiving prenatal care

Beliefs about pregnancy and childbirth; cultural beliefs about childbearing (antepartum, intrapartum, postpartum)

Racial, ethnic group

Beliefs about role of father during pregnancy and labor and in child care

Perception of needs of fetus

Perception of needs of infant and proposed methods to meet these needs

Contraceptive history: methods used, failures or problems, knowledge of alternate methods, willingness to use

Patterns of use of tobacco, alcohol, prescription and nonprescription drugs, illegal drugs; perception of effects on health of self and fetus

Patterns of nutrient intake: food dislikes, history and method of dieting

Planned method of infant feeding; why chosen

Occupation: present, former, how long, work requirements, hazards, amenities, plans regarding current occupation

Recreational activities: plans to continue, use of seat belt in car, pets in home

Community activities

Perception of and prior experiences with health care personnel and agencies

Date of last physical examination, including breast examination, Pap smear, chest x-ray films, dental checkup

Breast self-examination done regularly; if not, interested in learning about?

Aspects of support

Address: how long there, housing accommodations, phone, plans to move (when, where, why?)

Level of education and future plans regarding

Religious preference; normal or active involvement

Marital status: years married

Father of baby: age, occupation, educational level, racial and ethnic group, religious preference

Family composition: household members

Communication patterns with significant others

Communication patterns with health personnel

Perception of support system (mate, family, friends, community agencies): available and willingness to use

Perception of meaning of this pregnancy to significant others; mate's response to news of pregnancy

Type of prenatal service receiving and perception of its adequacy

Available transportation

Social service and community agencies involved with: how long and contact person

Self-concept and perceived ability to cope with life situations

Body-image concept: prepregnant and current; response to physiological changes of pregnancy

Mate's response to body changes in pregnancy

Feelings about parenting woman received as a child; history of separation from mother

Prior experiences with infants; knowledge of infant care

Feelings about previous pregnancies, labor, puerperium, and mothering skills

Knowledge of reproduction, labor and delivery, and puerperium

Evaluation of Normal Pregnancy by Trimester

First-trimester checklist
Diagnosis and expected date of birth
Schedule and events of visits
Counseling for self-care:
    Birth plan
    Adaptations/discomforts
        Breast changes
        Urinary frequency
        Nausea and vomiting
        Nasal stuffiness and epistaxis
        Gingivitis and epulis
        Leukorrhea
        Fatigue
        Psychosocial responses and family dynamics
    Exercise and rest
    Relaxation
    Nutrition
    Sexuality
Cultural variation
Warning signs of potential complications
Resources
    Education
    Dental evaluation
    Medical service
    Social service
    Emergency room
Diagnostic tests
    Specify
Other

Second-trimester checklist
Schedule of visits and events
Maternal assessment
Fetal growth and development
Diagnostic tests
    Specify
Counseling for self-care
    Birth plan

From Lowdermilk DL, Perry SE, Bobak IM: *Maternity and women's health care,* ed 6, St. Louis, 1997, Mosby.

Adaptations/discomforts
    Skin changes
    Palpitations
    Faintness
    Gastrointestinal distress
    Varicosities
    Neuromuscular and skeletal distress
  Safety (seat belts with shoulder harness and head rest)
  Exercise and rest
  Relaxation
  Nutrition
  Alcohol and other substances
  Sexuality
  Personal hygiene
  Warning signs of potential complications
Other

Third-trimester checklist

Schedule and events of visits
Counseling for self-care
  Adaptations/discomforts
    Dyspnea
    Insomnia
    Psychosocial responses and family dynamics
    Gingivitis and epulis
    Urinary frequency
    Perineal discomfort and pressure
    Braxton Hicks contractions
    Leg cramps
    Ankle edema
  Safety (balance)
  Exercise and rest
  Relaxation
  Nutrition
  Sexuality
  Warning signs of potential complications
  Warning signs—preterm labor
Fetal growth and development
Preparation for baby
  Feeding method
  Nipple preparation
Preparation for labor
  Recognition: false versus true

Prenatal classes
Control of discomfort
Hospital tour
Provision for other family members
Preparation for homecoming
Diagnostic tests
Specify
Other

How to Recognize Preterm Labor

Because the onset of preterm labor is subtle and often hard to recognize, it is important to know how to feel your abdomen for uterine contractions. You can feel for contractions in the following way. While lying down, place your fingertips on the top of your uterus. A contraction is the periodic tightening or hardening of your uterus. If your uterus is contracting, you will actually feel your abdomen get tight or hard and then feel it relax or soften when the contraction is over.

If you think you are having any of the other signs and symptoms of preterm labor, empty your bladder, drink three to four glasses of water for hydration, lie down tilted toward your side, and place a pillow at your back for support.

Check for contractions for 1 hour. To tell how often contractions are occurring, check the minutes that elapse from the beginning of one contraction to the beginning of the next.

It is *normal* to have some uterine contractions throughout the day. They usually occur when a woman changes positions. These usually irregular and mild contractions are called *Braxton Hicks contractions.* They help with uterine tone and uteroplacental perfusion.

It is *not normal* to have frequent uterine contractions (every 10 minutes or more often for 1 hour).

Contractions of labor are regular, frequent, and hard. They also may be felt as a tightening of the abdomen or a backache. This type of contraction causes the cervix to efface and dilate.

Call your primary health care provider clinic, or labor and birth unit, or go to the hospital, if any of the following signs occur:

- You have uterine contractions every 10 minutes or more often for 1 hour *or*

From Lowdermilk DL, Perry SE, Bobak IM: *Maternity and women's health care,* ed 6, St. Louis, 1997, Mosby.

- You have any of the other signs and symptoms for 1 hour *or*
- You have any bloody spotting or leaking of fluid from your vagina

It is often difficult to identify preterm labor. Accurate diagnosis requires assessment by the health care provider, usually in the hospital or clinic.

Post these instructions where they can be seen by everyone in the family.

Signs of Potential Complications by Trimester

First trimester

Signs/symptoms	Possible causes
Severe vomiting	Hyperemesis gravidarum
Chills, fever	Infection
Burning on urination	Infection
Diarrhea	Infection
Abdominal cramping, vaginal bleeding	Spontaneous abortion, miscarriage

Second and third trimesters

Sign/symptom	Possible causes
Persistent, severe vomiting	Hyperemesis gravidarum
Amniotic fluid discharge from vagina	Premature rupture of membranes
Vaginal bleeding, severe abdominal pain	Miscarriage, placental separation
Chills, fever, burning on urination, diarrhea	Infection
Change in fetal movements: absence of fetal movements after quickening, any unusual change in pattern or amount	Fetal jeopardy or intrauterine fetal death
Uterine contractions	Preterm labor
Visual disturbances: blurring, double vision, or spots	Hypertensive conditions, PIH
Swelling of face or fingers and over sacrum	Hypertensive conditions, PIH
Headaches: severe, frequent, or continuous	Hypertensive conditions, PIH
Muscular irritability or convulsions	Hypertensive conditions, PIH
Epigastric pain (perceived as severe stomachache)	Hypertensive conditions, PIH
Glucosuria, positive glucose tolerance test result	Gestational diabetes mellitus

From Lowdermilk DL, Perry SE, Bobak IM: *Maternity and women's health care,* ed 6, St. Louis, 1997, Mosby.

Symptoms of Impending Labor

Uterine contractions: The woman is instructed to report the frequency,
duration, and intensity of uterine contractions. True labor is characterized by an increase in frequency, strength, and duration of contractions. In true labor an increase in activity intensifies these symptoms. If the woman is in false labor, an increase in activity usually
causes the symptoms to diminish. Nulliparas are usually counseled
to remain at home until contractions are regular and 5 minutes apart.
Parous women are counseled to remain at home until the contractions are regular and 10 minutes apart. If the woman lives more than
20 minutes from the hospital or has a history of rapid labors, these
instructions are modified accordingly.

Rupture of the membranes: Fluid may leak slowly or may gush.

Bloody show: The show is scant, pink, and sticky (contains mucus).

From Lowdermilk DL, Perry SE, Bobak IM: *Maternity and women's health care,* ed 6,
St. Louis, 1997, Mosby.

Fetal Development

Fetal development at 13 weeks

Differentiation of tissues is complete as period of organogenesis ends.

Fetus has human appearance.

Fetus's sex is distinguishable externally.

Skeleton is ossifying.

Tooth buds are forming.

Respiratory activity is evident.

Insulin is being secreted (since eighth week).

Kidneys are secreting urine.

Intestine is returning to abdomen.

Head is one third of total length.

Length: 9 cm (3 1/2 in).

Weight 15 g (1/2 oz).

Fetus is less susceptible to malformation caused by teratogenic agents
after 8 to 10 weeks' gestation.

From Lowdermilk DL, Perry SE, Bobak IM: *Maternity and women's health care,* ed 6,
St. Louis, 1997, Mosby.

Fetal development at 26 weeks

Viable at 24 weeks.*

Fetal movements are obvious.

Fetal heartbeat is readily heard.

Scalp hair, eyebrows, and eyelashes have formed, and fine downy lanugo and vernix cover the skin.

Eyelids are still fused.

Skin is red, shiny, and thin.

Face is wrinkled, giving an "old man appearance."

Length is 30 cm (12 in).

Weight is 600 g (1 1/4 lb).

Uterus is at or just above level of umbilicus.

Fetal development at 40 weeks

Nutrients and maternal immunoglobulins are stored.

Subcutaneous fat is deposited.

Dramatic storage of iron, nitrogen, and calcium.

In male: testes are within well-wrinkled scrotum.

In female: labia are well developed and cover vestibule.

Lanugo has been shed, except for shoulders, generally.

Body contours are plump.

Decreased vernix.

Scalp hair is 2 to 3 cm (1 in) long.

Cartilage in nose and ears is well developed.

Fetus is 45 to 55 cm (18 to 22 in) long.

Fetus weighs 3400 g (7 1/2 lb) (average).

Fundal height is below xiphoid after lightening.

----

*In Canada the fetus is considered to achieve viability at 20 weeks' gestation or when it weighs 500 g.

Laboratory Tests in Prenatal Period

Laboratory test	Purpose
Hemoglobin/hematocrit/WBC, differential	Detects anemia and infection
Hemoglobin electrophoresis	Identifies hemoglobinopathies (for example, sickle cell anemia, thalassemia)
Blood type, Rh, irregular antibody	Identifies those fetuses at risk for developing erythroblastosis fetalis or hyperbilirubinemia in neonatal period
Rubella titer	Determines immunity to rubella
Tuberculin skin testing; chest film after 20 weeks gestation in women with reactive tuberculin tests	Screens high-risk population for exposure to tuberculosis
Urinalysis, including microscopic examination of urinary sediment; pH, specific gravity, color, glucose, albumin, protein, RBC, WBC, casts, acetone; hCG	Identifies unsuspected diabetes mellitus, renal disease, hypertensive disease of pregnancy, infection, pregnancy
Urine culture	Identifies asymptomatic bacteriuria

Continued.

From Lowdermilk DL, Perry SE, Bobak IM: *Maternity and women's health care*, ed 6, St. Louis, 1997, Mosby.

Laboratory Tests in Prenatal Period—cont'd

Laboratory test	Purpose
Renal function tests: BUN, creatinine, electrolytes, creatinine clearance, total protein excretion	Evaluates level of possible renal compromise in women with a history of diabetes, hypertension, or renal disease
Papanicolaou test	Screens for cervical intraepithelial neoplasia and herpes simplex virus type 2
Vaginal or rectal smear for *Neisseria gonorrhoeae*, *Chlamydia*, HPV, group B *Streptococcus*	Screens high-risk population for asymptomatic infection
VDRL/FTA-ABS	Identifies untreated syphilis
HIV* antibody, hepatitis B surface antigen, toxoplasmosis	Screens for infection
1-hour glucose tolerance	Screens for gestational diabetes; done at initial visit for women with risk factors; done at 28 weeks for all pregnant women
3-hour glucose tolerance	Screens for diabetes in women with elevated glucose level after 1-hour test; must have elevated fasting or two elevated readings for diagnosis
Cardiac evaluation: ECG, chest x-ray film, echocardiogram	Evaluates cardiac function in women with a history of hypertension or cardiac disease

BUN, Blood urea nitrogen; *ECG,* electrocardiogram; *FTA-ABS,* fluorescent treponemal antibody absorption test; *hCG,* human chorionic gonadotropin; *HPV,* human papillomavirus.

*After client counseling and consent obtained.

Developmental Tasks of Pregnant Adolescents

Developmental tasks	Actuality of pregnancy
Learn to accept and live comfortably with slowly changing body and associated sexual feelings and desires. Develop positive self-image.	Must deal with gross body changes, particularly huge abdomen and large breasts; skin is marred by chloasma and striae. Sexual feelings and desires may vary in intensity throughout pregnancy.
Reorganize thought processes, with thinking becoming less egocentric.	Because of individual's own growth as well as needs of pregnancy, large amounts of food are needed; this is in conflict with the slimness so highly valued in society. Huge hormonal increases as well as the tasks of pregnancy lead to progressive introspection, dependency, and egocentric thinking and behavior.
Become independent of parents and gradually develop interdependence.	Psychological dependency increases during pregnancy as young woman uses internal resources to cope with tasks of pregnancy. Because most adolescents are unable to support themselves, financial considerations increase dependency on parents; occasionally other extreme occurs—alienation from parents because of pregnancy.
Gain sense of identity through interaction, first with same-sex peers, then with heterosexual friends.	Being pregnant and thus different isolates adolescent from group. Firm foundation was established incompletely; if at all, with same-sex friends before physical relationship with opposite sex; thus adolescent often is left without peers of either sex.
Take increasing responsibility for own activities.	Critical difference between adolescent and adult is ability to be responsible for oneself and one's activities; financial consequences associated with pregnancy alone can prevent young woman from taking responsibility. Lack of knowledge and maturity also affect ability to parent an infant, although society still tends to hold the teenager more responsible for the pregnancy.

From Bishop B: *The maternity cycle: one nurse's reflections*, Philadelphia, 1980, FA Davis.

Risk Factors in Teen Parenting

- Early initiation of sexual activity
- No or inconsistent use of birth control
- Incorrect use or lack of understanding of birth control method
- Perceived or actual barriers to access to or availability of birth control
- Expense of over-the-counter birth control products
- School failure due to boredom, truancy, and/or dropping out
- Low self-esteem: may think that having a baby is something good to accomplish from both a male and a female point of view (e.g., male, "I can make someone pregnant"; female, "I am pregnant")
- Low socioeconomic status
- Depression, sexually acting out: may be indicative of depression and/or sex abuse
- Substance abuse: drugs, alcohol
- Sex abuse, rape, incest by male relative or "paramour" of teen's mother
- Prior pregnancy or forced termination of pregnancy: teenager may desire to replace loss
- Spontaneous miscarriage (teenager needs adequate counseling after pregnancy termination, whether voluntary or involuntary, to guard against depression and/or recidivism)
- Dysfunctional family/chaotic home life: teen may be responsible for younger siblings and may think that having her own baby is a "way out"
- History of sexually transmitted disease
- Older boyfriend (pressure on teen to have sex)
- New boyfriend, during pregnancy or after birth of infant, may want his own baby now—risk for second pregnancy
- High achievers
- Multiple sex partners

From Thomas JA: Teen parenting. In Fox J: *Primary health care of children,* St. Louis, 1997, Mosby.

Normal Discomforts Experienced During Pregnancy

First trimester

Discomfort	Physiology	Education for self-care
Breast changes, new sensations: pain, tingling	Hypertrophy of mammary glandular tissue and increased vascularization, pigmentation, and size and prominence of nipples and areolae caused by hormonal stimulation	Wear supportive maternity bras with pads to absorb discharge, may be worn at night; wash with warm water and keep dry; breast tenderness may interfere with sexual expression/foreplay but is temporary
Urgency and frequency of urination	Vascular engorgement and altered bladder function caused by hormones; bladder capacity reduced by enlarging uterus and fetal presenting part	Perform Kegel's exercises; limit fluid intake before bedtime; wear perineal pad; report pain or burning sensation to primary health care provider
Languor and malaise; fatigue (early pregnancy, usually)	Unexplained; may be caused by increasing levels of estrogen, progesterone, and hCG or by elevated BBT; psychologic response to pregnancy and its required physical/psychological adaptations	Rest as needed; eat well-balanced diet to prevent anemia

Continued.

From Lowdermilk DL, Perry SE, Bobak IM: *Maternity and women's health care*, ed 6, St. Louis, 1997, Mosby.

Normal Discomforts Experienced During Pregnancy—cont'd

First trimester—cont'd

Discomfort	Physiology	Education for self-care
Nausea and vomiting, morning sickness—occurs in 50% to 75% of pregnant women; starts between first and second missed periods and lasts until about fourth missed period; may occur any time during day; if mother does not have symptoms, expectant father may; may be accompanied by bad taste in mouth	Cause unknown; may result from hormonal changes, possibly hCG; may be partly emotional, reflecting pride in, ambivalence about, or rejection of pregnant state	Avoid empty or overloaded stomach; maintain good posture—give stomach ample room; stop or decrease smoking; eat dry carbohydrate on awaking; remain in bed until feeling subsides, or alternate dry carbohydrate one hour with fluids such as hot herbal decaffeinated tea, milk, or clear coffee the next hour until feeling subsides; eat five to six small meals per day; avoid fried, odorous, spicy, greasy, or gas-forming foods; consult primary health care provider if intractable vomiting occurs
Ptyalism (excessive salivation) may occur starting 2 to 3 weeks after first missed period	Possibly caused by elevated estrogen levels; may be related to reluctance to swallow because of nausea	Use astringent mouth wash; chew gum
Gingivitis and epulis (hyperemia, hypertrophy, bleeding, tenderness): condition will disappear spontaneously 1 to 2 months after delivery	Increased vascularity and proliferation of connective tissue from estrogen stimulation	Eat well-balanced diet with adequate protein and fresh fruits and vegetables; brush teeth gently and observe good dental hygiene; avoid infection
Nasal stuffiness; epistaxis (nosebleed)	Hyperemia of mucus membranes related to high estrogen levels	Use humidifier; avoid trauma; normal saline nose drops or spray may be used

Leukorrhea: often noted throughout pregnancy	Hormonally stimulated cervix becomes hypertrophic and hyperactive, producing abundant amount of mucus	Not preventable; *do not douche*; wear perineal pads; perform hygienic practices such as wiping front to back; report to primary health care provider if accompanied by pruritus, foul odor, or change in character or color
Psychosocial dynamics, mood swings, mixed feelings	Hormonal and metabolic adaptations; feelings about female role, sexuality, timing of pregnancy, and resultant changes in life and lifestyle	Participate in pregnancy support group; communicate concerns to partner, family, and others; request referral for supportive services if needed (financial assistance)
Second trimester		
Pigmentation deepens, acne, oil skin	Melanocyte-stimulating hormone (from anterior pituitary)	Not preventable; usually resolves during puerperium
Spider nevi (telangiectasias) appear over neck, thorax, face, and arms during second or third trimesters	Focal networks of dilated arterioles (end-arteries) from increased concentration of estrogens	Not preventable; they fade slowly during late puerperium; rarely disappear completely
Palmar erythema occurs in 50% of pregnant women; may accompany spider nevi	Diffuse reddish mottling over palms and suffused skin over thenar eminences and fingertips may be caused by genetic predisposition or hyperestrogenism	Not preventable; condition will fade within 1 week after giving birth
Pruritus (noninflammatory)	Unknown cause; various types as follows: nonpapular; closely aggregated pruritic papules	Keep fingernails short and clean; contact primary health care provider for diagnosis of cause

Continued.

Normal Discomforts Experienced During Pregnancy—cont'd

Second trimester—cont'd

Discomfort	Physiology	Education for self-care
Pruritus (noninflammatory)—cont'd	Increased excretory function of skin and stretching of skin possible factors	Not preventable; symptomatic: Keri baths; mild sedation Distraction; tepid baths with sodium bicarbonate or oatmeal added to water; lotions and oils; change of soaps or reduction in use of soap; loose clothing
Palpitations	Unknown; should not be accompanied by persistent cardiac irregularity	Not preventable; contact primary health care provider if accompanied by symptoms of cardiac decompensation
Supine hypotension (vena cava syndrome) and bradycardia	Induced by pressure of gravid uterus on ascending vena cava when woman is supine; reduces uterine-placental and renal perfusion	Side-lying position or semisitting posture, with knees slightly flexed
Faintness and, rarely, syncope (orthostatic hypotension) may persist throughout pregnancy	Vasomotor lability or postural hypotension from hormones; in late pregnancy may be caused by venous stasis in lower extremities	Moderate exercise, deep breathing, vigorous leg movement; avoid sudden changes in position* and warm crowded areas; move slowly and deliberately; keep environment cool; avoid hypoglycemia by eating 5 to 6 small meals per day; wear elastic hose; sit as necessary; if symptoms are serious, contact primary health care provider

Food cravings	Cause unknown; cravings determined by culture or geographical area	Not preventable; satisfy craving unless it interferes with well-balanced diet; report unusual cravings to primary health care provider
Heartburn (pyrosis or acid indigestion): burning sensation, occasionally with burping and regurgitation of a little sour-tasting fluid	Progesterone slows GI tract motility and digestion, reverses peristalsis, relaxes cardiac sphincter, and delays emptying time of stomach; stomach displaced upward and compressed by enlarging uterus	Limit or avoid gas-producing or fatty foods and large meals; maintain good posture; sip milk for temporary relief; hot herbal tea, chewing gum; primary health care provider may prescribe antacid between meals; contact primary health care provider for persistent symptoms
Constipation	GI tract motility slowed because of progesterone, resulting in increased resorption of water and drying of stool; intestines compressed by enlarging uterus; predisposition to constipation because of oral iron supplementation	Drink six glasses of water per day; include roughage in diet; moderate exercise; maintain regular schedule for bowel movements; use relaxation techniques and deep breathing; do *not* take stool softener, laxatives, mineral oil, other drugs, or enemas without first consulting primary health care provider
Flatulence with bloating and belching	Reduced GI motility because of hormones, allowing time for bacterial action that produces gas; swallowing air	Chew foods slowly and thoroughly; avoid gas-producing foods, fatty foods, large meals; exercise; maintain regular bowel habits

*Caution woman to rise slowly and sit on edge of bed or to assume hands-and-knees posture before rising, and to get up slowly after sitting or squatting.

Continued.

Normal Discomforts Experienced During Pregnancy—cont'd

Second trimester—cont'd

Discomfort	Physiology	Education for self-care
Varicose veins (varicosities): may be associated with aching legs and tenderness; may be present in legs and vulva; hemorrhoids are varicosities in the perianal area	Hereditary predisposition; relaxation of smooth muscle walls of veins because of hormones causing tortuous dilated veins in legs and pelvic vasocongestion; condition aggravated by enlarging uterus, gravity, and bearing down for bowel movements; thrombi from leg varices rare but may be produced by hemorrhoids	Avoid obesity, lengthy standing or sitting, constrictive clothing, and constipation and bearing down with bowel movements; moderate exercises; rest with legs and hips elevated; wear support stockings; thrombosed hemorrhoid may be evacuated; relieve swelling and pain with warm sitz baths, local application of astringent compresses
Leukorrhea: often noted throughout pregnancy	Hormonally stimulated cervix becomes hypertrophic and hyperactive, producing abundant amount of mucus	Not preventable; do *not* douche; maintain good hygiene; wear perineal pads; report to primary health care provider if accompanied by pruritus, foul odor, or change in character or color
Headaches (through week 26)	Emotional tension (more common than vascular migraine headache); eye strain (refractory errors); vascular engorgement and congestion of sinuses resulting from hormone stimulation	Conscious relaxation; contact primary health care provider for constant "splitting" headache, to assess for PIH

Carpal tunnel syndrome (involves thumb, second and third fingers, lateral side of little finger)	Compression of median nerve resulting from changes in surrounding tissues: pain, numbness, tingling, burning; loss of skilled movements (typing); dropping of objects	Not preventable; elevate affected arms; splinting of affected hand may help; regressive after pregnancy; surgery is curative
Periodic numbness, tingling of fingers (acrodysesthesia) occurs in 5% of pregnant women	Brachial plexus traction syndrome resulting from drooping of shoulders during pregnancy (occurs especially at night and early morning)	Maintain good posture; wear supportive maternity bra; condition will disappear if lifting and carrying baby does not aggravate it
Round ligament pain (tenderness)	Stretching of ligament caused by enlarging uterus	Not preventable; rest; maintain good body mechanics to avoid overstretching ligament; relieve cramping by squatting or bringing knees to chest
Joint pain, backache, and pelvic pressure; hypermobility of joints	Relaxation of symphyseal and sacroiliac joints because of hormones, resulting in unstable pelvis; exaggerated lumbar and cervicothoracic curves caused by change in center of gravity resulting from enlarging abdomen	Maintain good posture and body mechanics; avoid fatigue; wear low-heeled shoes; conscious relaxation; sleep on firm mattress; apply local heat or ice; get back rubs; do pelvic rock exercise; rest; condition will disappear 6 to 8 weeks after birth

Continued.

Normal Discomforts Experienced During Pregnancy—cont'd

Third trimester

Discomfort	Physiology	Education for self-care
Shortness of breath and dyspnea occur in 60% of pregnant women	Expansion of diaphragm limited by enlarging uterus; diaphragm is elevated about 4 cm (1½ in); some relief occurs after lightening	Maintain good posture; sleep with extra pillows; avoid overloading stomach; stop smoking; if symptoms worsen, consult health care provider to rule out anemia, emphysema, and asthma
Insomnia (later weeks of pregnancy)	Fetal movements, muscular cramping, urinary frequency, shortness of breath, or other discomforts	Perform conscious relaxation; have partner perform back massage or effeurage; support body parts with pillows; drink warm milk or take warm shower before retiring
Psychosocial responses: mood swings, mixed feelings, increased anxiety	Hormonal and metabolic adaptations; feelings about impending labor, birth, and parenthood	Seek reassurance and support from partner and nurse; improve communication with partner, family, and others
Gingivitis and epulis (hyperemia, hypertrophy, bleeding, tenderness): condition will disappear spontaneously 1 to 2 months after birth	Increased vascularity and proliferation of connective tissue resulting from estrogen stimulation	Eat well-balanced diet with adequate intake of protein, fresh fruits, and vegetables; gentle brushing and good dental hygiene; avoid infection
Urinary frequency and urgency return	Vascular engorgement and altered bladder function caused by hormones; bladder capacity reduced by enlarging uterus and fetal presenting part	Perform Kegel's exercises; limit fluid intake before bedtime; wear perineal pad; consult health care provider if pain or burning sensation occurs

Perineal discomfort and pressure	Pressure from enlarging uterus, especially when standing or walking; multifetal gestation	Rest, perform conscious relaxation, and maintain good posture; consult health care provider for assessment and treatment if pain is present; assess for onset of labor
Braxton Hicks contractions	Intensification of uterine contractions in preparation for work of labor	Rest; change position; practice breathing techniques when contractions are bothersome; effleurage; *assess for onset of labor*
Leg cramps (gastrocnemius spasm), especially when reclining	Enlarging uterus compresses nerves supplying lower extremities; reduced diffusible serum calcium level or elevated serum phosphorus level; aggravating factors: fatigue, poor peripheral circulation, pointing toes when stretching legs or when walking, drinking more than 1 L (1 qt) of milk per day	Have health care provider rule out blood clot; if clot ruled out, use massage and heat over affected muscle; dorsiflex foot until spasm eases; stand on cold surface; initiate oral supplementation with calcium carbonate or calcium lactate tablets; take aluminum hydroxide gel (1 oz) with each meal to remove phosphorus by absorbing it
Ankle edema (nonpitting) to lower extremities	Edema aggravated by prolonged standing, sitting, poor posture, lack of exercise, constrictive clothing (e.g., garters), or by hot weather	Maintain ample fluid intake for natural diuretic effect; put on support stockings before arising; rest periodically with legs and hips elevated; exercise moderately; consult health care provider if generalized edema develops; *diuretics are contraindicated*

INFANCY

An assessment of the infant in the home is an observational and educational function. The mother and family are taught about normal growth and development of the infant as the nurse is carrying out this assessment. The following tools will assist the nurse in this activity.

Postpartum Care for the High-Risk Family

The following represents possible orders for home care management of the postpartum and neonatal client.

Skilled nursing visits for assessment, intervention, and teaching
Laboratory services
Lactation support
Wound care
Durable medical equipment or supplies (dressings, bili lights)
Coordination of care and case management

Each client should have an individualized care plan based upon her specific needs; however, generic skilled nursing visits should include the assessments noted on pages 199-202.

Notes

Postpartum care

Assessment	Intervention
Vital Signs	Report T > 101°F, P > 120 or <60, R > 30 or <12 breaths/min, SBP > 140 mm Hg or <90 mm Hg, or DBP > 90 mm Hg or < 50 mm Hg.
Cardiovascular Heart rate and rhythm Homans' sign Postpartum diuresis	Report cardiac arrythmia, orthostatic blood pressure changes, + Homans' sign, headache, visual disturbances, edema, or excessive fatigue Administer and teach medications as ordered. Monitor cardiac functions as ordered.
Respiratory Respiratory effort Lung sounds Endurance	Report dyspnea, tachypnea, adventitious lung sounds, or poor oxygenation. Monitor oxygen saturation as ordered. Administer and teach medications as ordered.
Gastrointestinal Nutrition Bowel function Hepatic symptoms	Report signs of malnutrition or anorexia. Teach adequate nutrition and fluids. Teach therapy for constipation. Report jaundice, right upper quadrant pain, or intolerance to fatty foods.
Urological Amount and character of urine Flank pain	Report signs and symptoms of UTI or acute renal failure.
Reproductive Fundus Lochia	Teach self-fundal assessment and massage. Report signs of postpartum hemorrhage or infection. Teach periincision care.
Breasts Engorgement Milk production	Teach breast care and milk expression and storage. Teach adequate fluid intake. Report signs and symptoms of mastitis.

From *Health care resources: handbook of high-risk perinatal home care,* St. Louis, 1997, Mosby.   *Continued.*

Postpartum care—cont'd

Assessment	Intervention
Hematological	
Hematocrit	Replace iron as ordered.
Hemoglobin	Report laboratory results.
Endocrine	
Diabetes	Review and monitor blood sugar testing.
Hyperthyroidism	Review and monitor thyroid hormone level.
Hypothyroidism	Report results outside parameters or diabetic or thyroid crisis.
	Report depression, diarrhea, or fatigue.
Neurological	
Level of consciousness	Report change in mentation, syncope, significant
Affect	depression, seizure, or abnormal deep tendon
Seizure	reflexes.
Reflexes	
Psychosocial	
Coping	Refer to support services as needed for parenting
Support network	instruction, teen-mother support, drug or
Financial status	alcohol abuse, or domestic violence.
	Encourage venting of fears and feelings.
	Refer to Department of Social Services for financial or food assistance as needed.
	Coordinate care with other services.
Knowledge deficit	Teach self-care of periincision and breasts.
	Provide lactation support and teaching.
	Refer to support group as necessary for such things as twins or premature infant.
	Report signs and symptoms including:
	Bright red, heavy vaginal bleeding
	Signs of wound infection (redness, warmth, swelling, purulent drainage)
	Signs of endometritis (fever, chills, lower abdominal pain, purulent vaginal discharge)
	Danger signals particular to individual disease process.

Neonatal care

Assessment	Intervention
Vital signs	Report axillary T > 100°F, AP > 160 or < 100, or R >60 or <36 breaths/min.
Skin	
Jaundice	Administer phototherapy as ordered for hyperbilirubinemia.
Turgor	
Cord	Teach cord care.
Surgical incision	Perform and teach wound care.
	Teach hygiene.
	Report signs and symptoms of infection, unresolving jaundice, or umbilical bleeding.
Cardiovascular	
Heart sounds	Report cardiac arrythmia, signs of cardiac failure, poor peripheral pulses, or systemic edema.
Pulses	
Edema	
	Administer and teach medications as ordered.
Respiratory	
Respiratory rate or effort	Report grunting and nasal flaring or retracting.
	Report cyanosis.
Oxygenation	Monitor pulse oximetry as ordered.
Lung sounds	Administer and teach medications as ordered.
Gastrointestinal	
Weight each visit	Teach infant feeding, burping, and reflux precautions as ordered.
Nutritional status	
Bowel function	Teach relief of constipation by such means as water and rectal stimulation as ordered.
Abdominal girth or tenderness	Report significant increase in abdominal girth or apparent abdominal tenderness or absence of stool for 3 days.
Projectile vomiting	
Hydration	Report feeding difficulties or signs and symptoms of malnutrition or dehydration.
Feeding history	
	Teach formula preparation and storage as indicated.
Genitourinary	
Voiding	Report decreased urinary output.
Circumcision	Report signs and symptoms of circumcision infection or hemorrhage.
	Teach perineal and circumcision care.

Continued.

Neonatal care—cont'd

Assessment	Intervention
Neuromuscular	
Affect	Report irritability or lethargy.
Tone	Report hyper- or hypotonia and abnormal deep
Newborn reflexes	tendon reflexes.
Head circumference	Report poor root or suck or swallow.
and cranial sutures	Report significant increase in head
Sleeping patterns	circumference, widening cranial sutures, or
Seizures	seizure activity.
	Teach infant safety and stimulation.
Psychosocial	
Learning needs	Encourage family to vent feelings.
Safety	Teach infant care, sleep and hygiene needs,
Environment	feeding, axillary T, and bathing as necessary.
Bonding	Teach childproofing.
	Refer to support or parenting group as needed.
	Report signs and symptoms of feeding
	difficulties, elimination problems, or illness
	(fever, irritability or lethargy, vomiting,
	diarrhea).
	Report signs of neglect or abuse to child
	protective authorities.
	Teach care per specific disease, anomaly, or
	diagnosis as required.
Growth and development	
Weight gain	Report signs of developmental delay.
Milestones	Teach infant stimulation.
	Enroll in early intervention services as
	developmental testing requires.

Neonatal Perception Inventory

The Neonatal Perception Inventory is easily and quickly administered by telling the mother: "We are interested in learning more about the experiences of mothers and their babies during the first few weeks after delivery. The more we can learn about mothers and their babies, the better we will be able to help other mothers with their babies. We would appreciate it if you would help us to help other mothers by answering a few questions."

The procedures are identical for administering the Average Baby form of the NPI on the first or second postpartum day and the NPI at 1 month of age. The mother is handed the Average Baby form while the individual administering the inventory says: "Although this is your first baby, you probably have some ideas of what most little babies are like. Will you please check the blank you *think* best describes what *most* little babies are like."

The tester waits until the mother has completed the Average Baby form and takes it from the mother and then hands the mother the Your Baby form.*

The procedure for administering the Your Baby forms of the NPI is the same at Time I and Time II. However, the instructions given to the mother vary slightly to take into account the time factor. At Time I the tester tells the mother: "While it is not possible to know for certain what your baby will be like, you probably have some ideas of what your baby will be like. Please check the blank you *think* best describes what *your* baby will be like."

At Time II, she says:

"You have had a chance to live with your baby for a month now. Please check the blank you think best describes your baby."

Method of scoring

The Average Baby Perception form elicits the mother's concept of the average baby's behavior. The Your Baby Perception form elicits her rating of her own baby. Each of these instruments consists of six single-item scales. Values of 1 to 5 are assigned to each of these scales for each of the inventories. The blank signified none is valued as 1 and a great deal has a value of 5. The lower values on the scale represent the most desirable behavior.

---

*The tester remains with the mother during the entire administration procedure.

The six scales are totaled with no attempt at weighing the scales for each of the inventories separately. Thus a total score is obtained for the Average Baby and a total score is obtained for the Your Baby.

The total score of Your Baby Perception form is then subtracted from the Average Baby Perception form. The discrepancy constitutes the Neonatal Perception Inventory score.

The inventories have shown both construct and criterion validity.

Neonatal perception inventory I

Average baby

Although this is your first baby, you probably have some ideas of what most little babies are like. Please check the blank you think best describes the average baby.

How much crying do you think the average baby does?

a great deal	a good bit	moderate amount	very little	none

How much trouble do you think the average baby has in feeding?

a great deal	a good bit	moderate amount	very little	none

How much spitting up or vomiting do you think the average baby does?

a great deal	a good bit	moderate amount	very little	none

How much difficulty do you think the average baby has in sleeping?

a great deal	a good bit	moderate amount	very little	none

How much difficulty does the average baby have with bowel movements?

a great deal	a good bit	moderate amount	very little	none

How much trouble do you think the average baby has in settling down to a predictable pattern of eating and sleeping?

a great deal	a good bit	moderate amount	very little	none

Your baby

While it is not possible to know for certain what your baby will be like, you probably have some ideas of what your baby will be like. Please check the blank that you think best describes what your baby will be like.

How much crying do you think your baby will do?

| a great deal | a good bit | moderate amount | very little | none |

How much trouble do you think your baby will have feeding?

| a great deal | a good bit | moderate amount | very little | none |

How much spitting up or vomiting do you think your baby will do?

| a great deal | a good bit | moderate amount | very little | none |

How much difficulty do you think your baby will have sleeping?

| a great deal | a good bit | moderate amount | very little | none |

How much difficulty do you expect your baby to have with bowel movements?

| a great deal | a good bit | moderate amount | very little | none |

How much trouble do you think your baby will have settling down to a predictable pattern of eating and sleeping?

| a great deal | a good bit | moderate amount | very little | none |

Neonatal perception inventory II

Note: Same inventory for average baby is given again.

Your baby

You have had a chance to live with your baby for a month now. Please check the blank you think best describes your baby.

How much crying has your baby done?

| a great deal | a good bit | moderate amount | very little | none |

How much trouble has your baby had feeding?

| a great deal | a good bit | moderate amount | very little | none |

How much spitting up or vomiting has your baby done?

| a great deal | a good bit | moderate amount | very little | none |

How much difficulty has your baby had sleeping?

| a great deal | a good bit | moderate amount | very little | none |

How much difficulty has your baby had with bowel movements?

a great deal	a good bit	moderate amount	very little	none

How much trouble has your baby had in settling down to a predictable pattern of eating and sleeping?

a great deal	a good bit	moderate amount	very little	none

Degree of bother inventory

Listed below are some of the things that have sometimes bothered mothers in caring for their babies. We would like to know if you were bothered about any of these. Please place a check in the blank that best describes how much you were bothered by your baby's behavior in regard to these.

Crying

a great deal	somewhat	very little	none

Spitting up or vomiting

a great deal	somewhat	very little	none

Sleeping

a great deal	somewhat	very little	none

Feeding

a great deal	somewhat	very little	none

Elimination

a great deal	somewhat	very little	none

Lack of a predictable schedule

a great deal	somewhat	very little	none

Other (specify):

_____

a great deal	somewhat	very little	none

_____

a great deal	somewhat	very little	none

_____

a great deal	somewhat	very little	none

Assessment of Infant Reflexes

Reflex	Expected behavioral response	Deviation
Localized		
Eyes		
Blinking or corneal reflex	Infant blinks at sudden appearance of a bright light or at approach of an object toward the cornea; should persist throughout life	Absent or asymmetric blink suggests damage to cranial nerves II, IV, and V
Pupillary	Pupil constricts when a bright light shines toward it, should persist throughout life	Unequal constriction Fixed dilated pupil
Doll's eye	As the head is moved slowly to the right or left, eyes normally do not move, should disappear as fixation develops	Asymmetric in abducens paralysis
Nose		
Sneeze	Spontaneous response of nasal passages to irritation or obstruction; should persist throughout life	Absent or continuous sneezing
Glabellar	Tapping briskly on glabella (bridge of nose) causes eyes to close tightly	Absence
Mouth and throat		
Sucking	Infant should begin strong sucking movements of circumoral area in response to stimulation; should persist throughout infancy, even without stimulation, such as during sleep	Weak or absent suck

From Wong DL: *Clinical manual of pediatric nursing*, ed 5, St. Louis, 1997, Mosby.

Continued.

Assessment of Infant Reflexes—cont'd

Reflex	Expected behavioral response	Deviation
Mouth and throat—cont'd		
Gag	Stimulation of posterior pharynx by food, suction, or passage of a tube should cause infant to gag; should persist throughout life	Absence of gag suggests damage to glossopharyngeal nerve
Rooting	Touching or stroking the cheek along the side of the mouth will cause infant to turn the head toward that side and begin to suck; should disappear at about age 3 to 4 months, but may persist for up to 12 months	Absence, especially when infant is not satiated
Extrusion	When tongue is touched or depressed, infant responds by forcing it outward; should disappear by age 4 months	Constant protrusion of tongue may suggest Down syndrome
Yawn	Spontaneous response to decreased oxygen by increasing amount of inspired air; should persist throughout life	Absence
Cough	Irritation of mucous membranes of larynx or tracheobronchial tree causes coughing; should persist throughout life; usually present after first day of birth	Absence

Extremities

Grasp — Touching palms of hands or soles of feet near base of digits causes flexion of hands and toes; palmar grasp should lessen after age 3 months, to be replaced by voluntary movement; plantar grasp lessens by 8 months of age — Asymmetric flexion may indicate paralysis

Babinski — Stroking outer sole of foot upward from heel and across ball of foot causes toes to hyperextend and hallux to dorsiflex; should disappear after age 1 year — Persistence indicates a pyramidal tract lesion

Ankle clonus — Briskly dorsiflexing foot while support knee in partially flexed position results in one to two oscillating movements ("beats"); eventually no beats should be felt — Several beats

Mass

Moro — Sudden jarring or change in equilibrium causes sudden extension and abduction of extremities and fanning of fingers, with index finger and thumb forming a C shape, followed by flexion and abduction of extremities; legs may weakly flex; infant may cry; should disappear after age 3 to 4 months, usually strongest during first 2 months — Persistence of Moro reflex past age 6 months may indicate brain damage

Asymmetric Moro reflex may suggest injury to brachial plexus, clavicle, or humerus

Continued.

Assessment of Infant Reflexes—cont'd

Reflex	Expected behavioral response	Deviation
Mass—cont'd		
Startle	A sudden loud noise causes abduction of the arms with flexion of the elbows; the hands remain clenched; should disappear by age 4 months	Absence indicates hearing loss
Perez	While infant is prone on a firm surface, thumb is pressed along spine from sacrum to neck; infant responds by crying, flexing the extremities, and elevating the pelvis and head; lordosis of the spine, as well as defecation and urination, may occur; should disappear by age 4 to 6 months	Significance is similar to that of Moro reflex
Asymmetric tonic neck	When infant's head is quickly turned to one side, arm and leg extends on that side, and opposite arm and leg flex; should disappear by age 3 to 4 months, to be replaced by symmetric positioning of both sides of body	Absence or persistence may indicate central nervous system damage
Neck-righting	While infant is supine, head is turned to one side; shoulder and trunk turns toward that side, followed by pelvis; disappears at age 10 months	Absence; significance is similar to that of asymmetric tonic neck reflex

Mass—cont'd

Otolith-righting	When body of an erect infant is tilted, head is returned to upright, erect position	Absence; significance is similar to that of asymmetric tonic neck reflex
Trunk incurvation (Galant)	Stroking infant's back alongside spine causes hips to move toward stimulated side; should disappear by age 4 weeks	Absence may indicate spinal cord lesion
Dance or step	If infant is held so that sole of foot touches a hard surface, there is a reciprocal flexion and extension of the leg, simulating walking; should disappear after age 3 to 4 weeks, to be replaced by deliberate movement	Asymmetry of stepping
Crawling	Infant, when placed on abdomen, makes crawling movements with the arms and legs; should disappear at about age 6 weeks	Asymmetry of movement
Placing	When infant is held upright under arms and dorsal side of foot is briskly placed against hard object, such as table, leg lifts as if foot is stepping on table; age of disappearance varies	Absence

Nursing Interventions to Assist in Stressful Situations During Infancy

Attempt to meet the infant's needs promptly.

Allow favorite toy or item of security to be present during stressful experiences.

Allow familiar caregiver to be present to calm infant.

Attempt to keep the number of strangers interacting with infant to a minimum.

Attempt to provide a warm and accepting environment for the infant.

Allow freedom of expression (crying) to reduce tension in the infant.

Identify the infant's established daily routine and try to follow through.

Reinforce the infant's need for expression.

Establish a trust relationship with the infant.

Provide opportunity for play so that the infant can "vent" fears.

Provide emotional support for the parents so they may in turn give support to their infant.

From Edelman CL, Mandle CL: *Health promotion throughout the lifespan,* ed 4, St. Louis, 1998, Mosby.

Nursing Interventions to Prevent Aspiration of Foreign Objects by Infants

Keep all small objects out of an infant's reach.

Avoid propping bottles and making large holes in nipples to prevent aspiration of formula into the infant's lungs.

Discourage the use of powder for infants to reduce risk of aspiration pneumonia from inhalation of zinc stearate.

Burp the infant well before placing into the crib; place on abdomen or prop on right side.

Older children should not give food to the infant, who may choke on it. An adult should be close by to supervise children around infants.

Adults should not set a bad example by putting pins or other objects in their mouths; older infants mimic them and may do likewise.

Inspect all toys for loose, removable parts that potentially could reach the infant's mouth.

From Edelman CL, Mandle CL: *Health promotion throughout the lifespan,* ed 4, St. Louis, 1998, Mosby.

Clues to Difficulty in Parent-Infant Bond Formation

The nurse will be alerted to potential problems in mother-infant bond formation if:

- The mother is young or immature.
- The mother must struggle against a nonsupportive or isolated environment.
- The mother is beset by stress-causing situations (e.g., poor environmental conditions, serious illness in the family, severe disappointment, or rapid and repeated pregnancies) in addition to the birth of the new infant.
- The mother is separated from her infant for a prolonged period after birth (e.g., prematurity, maternal illness).

The nurse will strongly suspect that there is a problem in parent-infant attachment if:

- The parent expresses inappropriate feelings (e.g., anger, frustration, or helplessness) in response to the infant's crying.
- The parent fails to express anything about the infant that she or he likes (i.e., the parent has not found in the infant a claiming clue—a physical or psychological attribute valued in self).
- The parent expresses unresolved feelings over a "dream" child (e.g., disappointment over the sex of the infant).
- The parent expresses mostly negative feelings about the infant (e.g., disgust over messy diapers or a perception that the infant is too demanding).
- The parent expresses expectations of the infant far beyond the infant's developmental stage.
- The parent fails to exhibit close, gentle, physical contact with the infant (e.g., holds infant away from body, plays roughly, or avoids eye contact and the *en face* position).

From Dickason E, Silverman B, Kaplan J: *Maternal-infant nursing care,* ed 3, St. Louis, 1998, Mosby.

Clinical Manifestations of Dehydration

	Isotonic (loss of water and salt)	Hypotonic (loss of salt in excess of water)	Hypertonic (loss of water in excess of salt)
Skin			
Color	Gray	Gray	Gray
Temperature	Cold	Cold	Cold or hot
Turgor	Poor	Very poor	Fair
Feel	Dry	Clammy	Thickened, doughy
Mucous membranes	Dry	Slightly moist	Parched
Tearing and salivation	Absent	Absent	Absent
Eyeball	Sunken	Sunken	Sunken
Fontanel	Sunken	Sunken	Sunken
Body temperature	Subnormal or elevated	Subnormal or elevated	Subnormal or elevated
Pulse	Rapid	Very rapid	Moderately rapid
Respirations	Rapid	Rapid	Rapid
Behavior	Irritable to lethargic	Lethargic to comatose; convulsions	Marked lethargy with extreme hyperirritability on stimulation

From Wong D: *Whaley and Wong's nursing care of infants and children*, ed 6, St. Louis, 1999, Mosby.

POSTNATAL CARE

Ideally a woman should be followed prenatally through home visits, but frequently the nurse first meets a woman postnatally, especially if the pregnancy is uneventful. The following tools will assist the nurse in making appropriate observations during the postnatal period.

MIST: Mother/Infant Screening Tool

The Mother/Infant Screening Tool assesses mother-infant bonding. It includes four areas for evaluation: tactile, visual, auditory, and feeding. Circle the answer under A, B, C, D that best describes the *mother's* behavior. Circle the answer under A, B, C, D that best describes the *infant's* behavior. Add the numbers under each A, B, C, D for mothers and infants separately. The more A's mother and baby have, the more attachment that has occurred. The more D's mother and baby have, the less attachment. Use as a guide for planning care.

Notes

		A	B	C	D
T	**Mother**	Holds infant close to her body	Holds infant on forearm	Holds infant away from body	Does not hold infant
A	**Infant**	Curls up close to mother	Keeps some distance	Moves away when touched	Stiffens up when held
C					
T	**Mother**	Comfortable touching infant, strokes head or face	Looks comfortable, pats infant's back	Tentative when touching infant	Avoids touching infant
I					
L	**Infant**	At ease; turns toward mother's touch	Looks at ease	Looks tense	Cries when touched
E					
V	**Mother**	Establishes eye contact	Looks at infant's face	Does not look at infant's face	Does not look at infant
I	**Infant**	Establishes eye contact	Looks at mother's face	Does not look at mother's face	Does not look at mother
S					
U	**Mother**	Smiles and makes faces in play	Smiles	No special facial expressions	Looks unhappy
A					
L	**Infant**	Laughs or big smile	Smiles	No special facial expressions	Looks unhappy

From Reiser SL: A tool to facilitate mother-infant attachment, *JOGN Nursing* 10:297, 1981.

	A	B	C	D
A **U**	**Mother** Talks to infant in soothing or playful way	Talks to infant in calm way	Talks but just gives directions	Does not talk to infant
D **I**	**Infant** Infant makes happy sounds, coos and goos	Makes ah-ah sounds	Cries	Does not talk
T **O** **R**	**Mother** Understands meaning of infant's cries	Differentiates most of infant's cries	Seldom differentiates infant's cries	Never differentiates infant's cries
Y	**Infant** Exhibits different cries	Usually exhibits different cries	Seldom exhibits different cries	Never exhibits different cries
F **E** **E**	**Mother** Shows signs of pleasure during feeding—smiles, rocks, sings	Looks content during feeding	Acts unsure during feeding—stops and starts	Agitated or irritable
D **I**	**Infant** Shows pleasure in being fed—smiles, coos	Looks content during feeding	Restless during feeding	Agitated—cries during feeding
N **G**	**Mother** Looks pleased after feeding	Looks satisfied after feeding	Looks uneasy after feeding	Looks agitated after feeding
	Infant Looks happy after feeding	Looks satisfied after feeding	Looks restless after feeding	Looks agitated after feeding

Total score   Mother

           Infant

Date

Psychosocial Perinatal Warning Indicators for Families at High Risk for Abnormal Parenting Practices

Pregnancy	Labor and birth	Postpartum
Parent's physical and psychological well-being		
Pregnancy is perceived as very difficult or burdensome	Mother experiencing excessive discomfort, fatigue, drug effects, or physical complications immediately after birth	Mother does not see attention focused on infant as something positive for herself
Mother feels her health will suffer from childbearing or child rearing	Mother or father perceive labor or birth as traumatic or unsatisfactory	Mother bothered by infant's crying; makes her feel helpless, hopeless, or unloved
Mother intellectually subnormal	Obvious lack of supportive interaction between couple	Mother relinquishes control to physicians and nurses for meeting needs of infant
Mother shows great depression over pregnancy	Hostile interaction between couple	Evidence of low self-esteem ("I'm no good"), especially in parenting ability
Mother persists in feeling frightened and alone, especially before birth; careful explanations do not dissipate the fear		Parents express excessive feelings of failure concerning performance during labor or birth
Excessive visits for health care or expresses multiple psychosomatic complaints		Parents express resentment or anger toward infant over childbirth experience
Evidence of emotional instability or mental illness		Express excessive doubt about ability to care for infant
History of drug or alcohol abuse		
Child wanted to fill unmet need in parents' lives		
Evidence of low self-esteem ("I'm no good"), particularly in parenting ability		
Mother's age under 20 years		
Previous pregnancy terminating in spontaneous abortion, fetal or neonatal death, or birth of a damaged child		

History of previous child's death or removal from home because of abuse or neglect

Characteristics of child

	Preterm	As in column 2
	Physically or mentally defective	Perceived by parent as being different or "not normal" despite normal findings
	Immature or defective reflex behaviors	Sex of infant remains unacceptable to parent
	Unresponsive	Denies or exaggerates handicapped infant's capabilities
	Condition necessitates separation from parents	Difficult feeder
	"Wrong" sex	Unresponsive, e.g., sleepy baby
	Looks or behavior perceived in negative way by parents	Irritable or difficult to console
		Hyperreflexive infant
		Rigid or noncuddly infant

Parent-child attachment

	Pregnancy unplanned or unwanted	Does not comfort crying infant and does not heed physical needs
	Parents considered abortion or relinquishment	Appears apathetic toward or disinterested in infant
	Denial of pregnancy, e.g., unwilling to gain weight, refusal to talk about pregnancy	Expresses excessive doubt about ability to care for infant
	Mother looks distressed, disappointed	
	Does not talk to infant in affectionate terms	
	Makes negative or hostile remarks to infant	
	Expresses disappointment with sex of infant	

Modified from Ledger KE, Williams DL: *Parents at risk: an instructional program for perinatal assessment and preventive intervention*, Victoria, BC, Canada, 1981, Ministry of Health and Queen Alexandra Solarium for Crippled Children Society. *Continued.*

Psychosocial Perinatal Warning Indicators for Families at High Risk for Abnormal Parenting Practices—cont'd

Pregnancy	Labor and birth	Postpartum
Parent-child attachment—cont'd		
In advanced pregnancy, mother dresses and acts as though she is not pregnant	Mother makes inappropriate verbalizations, glances, or disparaging remarks about or toward infant	Remains disappointed over sex of infant
Absent or disturbed response to quickening		Frequently voices negative feelings about or toward infant
Mother perceives fetal movement as abusive or aggressive actions	Avoids eye contact and direct *en face* position	Repelled by messiness and diaper changing
Mother reports an experience she fears will damage baby (e.g., a "scare," accident)	Mother does not hold, touch, or examine infant	Negative identification of infant by name or association with someone disliked
Undue concern about infant's sex or performance	Mother handles infant in rough manner	No feelings of attachment or bonding toward infant after 1 month
Absence of any fantasies about what baby will be like or predominantly negative fantasies		Mother does not appear to enjoy playing with infant
Mother attributes negative characteristics to fetus		
Apparent lack of concern for physical well-being of unborn fetus, as evidenced by refusal to make health and lifestyle changes (e.g., poor nutrition, excessive use of drugs and alcohol)		
Absence of "nesting" behavior in the third trimester (e.g., preparation of clothing, equipment, space for infant)		

Parenting knowledge, beliefs, and expectations

Perceive own upbringing as abusive or neglectful	As in column 1
Experienced harsh physical punishment during childhood	Unaware of infant's characteristics and ability
Express belief that physical force is necessary in rearing and disciplining children	See infant as demanding or manipulative
Express a strong desire to parent in manner different from that of own parents	Inadequate preparation for child rearing
Express inaccurate knowledge of infant care and development	Express expectations developmentally far beyond infant's capabilities
Express rigid or unrealistic expectations for infant's physical characteristics, behavior, development	Express fear of "spoiling" the infant

Support systems

No spouse, mate, or significant other	Mother expresses hostility toward father, who "put her through all this"
Express dissatisfaction with spouse or mate relationship	As in column 1
Chronic marital discord, especially if focus of conflict is around childbearing or child rearing	
Chronic conflict with or alienation from one's own mother or other female relatives	
History of loss of mother's own mother before her own puberty	

Continued.

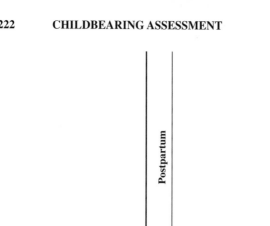

Psychosocial Perinatal Warning Indicators for Families at High Risk for Abnormal Parenting Practices—cont'd

Pregnancy	Labor and birth	Postpartum
Mate's or family's reaction to pregnancy is negative or nonsupportive		
Lack or loss of support systems, e.g., no supportive friends or relatives nearby		
Show evidence of social isolation, i.e., no telephone, outside interests, use of community resources		
Family circumstances		
Parent seems unaware or denies impact of new baby on relationship with mate, own time, other siblings	As in column 1	As in column 1
Express concern that this child is going to be "one too many"		

Inadequate housing for family's needs

Children too closely spaced

Recent death or loss of loved one

Have recently moved

Financial, health, social, or interpersonal problems in the family

Parents describe stresses of chaotic nature (e.g., physical fights, heavy drinking, arguments among immediate family members, abandonment by mate)

Parents exhibit few skills for dealing with stress

Express inability to cope with present life circumstances

Dissatisfied with career or career change

Progression of Puerperal Changes

Assessment	2-24 hours (day 1)	25-48 hours (day 2)	49-72 hours (day 3)
Temperature	97.1° F (36.2° C) 100.4° F (38° C)	Within normal range	Within normal range
Pulse	Bradycardia: 50-70 beats/min	Bradycardia may persist or rate may return to within normal range	Bradycardia may persist or rate may return to within normal range
Blood pressure	Within normal range	Within normal range	Within normal range
Energy level	Euphoric, happy, excited, or fatigued; may show need for sleep	Often tired, slow moving	Anxious to go home; level within normal range but variable
Uterus	At umbilicus or just below; firm	1 cm or more below umbilicus; firm	2 cm or more below umbilicus; firm
Lochia	Rubra; moderate; few clots, if any; fleshy odor of normal menstrual flow	Rubra to serosa; moderate to scant; odor continues to be "fleshy" or absent	Rubra to serosa: scant; odor continues to be "fleshy" or absent
Perineum	Edematous; clean, healing, intact	Edema lessening; clean, healing	Edema lessening or absent; clean, healing
Legs	Pretibial or pedal edema; Homans' sign negative	Edema lessening; Homans' sign negative	Edema minimal or absent; Homans' sign negative

Breasts	Remain soft to palpation; colostrum can be expressed	Begin to feel firmer; occasionally feel lumpy	Increase in vacularity and initiation of swelling; feel firmer and warmer to touch; milk expected within 2-4 days after birth
Appetite	Excellent; may ask for double helpings, snacks	Usually remains excellent	Varies; appetite may have returned to normal range or may lessen (especially if client is constipated)
Elimination			
Voiding	Up to 3000 mL	Large amounts	Amount/24 hour is lessening
Defecation	None expected	None expected	Usually defecates; may need enema, etc.
Discomfort	Generalized aching; perineal area: episiotomy, hemorrhoids	Muscle aches; perineal area: episiotomy, hemorrhoids	Possible tension headache, perineal area: usually lessening; breasts, nipples

From Bobak I, Jensen M: *Maternity and gynecologic care*, ed 5, St. Louis, 1993, Mosby.

Signs of Potential Physiological Problems

Temperature	More than 100.4° F (38° C) after the first 24 hours
Pulse	Tachycardia, marked bradycardia
Blood pressure	Hypotension or hypertension
Energy level	Lethargy, extreme fatigue
Uterus	Deviated from the midline, boggy, remains above the umbilicus after 24 hours
Lochia	Heavy, foul odor
Perineum	Pronounced edema, not intact, signs of infection, marked discomfort
Legs	Homans' sign positive; painful, reddened area; warmth on posterior aspect of calf
Breasts	Redness, heat, pain, cracked and fissured nipples, inverted nipples, palpable mass
Appetite	Lack of appetite
Elimination	*Urine:* inability to void, urgency, frequency, dysuria; *bowel:* constipation, diarrhea
Rest	Inability to rest or sleep

From Bobak I, Jensen M: *Maternity and gynecologic care,* ed 5, St. Louis, 1993, Mosby.

Protocol for Postpartum Home Visit

Previsit interventions

1. Contact family to arrange details for home visit.
   a. Identify self, credentials, and agency role.
   b. Review purpose of home visit follow-up.
   c. Schedule convenient time for visit.
   d. Confirm address and route to family home.
2. Review and clarify appropriate data.
   a. All available assessment data for mother and infant (e.g., referral forms, hospital discharge summaries, family-identified learning needs).
   b. Review records of any previous nursing contacts.
   c. Contact other professional caregivers, as necessary to clarify data (e.g., obstetrician, nurse midwife, pediatrician, referring nurse).

From Lowdermilk DL, Perry SE, Bobak IM: *Maternity and women's health care,* ed 6, St. Louis, 1997, Mosby.

3. Identify community resources and teaching materials appropriate to meet needs already identified.
4. Plan the visit and prepare bag with equipment, supplies, and materials necessary for assessments of mother and infant, actual care anticipated for mother and infant, and client teaching.

In-home interventions: establishing a relationship

1. Reintroduce self and establish purpose of postpartum follow-up visit for mother, infant, and family; offer family opportunity to clarify their expectations of contact.
2. Spend brief time socially interacting with family to become acquainted and establish trusting relationship.

In-home interventions: working with family

1. Conduct systematic assessment of mother and newborn to determine physiological adjustment and any existing complications.
2. Throughout visit, collect data to assess the emotional adjustment of individual family members to newborn and lifestyle changes. Note evidence of family-newborn bonding and sibling rivalry; note relationships among mother, father, children, and grandparents.
3. Determine adequacy of support system.
   a. To what extent does someone help with cooking, cleaning, and other home-management tasks?
   b. To what extent is help being provided in caring for the newborn and any other children?
   c. Are support persons encouraging the new mother to care for herself and get adequate rest?
   d. Who is providing helpful information? Emotional support?
4. Throughout the visit, observe home environment for adequacy of the following resources:
   a. Space: privacy, safe play of children, sleeping
   b. Overall cleanliness and state of repair
   c. Number of steps new mother must climb
   d. Adequacy of cooking arrangements
   e. Adequacy of refrigeration and other food storage areas
   f. Adequacy of bathing, toileting, and laundry facilities
   g. Arrangements in home for newborn: sleeping, bathing, formula preparation (if needed), layette items, and diapers
5. Throughout the visit, observe home environment for overall state of repair and existence of the following safety hazards:
   a. Storage of medications, household cleaners, and other substances hazardous to children

  b. Presence of peeling paint on furniture, walls, or pipes
  c. Factors that contribute to falls, such as dim lighting, broken steps, scatter rugs
  d. Presence of vermin
  e. Use of crib or playpen that fails to meet safety guidelines
  f. Existence of emergency plan in case of fire; fire alarm or extinguisher

 6. Provide care to mother or newborn as prescribed by their respective primary caregiver or in accord with agency protocol.
 7. Provide client teaching on basis of previously identified needs.
 8. Refer family to appropriate community agencies or resources, such as warm lines and support groups.
 9. Ascertain that client knows potential problems to watch for and whom to call if they occur.
 10. Ensure that used disposable items have been handled appropriately and that reusable items are cleaned and repacked appropriately in the nurse's bag.

In-home interventions: ending the visit*

1. Summarize the activities and main points of the visit.
2. Clarify future expectations, including schedule of next visit.
3. Review teaching plan, and provide major points in writing.
4. Provide information about reaching the nurse or agency if needed before the next scheduled visit.

Postvisit interventions

1. Document the visit thoroughly, using the necessary agency forms to serve as a legal record of the visit and to allow third-party reimbursement, as possible.
2. Initiate the plan of care on which the next encounter with the client/family will be based.
3. Communicate appropriately (by telephone, letter, progress notes, or referral form) with primary caregiver, other health professionals, or referral agencies on behalf of client/family.

---

*If this is the nurse's final planned encounter with the client/family, it is important to recognize that both the client and nurse may have feelings evoked by ending a meaningful relationship and by saying goodbye. Such feelings as anger, denial, and sadness are normal in this situation. Freely expressing these feelings at the end of the relationship is encouraged. Often clients are encouraged to do so if the nurse shares such feelings first.

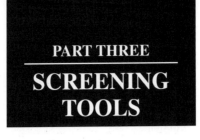

PART THREE

SCREENING TOOLS

Screening tools are valuable instruments for identifying and planning appropriate interventions for clients of all ages. The instruments in this section primarily address mechanisms for the nurse to diagnose client problems that are seen in the community as a basis for assessing client needs and planning care. They may be used or adapted to the practice of the nurse in ways that are most useful to a specific setting or agency.

CLINICAL DECISION-MAKING GUIDES

The nurse often finds it necessary to plan care based on physiological changes that occur suddenly or insidiously. Appropriate clinical decision making is essential to initiate proper referrals or to plan interventions. The following selected tools will assist the nurse in the home.

Signs and Symptoms of Congestive Heart Failure

Right ventricular failure
  Peripheral edema (pitting)
  Liver enlargement with right upper quadrant pain
  Ascites
  Distended neck veins
Left ventricular failure
  Dyspnea
  Orthopnea
  Paroxysmal nocturnal dyspnea (PND)
  Cheyne-Stokes respirations
  Fatigue
  Auscultatory crackles

From Phipps WJ et al.: *Medical-surgical nursing: concepts and clinical practice,* ed 5, St. Louis, 1995, Mosby.

Assessment

Subjective data

Data to be collected to assess the client with congestive heart failure concern the person's perception of breathing ability, fluid retention, response to activity, and knowledge of and response to the cardiac failure, including the following:

Shortness of breath and presence of cough
Presence of orthopnea (number of pillows needed for sleep)
Recent weight gain
Edema, especially pedal
Dizziness or confusion
Fatigue
Exercise or heat intolerance
Discomfort: anginal or abdominal pain
Appetite
Usual bowel patterns
Concerns, anxieties
Knowledge of condition
Usual coping skills

Objective data

Objective data focus primarily on signs of fluid retention and include the following:

Respiratory distress, increased effort, and respiratory rate
Neck vein distention: presence, degree
Adventitious breath sounds
Heart sounds: presence of S_3 or gallop rhythm
Edema: site and degree of pitting
Coolness of extremities
Pulse changes
Abdominal distention
Daily weights
Level of consciousness
Character of stools

Signs and Symptoms of TIA

The major importance of TIAs is that they warn the client and health care professional of the existence of an underlying pathological condition. At least one third of clients who have TIAs will have a CVA in 2 to 5 years. A person with a TIA needs to be aggressively assessed to determine if preventive measures can be taken.

Assessment

Subjective data

1. Client's understanding of disease or symptoms
2. Characteristics of onset of symptoms
3. Presence of headache—nature and location
4. Any sensory deficits
5. Visual ability—presence of diplopia, blurred vision
6. Ability to think clearly
7. Any other concomitant symptom

Objective data

1. Motor strength—paresis or plegia is common
2. Change in level of consciousness, including unconsciousness
3. Signs of increased intracranial pressure
4. Respiratory status
5. Ability to verbalize—presence of aphasia

The exact clinical picture varies depending on the area of the brain affected. The most common focal signs and symptoms are caused by disruption of flow through the midcerebral artery. These symptoms include the following:

1. Contralateral paralysis or paresis
2. Contralateral sensory loss
3. Sensory and motor loss most noticeable in face, neck, and upper extremities
4. Dysphasia or aphasia; occurs if dominant hemisphere is affected (left hemisphere in right-handed persons and most left-handed persons)
5. Spatial-perceptual problems, changes in judgment and behavior, neglect of paralyzed side, and inability to recognize paralyzed extremity as own *(anosognosia)* if nondominant hemisphere is affected
6. Contralateral *homonymous hemianopsia*

Aphasia is a disorder of language caused by damage to the speech-controlling areas of the brain. It includes all areas of language, including speech, reading, writing, and understanding. These abnormalities can occur in a variety of ways as follows:

1. **Sensory aphasia**—inability to comprehend spoken word (also called receptive aphasia)
2. **Motor aphasia**—inability to use the symbols of speech (also called expressive aphasia)
3. **Global aphasia**—inability to understand the spoken word, as well as to speak

Warning Signs of a Stroke

If you notice one or more of these warning signs, seek medical treatment immediately. Your body may be trying to tell you something.

1. Sudden weakness or numbness of the face, arm, and leg on one side of the body
2. Loss of speech, or trouble talking or understanding speech
3. Dimness or loss of vision, particularly in only one eye
4. Unexplained dizziness, unsteadiness, or sudden falls, especially along with any of the previous symptoms

About 10% of brain attacks are preceded by "temporary strokes," or transient ischemic attacks (TIAs). These can occur days, weeks, or even months before a major stroke. TIAs result when a blood clot temporarily clogs an artery and part of the brain does not get the supply of blood that is required. The symptoms occur rapidly and last a relatively short time, usually from a few minutes to several hours. The usual symptoms are like those of a full-fledged brain attack, except that they are temporary, lasting 24 hours or less.

From *What you should know about stroke,* 1994, Copyright American Heart Association.

Classification of Cerebral Aneurysms

Grade I—minimal bleed	Asymptomatic or minimal headache, slight nuchal rigidity
Grade II—mild bleed	Moderate to severe headache, nuchal rigidity, minimal neurological deficits
Grade III—moderate bleed	Drowsiness, confusion, mild focal neurological deficits
Grade IV—moderate to severe bleed	Stupor, moderate to severe hemiparesis, early decerebrate posturing
Grade V—severe bleed	Deep coma, decerebrate rigidity, disruption of vegetative functions

From Phipps WJ et al.: *Medical-surgical nursing: concepts and clinical practice,* ed 6, St. Louis, 1999, Mosby.

Comparison of Expressive and Receptive Aphasia

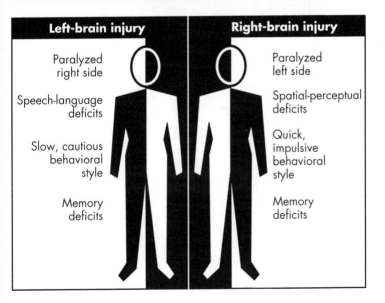

Receptive and expressive aphasia arising from right and left brain damage.

From *American Heart Association: how stroke affects behavior,* Dallas, 1994, The Association. Copyright American Heart Association.

Types of Aphasia

Type	Definition	Site of lesion
Motor (expressive)	Impairment of ability to speak and write; client can understand written and spoken words	Insula and surrounding region including Broca's motor area
Anomic	Inability to name objects, qualities, and conditions although speech is fluent	Area of angular gyrus
Fluent	Speech is well articulated and grammatically correct but is lacking in content and meaning	
Nonfluent	Problems in selecting, organizing, and initiating speech patterns May also affect writing	Motor cortex at Broca's area
Sensory (receptive)	Impairment of ability to understand written or spoken language	Disease of auditory and visual word centers
Wernicke's	See fluent aphasia above	Wernicke's area of left hemisphere
Mixed aphasia	Combined expressive and receptive aphasia deficits	Damage to various speech and language areas
Global aphasia	Total aphasia involving all functions that make up speech and communication Few if any intact language skills	Severe damage to speech areas

From Phipps WJ et al.: *Medical-surgical nursing: concepts and clinical practice*, ed 6, St. Louis, 1999, Mosby.

Communicating With Aphasic Clients

- Explain situations, treatments, and anything else that is pertinent to client as he or she may understand; the sounds of normal speech tend to be rehabilitative even if the words are not understood. Talk as if the person understands.
- Avoid patronizing and childish phrases.
- The aphasic client may be especially sensitive to feelings of annoyance; remain calm and patient.
- Speak slowly, ask one question at a time, and wait for a response.
- Ask questions in a way that can be answered with a nod or the blink of an eye; if the client cannot verbally respond instruct him or her in nonverbal responses.
- Speak of things familiar and of interest to client.
- Use visual cues, objects, pictures, and gestures, as well as words.
- Organize environment to be as predictable as possible.
- Encourage articulation even if words convey no meaning.
- Show interest in the client as an individual.

From Ebersole P, Hess P: *Toward healthy aging: human needs and nursing response,* ed 5, St. Louis, 1998, Mosby.

Notes

Comparison of Delirium, Depression, and Dementia

	Delirium	Depression	Dementia
Onset	Rapid (hours to days)	Rapid (weeks to months)	Gradual (years)
Course	Wide fluctuations; may continue for weeks if cause not found	May be self-limited or may become chronic without treatment	Chronic; slow but continuous decline
Level of consciousness	Fluctuates from hyperalert to difficult to arouse	Normal	Normal
Orientation	Client is disoriented, confused	Client may seem disoriented	Client is disoriented, confused
Affect	Fluctuating	Sad, depressed, worried, guilty	Labile; apathy in later stages
Attention	Always impaired	Difficulty concentrating; client may check and recheck all actions	May be intact; client may focus on one thing for long periods
Sleep	Always disturbed	Disturbed; excess sleeping or insomnia, especially early-morning waking	Usually normal
Behavior	Agitated, restless	Client may be fatigued, apathetic; may occasionally be agitated	Client may be agitated or apathetic; may wander
Speech	Sparse or rapid; client may be incoherent	Flat, sparse, may have outbursts; understandable	Sparse or rapid; repetitive; client may be incoherent

	Delirium	Depression	Dementia
Memory	Impaired, especially for recent events	Varies day to day; slow recall; often short-term deficit	Impaired, especially for recent events
Cognition	Disordered reasoning	May seem impaired	Disordered reasoning and calculation
Thought content	Incoherent, confused, delusions, stereotyped	Negative, hypochondriacal, thoughts of death, paranoid	Disorganized, rich content, delusional, paranoid
Perception	Misinterpretations, illusions, hallucinations	Distorted; client may have auditory hallucinations; negative interpretation of people and events	No change
Judgment	Poor	Poor	Poor; socially inappropriate behavior
Insight	May be present in lucid moments	May be impaired	Absent
Performance on mental status exams	Poor but variable; improves during lucid moments and with recovery	Memory impaired; calculation, drawing, following directions usually not impaired; frequent "I don't know" answers	Consistently poor; progressively worsens; client attempts to answer all questions

From Holt J: *Am J Nurs* 93:32, 1993.

Four Phases of Alzheimer's Disease

Phase	Observable changes
I	Onset is insidious. Spontaneity, energy, and initiative are decreased; slowness is increased. Word-finding is difficult. Learning times and reacting are slower. Anger is easier. Familiarity is sought and preferred.
II	Supervision with detailed activities such as banking is needed. Speech and understanding are much slower. Train of thought is lost.
III	Personality change is marked (can be depressed). Directions must be specific and repeated for safety. Recent memory is poor. Disorientation is easy. People are incorrectly identified. Behavior is lethargic.
IV	Apathy is noticeable. Memory is poor or absent. Person cannot be alone. Urinary incontinence is present. Individuals are not recognized.

From Edelman CL, Mandle CL: *Health promotion throughout the lifespan*, ed 3, St. Louis, 1994, Mosby.

Notes

Criteria for Clinical Diagnosis of Alzheimer's Disease

I. The criteria for the clinical diagnosis of *probable* Alzheimer's disease include the following:

Dementia established by clinical examination and documented by the Mini-Mental Test, Blessed Dementia Scale, or some similar examination and confirmed by neuropsychological tests

Deficits in two or more areas of cognition

Progressive worsening of memory and other cognitive functions

No disturbance of consciousness

Onset between ages 40 and 90, most often after age 65

Absence of systemic disorders or other brain diseases that in and of themselves could account for the progressive deficits in memory and cognition

II. The diagnosis of *probable* Alzheimer's disease is supported by the following:

Progressive deterioration of specific cognitive functions such as language (aphasia), motor skills (apraxia), and perception (agnosia)

Impaired activities of daily living and altered patterns of behavior

Family history of similar disorders, particularly if confirmed neuropathologically

Laboratory results of normal lumbar puncture as evaluated by standard techniques; normal pattern or nonspecific changes in EEG, such as increased slow-wave activity; and evidence of cerebral atrophy on CT with progression documented by serial observation

III. Other clinical features consistent with the diagnosis of *probable* Alzheimer's disease, after exclusion of causes of dementia other than Alzheimer's disease, include the following:

Plateaus in the course of progression of the illness

Associated symptoms of depression, insomnia, incontinence, delusions, illusions, hallucinations, catastrophic verbal, emotional, or physical outbursts, sexual disorders, and weight loss

From McKhann G et al.: Clinical diagnosis of Alzheimer's disease: a report of the NINCDS-ADRDA work group under the auspices of the Department of Health and Human Services Task Force on Alzheimer's disease, *Neurology* 34:939, 1984.

Other neurological abnormalities in some clients, especially with more advanced disease and including motor signs such as increased muscle tone, myoclonus, or gait disorder

Seizures in advanced disease

CT normal for age

IV. Features that make the diagnosis of *probable* Alzheimer's disease uncertain or unlikely include the following:

Sudden, apoplectic onset

Focal neurological findings such as hemiparesis, sensory loss, visual field deficits, and incoordination early in the course of the illness

Seizures or gait disturbances at the onset or very early in the course of the illness

V. Clinical diagnosis of *possible* Alzheimer's disease:

May be made on the basis of the dementia syndrome, in the absence of other neurological, psychiatric, or systemic disorders sufficient to cause dementia, and in the presence of variations in the onset, in the presentation, or in the clinical course

May be made in the presence of a second systemic or brain disorder sufficient to produce dementia, which is not considered to be *the* cause of the dementia

Should be used in research studies when a single, gradually progressive severe cognitive deficit is identified in the absence of other identifiable cause

VI. Criteria for diagnosis of *definite* Alzheimer's disease are as follows:

The clinical criteria for probable Alzheimer's disease

Histopathological evidence obtained from a biopsy or autopsy

VII. Classification of Alzheimer's disease for research purposes should specify features that may differentiate subtypes of the disorder, such as the following:

Familial occurrence

Onset before age of 65

Presence of trisomy-21

Coexistence of other relevant conditions such as Parkinson's disease

Classification of Seizures

Type of seizure	Effect on consciousness	Signs and symptoms	Postictal state
Partial seizures			
Simple partial (focal)	Not impaired	Focal twitching of extremity Speech arrest Special visual sensations (e.g., seeing lights), feeling of fear or doom	No
Complex partial (formerly psychomotor or temporal lobe seizures)	Impaired	May begin as simple partial and progress to complex Automatic behavior (e.g., lip smacking, chewing, or picking at clothes)	Yes
Complex partial generalizing to generalized tonic-clonic seizures	Impaired	Begins as complex partial as above, then progresses to tonic-clonic as described below	Yes
Generalized seizures			
Absence (formerly petit mal)	Impaired	Brief loss of consciousness, staring, unresponsive	No
Tonic-clonic (formerly grand mal)	Impaired	Tonic phase involves rigidity of all muscles, followed by clonic phase, which involves rhythmic jerking of muscles, possibly tongue biting and urinary and fecal incontinence May be any combination of tonic and clonic movements	Yes
Atonic	Impaired for only a few seconds	Brief loss of muscle tone, which may cause client to fall or drop something; referred to as drop attacks	No
Myoclonic	Impaired for only a few seconds or not at all	Brief jerking of a muscle group, which may cause the client to fall	No

Modified from Phipps WJ et al.: *Medical-surgical nursing: concepts and clinical practice*, ed 6, St. Louis, 1999, Mosby.

Common Causes of Transient Urinary Incontinence

Potential causes	Comment
Delirium (confusional state)	In the delirious client, incontinence is usually an associated symptom that will abate with proper diagnosis and treatment of the underlying cause of confusion.
Infection (symptomatic urinary tract infection)	Dysuria and urgency from symptomatic infection may defeat the older person's ability to reach the toilet in time. Asymptomatic infection, although more common than symptomatic infection, is rarely a cause of incontinence.
Atrophic urethritis or vaginitis	Atrophic urethritis may present as dysuria, dyspareunia, burning on urination, urgency, agitation (in demented clients), and occasionally as incontinence. Both disorders are readily treated by conjugated estrogen administered either orally (0.3 to 1.25 mg/day) or locally (2 g or fraction/day).
Pharmaceuticals Sedative hypnotics	Benzodiazepines, especially long-acting agents such as flurazepam and diazepam, may accumulate in elderly clients and cause confusion and secondary incontinence. Alcohol, frequently used as a sedative, can cloud the sensorium, impair mobility, and induce a diuresis, resulting in incontinence.
Diuretics	A brisk diuresis induced by loop diuretics can overwhelm bladder capacity and lead to polyuria, frequency, and urgency, thereby precipitating incontinence in a frail older person. The loop diuretics include furosemide, ethacrynic acid, and bumetanide.

From DHHS, PNS, AHCPR: *Urinary incontinence in adults: the quick reference guide for clinicians,* Publication #AHCRR 92-0041, Rockville, Md, 1992.

Common Causes of Transient Urinary Incontinence—cont'd

Potential causes	Comment
Anticholinergic agents Antihistamines Antidepressants Antipsychotics Disopnamide Opiates Antispasmodics (dicyclomine and Donnatal) Antiparkinsonian agents (trihexyphenidyl and benztropine mesylate)	Nonprescription (over-the-counter) agents with anticholinergic properties are taken commonly by older clients for insomnia, coryza, pruritus, and vertigo, and many prescription medications also have anticholinergic properties. Anticholinergic side effects include urinary retention with associated urinary frequency and overflow incontinence. Besides anticholinergic actions, antipsychotics such as thioridazine and haloperidol may cause sedation, rigidity, and immobility.
Alpha-adrenegic agents Sympathomimetics (decongestants) Sympatholytics (e.g., prazosin, terazosin, and doxazosin)	Sphincter tone in the proximal urethra can be decreased by alpha antagonists and increased by alpha agonists. An older woman, whose urethra is shortened and weakened with age, may develop stress incontinence when taking an alpha antagonist for hypertension. An older man with prostate enlargement may develop acute urinary retention and overflow incontinence when taking multicomponent "cold" capsules, which contain alpha agonists and anticholinergic agents, especially if a nasal decongestant and a nonprescription hypnotic antihistamine are added.
Calcium-channel blockers	Calcium-channel blockers can reduce smooth muscle contractility in the bladder and occasionally can cause urinary retention and overflow incontinence.
Psychological	Severe depression may occasionally be associated with incontinence, but is probably less frequently a cause in older clients.

Continued.

Common Causes of Transient Urinary Incontinence—cont'd

Potential causes	Comment
Excessive urine production	Excess intake, endocrine conditions that cloud the sensorium and induce a diuresis (e.g., hypercalcemia, hyperglycemia, and diabetes insipidus); expanded volume states such as congestive heart failure, lower extremity venous insufficiency, drug-induced ankle edema (e.g., nifedipine, indomethacin); and low albumen states cause polyuria and can lead to incontinence.
Restricted mobility	Limited mobility is an aggravating or precipitating cause of incontinence that can frequently be corrected or improved by treating the underlying condition (e.g., arthritis, poor eyesight, Parkinson's disease, or orthostatic hypotension). A urinal or bedside commode and scheduled toileting often help resolve the incontinence that results from hospitalization and its environmental barriers (e.g., bed rails, restraints, and poor lighting).
Stool impaction	Clients with stool impaction have either urge or overflow incontinence and may have fecal incontinence as well. Disimpaction restores continence.

Types of Urinary Incontinence

Description	Causes	Symptoms
Total Total uncontrolled and continuous loss of urine	Neuropathy of sensory nerves; trauma or disease of spinal nerves or urethral sphincter; fistula between bladder and vagina	Constant flow of urine at unpredictable times, nocturia, unawareness of bladder filling or incontinence
Functional Involuntary, unpredictable passage of urine in client with intact urinary and nervous systems	Change in environment; sensory, cognitive, or mobility deficits	Strong urge to void that causes loss of urine before reaching appropriate receptacle
Stress Increased intra-abdominal pressure that causes leakage of small amount of urine	Coughing, laughing, vomiting, or lifting with full bladder; obesity; full uterus in third trimester; incompetent bladder outlet; weak pelvic musculature	Dribbling of urine with increased intraabdominal pressure, urinary urgency and frequency
Urge Involuntary passage of urine after strong sense of urgency to void	Decreased bladder capacity; irritation of bladder stretch receptors; alcohol or caffeine ingestion; increased fluid intake	Urinary urgency, abdominal frequency (more often than every 2 hours), bladder contracture or spasm, nocturia, voiding in small (less than 100 ml) or large (more than 550 ml) amounts
Reflex or overflow Involuntary loss of urine occurring at somewhat predictable intervals when specific bladder volume is reached	Upper spinal cord injury or disease involving area above reflex arc, blocking cerebral awareness Lower spinal cord injury blocking impulses to reflex arc	Unawareness of bladder filling, lack of urge to void, uninhibited bladder contraction or spasm at regular intervals

From Potter PA, Perry AG: *Basic nursing: a critical thinking approach,* ed 4. St. Louis, 1999, Mosby.

Elements of an Incontinence Assessment

History	Details of present problem
	Medical history
	Surgical history
	Urological procedures/problems
	Dietary and bowel patterns
	Fluid intake
Environmental review	Location of toilet facility
	Assistive devices needed
	Factors that impede (rugs, stairs, layout of living area)
Medications	
Physical examination with limited neurological examination	Gross motor functions
	Fine motor movement
	Mental status
	Rectal tone
	Presence/absence fecal impaction
Females	Inspection outer perineal area
	Look for pelvic descent
	Internal examination
Males	Check prostate
Functional examination	Determine mobility; ability to handle devices
	Observe clothing, how client manages now—*important to see how individual functions*
Urinalysis	Detect associated conditions such as hematuria, glycosuria, proteinuria, bacteria, or white cells

From *Clinical practice guidelines: urinary incontinence in adults,* USDHHS, AHCPR, Rockville, Md, 1992.

Elements of a Supplemental Urinary Incontinence Assessment

Use of a voiding record
Evaluation of environmental and social factors
Observing voiding
Blood tests
Urine cytology
Urodynamic tests
Endoscopic tests
Imaging tests of upper tract and/or lower tract with and without voiding

From *Clinical practice guidelines: urinary incontinence in adults,* USDHHS, AHCPR, Rockville, Md, 1992.

Focused Physical Examination for Bowel Function Evaluation

Parameter	Assessment strategy
Chewing	Inspect condition of teeth and gums. Poor dentition or poorly fitting dentures influence the ability to chew.
Mobility	*In ambulatory clients*—Observe gait; determine need for assistive devices or personnel. *In wheelchair-bound clients*—Note degree of needed assistance to transfer from chair to commode or toilet.
Dexterity	Ask client to demonstrate hand motions that would be required to insert suppository or perform digital stimulation (e.g., grasping a pencil, rotation of forefinger).
Anal sphincter function	Inspect anus at rest. Then perform digital examination while asking client to contract and relax sphincter followed by Valsalva maneuver. The inability to sense rectal distention, to voluntarily contract anus, or to "bear down" is indicative of impaired function.
Abdominal muscle contractility	Instruct client to "bear down" (or to push against the examiner's hand) while lightly palpating the abdominal wall. Check for presence, volume, and consistency of stool in rectum. The presence of large amounts of stool is indicative of decreased sensation and/or impaired emptying.

From Potter PA, Perry AG: *Basic nursing: a critical thinking approach,* ed 4, St. Louis, 1999, Mosby. Based on data from Doughty D: A step-by-step approach to bowel training, *Progressions* 4(2):18, 1992.

Notes

Causes of Fecal Incontinence in the Aged

Fecal impaction
Functional impairment
Mental
  Dementia
  Mental retardation
  Confusion
Physical
  Weakness
  Immobility

Decreased reservoir capacity
Aging
Radiation
Proctitis
Tumor
Ischemia
Surgical resection

Decreased rectal sensation
Diabetes mellitus
Megacolon
Fecal impaction
Central nervous system
  Stroke
  Multiple sclerosis
  Meningomyelocele
  Degenerative diseases
  Severe B_{12} deficiency
Peripheral nervous system
  Diabetes mellitus
  Shy-Drager syndrome
  Toxic neuropathy
  Perineal descent syndrome
Drug reaction/intoxication

Impaired anal sphincter and puborectal muscle function
Idiopathic
Trauma (disruption of nerves and musculature)
Surgery
Spinal cord or pudendal lesions
Diabetes mellitus

Abnormal delivery of feces to rectum
Drug-induced
Diarrhea
Blind loop syndrome
Inflammatory bowel disease
Infectious disease
Celiac sprue

From Ebersole P, Hess P: *Toward healthy aging*, ed 5, St. Louis, 1998, Mosby.

Fecal Incontinence Assessment

History
Characteristics of incontinence
Relevant medical history
Medication review
Diet history
Activity patterns
Client/caregiver perception
Environmental characteristics
Physical examination
Abdomen
Neurological
Rectal

Functional assessment of mobility status

Bowel record (1 week)

Laboratory and other tests as needed

From Ebersole P, Hess P: *Toward healthy aging: human needs and nursing response,* ed 5, St. Louis, 1998, Mosby.

Notes

Types of Skin Lesions

Observed skin changes	Differentiation	Term	Example
Change in color or texture			
Spot	Circumscribed; flat; color change	Macule	Freckle
Discoloration (reddish purple)	Bleeding beneath the surface; injury to tissue	Contusion	Bruise
Soft whitening	Caused by repeated wetting of skin	Maceration	Between toes after soaking
Flake	Dry cells of surface	Scale	Dandruff; psoriasis
Roughness from dried fluid	Dry exudate over lesions	Crust	Eczema, impetigo
Roughness from cells	Leathery thickening of outer skin layer	Lichenification	Callus on foot
Change in shape			
Fluid-filled lesions	Less than 1 cm; clear fluid	Vesicle	Blister; chicken pox
	Greater than 1 cm; clear fluid	Bulla	Large blister; pemphigus
	Small, thick yellowish fluid (pus)	Pustule	Acne
Solid mass, *cellular* growth	Less than 5 mm	Papule	Small mole; raised rash
	5 mm to 2 cm	Nodule	Enlarged lymph node
	Greater than 2 cm	Tumor	Benign or malignant tumor
	Excess connective tissue over scar	Keloid	Overgrown scar
Swelling of tissue	Generalized swelling; fluid between cells	Edema	Inflammation; swelling of feet
	Circumscribed surface edema; transient; some itching	Wheal ("hive")	Allergic reaction

Breaks in skin surfaces

Oozing, scraped surface	Abrasion	Loss of superficial structure of skin	"Floor burn"; scrape
Scooped-out depression	Ulcer	Loss of deeper layers of skin	Decubitus or stasis ulcer
Superficial linear skin breaks	Excoriations	Scratch marks, frequently by fingernails	Scratching
Linear cracks or cleft	Fissure	Slit or splitting of skin layers	Athlete's foot
Jagged cut	Laceration	Tearing of skin surface	Accidental cut by blunt object
Linear cut, edges approximated	Incision	Cutting by sharp instrument	Knife cut

Vascular lesions

Small, flat, round, purplish, red spot	Petechia	Intradermal or submucous hemorrhage	Bleeding tendency; vitamin C deficiency
Spiderlike, red, small	Telangiectasis	Dilation of capillaries, arterioles, or venules	Liver disease, vitamin B deficiency
Discoloration, reddish purple	Ecchymosis	Escape of blood into tissue	Trauma to blood vessels

From Weaver V: Assessment of the skin. In Phipps WJ et al., editors: *Medical-surgical nursing: concepts and clinical practice*, ed 6, St. Louis, 1999, Mosby.

Characteristics of Pressure Sores—Ulcer Sites

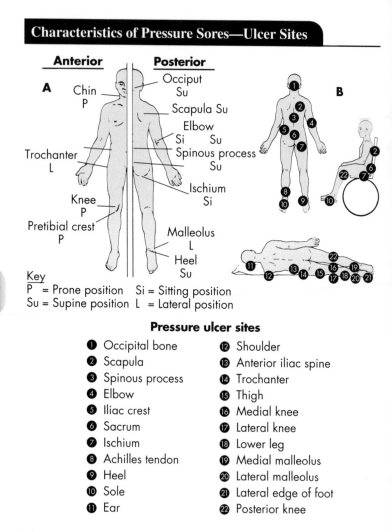

Key
P = Prone position   Si = Sitting position
Su = Supine position   L = Lateral position

Pressure ulcer sites

1. Occipital bone
2. Scapula
3. Spinous process
4. Elbow
5. Iliac crest
6. Sacrum
7. Ischium
8. Achilles tendon
9. Heel
10. Sole
11. Ear
12. Shoulder
13. Anterior iliac spine
14. Trochanter
15. Thigh
16. Medial knee
17. Lateral knee
18. Lower leg
19. Medial malleolus
20. Lateral malleolus
21. Lateral edge of foot
22. Posterior knee

Figure 2   **A,** Bony prominences most frequently underlying pressure ulcers. **B,** Pressure ulcer sites. *(From Trelease CC: Pressure ulcer sites, Ostomy/Wound Manage 20:46, 1988.)*

Bates-Jensen Pressure Sore Status Tool

NAME _____

Complete the rating sheet to assess pressure sore status. Evaluate each item by picking the response that best describes the wound and entering the score in the item score column for the appropriate date.

Location: Anatomical site. Circle, identify right (**R**) or left (**L**), and use "**X**" to mark site on body diagrams:

____ Sacrum & coccyx   ____ Ischial tuberosity   ____ Medial ankle

____ Trochanter   ____ Lateral ankle   ____ Heel   Other site ____

Shape: Overall wound pattern; assess by observing perimeter and depth.
Circle and *date* appropriate description:

____ Irregular   ____ Square/rectangle   ____ Bowl/boat

____ Round/oval   ____ Linear or elongated   ____ Butterfly   Other shape ____

Item	Assessment	Date	Date	Date
		Score	Score	Score
1. **Size**	1 = Length × width <4 sq cm 2 = Length × width 4-16 sq cm 3 = Length × width 16.1-36 sq cm 4 = Length × width 36.1-80 sq cm 5 = Length × width >80 sq cm			
2. **Depth**	1 = Nonblanchable erythema on intact skin 2 = Partial thickness skin loss involving epidermis and/or dermis 3 = Full thickness skin loss involving damage or necrosis of subcutaneous tissue; may extend down to but not through underlying fascia; and/or mixed partial and full thickness and/or tissue layers obscured by granulation tissue 4 = Obscured by necrosis 5 = Full thickness skin loss with extensive destruction, tissue necrosis, or damage to muscle, bone, or supporting structures			

Continued.

© 1990 Barbara Bates-Jensen.

Bates-Jensen Pressure Sore Status Tool—cont'd

Item	Assessment	Date Score	Date Score	Date Score	Date Score
3. Edges	1 = Indistinct, diffuse, none clearly visible 2 = Distinct, outline clearly visible, attached, even with wound base 3 = Well-defined, not attached to wound base 4 = Well-defined, not attached to base, rolled under, thickened 5 = Well-defined, fibrotic, scarred, or hyperkeratotic				
4. Undermining	1 = Undermining <2 cm in any area 2 = Undermining 2-4 cm involving <50% wound margins 3 = Undermining 2-4 cm involving >50% wound margins 4 = Undermining >4 cm in any area 5 = Tunneling and/or sinus tract formation				
5. Necrotic tissue type	1 = None visible 2 = White/grey nonvariable tissue and/or nonadherent yellow slough 3 = Loosely adherent yellow slough 4 = Adherent, soft, black eschar 5 = Firmly adherent, hard, black eschar				
6. Necrotic tissue amount	1 = None visible 2 = <25% of wound bed covered 3 = 25-50% of wound covered 4 = >50% and <75% of wound covered 5 = 75-100% of wound covered				

7. **Exudate type**	1 = None or bloody 2 = Serosanguineous: thin, watery, pale red/pink 3 = Serous: thin, watery, clear 4 = Purulent: thin or thick, opaque tan/yellow 5 = Foul purulent: thick, opaque, yellow/green with odor	
8. **Exudate amount**	1 = None 2 = Scant 3 = Small 4 = Moderate 5 = Large	
9. **Skin color surrounding wound**	1 = Pink or normal for ethnic group 2 = Bright red and/or blanches to touch 3 = White or grey pallor or hypopigmented 4 = Dark red or purple and/or nonblanchable 5 = Black or hyperpigmented	
10. **Peripheral tissue edema**	1 = Minimal swelling around wound 2 = Nonpitting edema extends <4 cm around wound 3 = Nonpitting edema extends ≥4 cm around wound 4 = Pitting edema extends <4 cm around wound 5 = Crepitus and/or pitting edema extends ≥4 cm	
11. **Peripheral tissue induration**	1 = Minimal firmness around wound 2 = Induration <2 cm around wound 3 = Induration 2-4 cm extending <50% around wound 4 = Induration 2-4 cm extending ≥50% around wound 5 = Induration <4 cm in any area	

Continued.

Bates-Jensen Pressure Sore Status Tool—cont'd

Item	Assessment	Date Score	Date Score	Date Score
12. **Granulation tissue**	1 = Skin intact or partial thickness wound 2 = Bright, beefy red; 75-100% of wound filled and/or tissue overgrowth 3 = Bright, beefy red; <75% and >25% of wound filled 4 = Pink and/or dull, dusky red and/or fills ≤25% of wound 5 = No granulation tissue present			
13. **Epithelialization**	1 = 100% wound covered, surface intact 2 = 75% to <100% wound covered and/or epithelial tissue 3 = 50% to <75% wound covered and/or epithelial tissue extends to >0.5 cm into wound bed 4 = 25% to <50% wound covered 5 = <25% wound covered			
Total Score				
Signature				

Pressure Sore Status Continuum

1　　10　5　20　25　30　35　40　45　50　55　60　65

Tissue health　Wound regeneration　　　　Wound degeneration

Plot the total score on the Pressure Sore Status Continuum by putting an "**X**" on the line and the date beneath the line. Plot multiple scores with their dates to see at a glance regeneration or degeneration of the wound.

Pressure Sore Status Tool

Instructions for use

General Guidelines:

Fill out the attached rating sheet to assess a pressure sore's status after reading the definitions and methods of assessment described below. Evaluate once a week and whenever a change occurs in the wound. Rate according to each item by picking the response that best describes the wound and entering that score in the item score column for the appropriate date. When you have rated the pressure sore on all items, determine the total score by adding together the 13-item scores. The HIGHER the total score, the more severe the pressure sore status. Plot total score on the Pressure Sore Status Continuum to determine progress.

Specific Instructions:

1. **Size:** Use ruler to measure the longest and widest aspect of the wound surface in centimeters; multiply length × width.
2. **Depth:** Pick the depth, thickness, most appropriate to the wound using these additional descriptions:

   1 = Tissues damaged but no break in skin surface

   2 = Superficial, abrasion, blister, or shallow crater; even with and/or elevated above skin surface (e.g., hyperplasia)

   3 = Deep crater with or without undermining of adjacent tissue

   4 = Visualization of tissue layers not possible due to necrosis

   5 = Supporting structures include tendon, joint capsule

3. **Edges:** Use this guide:

   Indistinct, diffuse   = unable to clearly distinguish wound outline

   Attached   = even or flush with wound base, *no* sides or walls present; flat

   Not attached   = sides or walls *are* present: floor or base of wound is deeper than edge

   Rolled under, thickened   = soft to firm and flexible to touch

   Hyperkeratosis   = callouslike tissue formation around wound and at edges

   Fibrotic, scarred   = hard, rigid to touch

Continued.

Bates-Jensen Pressure Sore Status Tool—cont'd

4. **Undermining:** Assess by inserting a cotton tipped applicator under the wound edge; advance it as far as it will go without using undue force; raise the tip of the applicator so it may be seen or felt on the surface of the skin; mark the surface with a pen; measure the distance from the mark on the skin to the edge of the wound. Continue process around the wound. Then use a transparent metric measuring guide with concentric circles divided into 4 (25%) pie-shaped quadrants to help determine percent of wound involved.

5. **Necrotic tissue type:** Pick the type of necrotic tissue that is *predominant* in the wound according to color, consistency, and adherence using this guide:

White/gray nonviable tissue	= may appear before wound opening; skin surface is white or gray
Nonadherent, yellow slough	= thin, mucinous substance; scattered throughout wound bed; easily separated from wound tissue
Loosely adherent, yellow slough	= thick, stringy, clumps or debris; attached to wound tissue
Adherent, soft, black eschar	= soggy tissue; strongly attached to tissue in center or base of wound
Firmly adherent, hard/black eschar	= firm, crusty tissue; strongly attached to wound base *and* edges (like a hard scab)

6. **Necrotic tissue amount:** Use a transparent metric measuring guide with concentric circles divided into 4 (25%) pie-shaped quadrants to help determine percent of wound involved.

7. **Exudate type:** Some dressings interact with wound drainage to produce a gel or trap liquid. Before assessing exudate type, gently cleanse wound with normal saline or water. Pick the exudate type that is *predominant* in the wound according to color and consistency, using this guide:

Bloody	= thin, bright red
Serosanguineous	= thin, watery pale red to pink
Serous	= thin, watery, clear
Purulent	= thin or thick, opaque tan to yellow
Foul purulent	= thick, opaque yellow to green with offensive odor

8. **Exudate amount:** Use a transparent metric measuring guide with concentric circles divided into 4 (25%) pre-shaped quadrants to determine percent of dressing involved with exudate. Use this guide:

   None = wound tissues dry
   Scant = wound tissues moist; no measurable exudate
   Small = wound tissues wet; moisture evenly distributed in wound; drainage involves ≤25% dressing
   Moderate = wound tissues saturated; drainage may or may not be evenly distributed in wound; drainage involves >25% to ≤75% dressing
   Large = wound tissues bathed in fluid; drainage freely expressed; may or may not be evenly distributed in wound; drainage involves >75% of dressing

9. **Skin color surrounding wound:** Assess tissues within 4 cm of wound edge. Dark-skinned persons show the colors "bright red" and "dark red" as a deepening or normal ethnic skin color or a purple hue. As healing occurs in dark-skinned persons, the new skin is pink and may never darken.

10. **Peripheral tissue edema:** Assess tissues within 4 cm of wound edge. Nonpitting edema appears as skin that is shiny and taut. Identify pitting edema by firmly pressing a finger down into the tissues and waiting for 5 seconds. On release of pressure, tissues fail to resume previous position and an indentation appears. Crepitus is accumulation of air or gas in tissues. Use a transparent metric measuring guide to determine how far edema extends beyond wound.

11. **Peripheral tissue induration:** Assess tissues within 4 cm of wound edge. Induration is abnormal firmness of tissues with margins. Assess by gently pinching the tissues. Induration results in an inability to pinch the tissues. Use a transparent metric measuring guide with concentric circles divided into 4 (25%) pie-shaped quadrants to determine percent of wound and area involved.

12. **Granulation tissue:** Granulation tissue is the growth of small blood vessels and connective tissue to fill in full thickness wounds. Tissue is healthy when bright, beefy red, shiny, and granular with a velvety appearance. Poor vascular supply appears as pale pink or balanced to dull, dusky red color.

13. **Epithelialization:** Epithelialization is the process of epidermal resurfacing and appears as pink or red skin. In partial thickness wounds it can occur throughout the wound bed, as well as from the wound edges. In full thickness wounds it occurs from the edges only. Use a transparent metric measuring guide with concentric circles divided into 4 (25%) pie-shaped quadrants to help determine percent of wound involved and to measure the distance the epithelial tissue extends into the wound.

Norton Scale Pressure Sore Risk Assessment

Norton Scale

A Physical condition	B Mental state	C Activity	D Mobility	E Incontinence	Total score
4 Good	4 Alert	4 Ambulant	4 Full	4 Not	
3 Fair	3 Apathetic	3 Walks with help	3 Slightly limited	3 Occasional	
2 Poor	2 Confused	2 Chairbound	2 Very limited	2 Usually urine	
1 Bad	1 Stupor	1 Bed rest	1 Immobile	1 Double incontinence	

Norton Plus Scale

(For determining high risk for pressure sores)

Check ONLY if YES   *YES*

Diagnosis of diabetes

Diagnosis of hypertension

Hematocrit (M) <41%
         (F) <36%

Hemoglobin (M) <14 g/dl
              (F) <12 g/dl

Albumin level <3.3 g/dl

Febrile >99.6° F

5 or more medications

Changes in mental status to confused, lethargic within 24 hours

TOTAL Number of Checkmarks

Norton Scale Score

Minus total from above

Norton Plus Score

From Norton D, McLaren R, Exton-Smith AN: *An investigation of geriatric nursing problems in hospital*, Edinburgh, 1975, Churchill Livingstone. Maximum score = 20 (good physical condition); minimum score = 5; high risk for pressure ulcers = 12 or below.

Stages of Pressure Sores

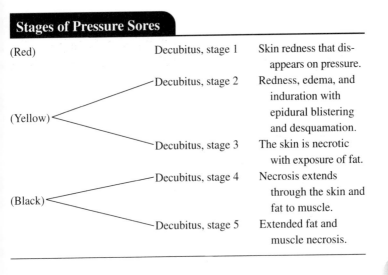

(Red)   Decubitus, stage 1   Skin redness that disappears on pressure.

(Yellow)

Decubitus, stage 2   Redness, edema, and induration with epidural blistering and desquamation.

Decubitus, stage 3   The skin is necrotic with exposure of fat.

(Black)

Decubitus, stage 4   Necrosis extends through the skin and fat to muscle.

Decubitus, stage 5   Extended fat and muscle necrosis.

Prevention of Pressure Sores

- Inspect the skin daily in good light.
- Keep the skin clean and dry.
- Consult a nutritionist for information on proper nutrition.
- Help the client exercise joints, arms, and legs, if possible.
- Turn the client often (every 1/2 hour to every 2 or more hours, depending on the person's condition), or arrange a trapeze over the bed to enable the person to shift positions.
- Use a footboard and keep the bed at less than a 30-degree angle to prevent "shearing" (damage from the skin's being stretched and torn from sliding down the bed or wheelchair).
- Use pull and draw sheets for turning or lifting.
- Make sure bed linen is smooth and soft, without crumbs, wrinkles, or folds to irritate the skin.
- Contact a medical supply dealer for information on pressure- and friction-relieving products, such as sheepskin, elbow and heel protectors, cushions, and pads that provide equal weight and pressure distribution for wheelchair users.

Aspects of Care for Pressure Ulcers

Diagnostic tests
There are no specific laboratory tests to assist with diagnosis of pressure ulcers. Related laboratory examinations pertinent to risk factors have been included in the previous discussion of risk factors.

Medication
There are no particular medications for pressure ulcers. Antibiotics are used if an infection is present.

Treatment
More than 100 products exist as purported treatment measures for pressure ulcers.

Diet
Clients with wounds require additional protein and calorie intake to assist with tissue regeneration on a cellular level. A well-balanced diet is sufficient to maintain healthy skin; however, most clients with any identified risk factors are not eating a well-balanced diet. Protein supplementation in balanced amounts is helpful. Only a registered dietitian can determine accurately a balance of demand and replacement that will be therapeutic for the client. Research also suggests that supplemental vitamin C and zinc, as well as a multiple vitamin with iron, help stimulate wound healing on a cellular level.

Activity
The more independently active the client is, the lower the risk of pressure sore formation and the greater the chances of wound healing. If the client is unable to assume an active role in mobility, it *must* be assumed by the nurse for the client. The key factor related to wound healing is the removal of the causative agent(s). Regardless of the treatment prescribed for wound care, if the pressure is not relieved by the client or passively by the nurse, wound healing will not occur.

Modified from Phipps WJ et al.: *Medical-surgical nursing: concepts and clinical practice,* ed 6, St. Louis, 1999, Mosby.

Braden Scale for Predicting Pressure Ulcer Risk*

	1 Point	2 Points	3 Points	4 Points
Sensory perception Ability to respond meaningfully to pressure-related discomfort	*Completely limited:* Unresponsive (does not moan, flinch, or grasp) to painful stimuli due to diminished level of consciousness or sedation. OR Limited ability to feel pain over most of body surface.	*Very limited:* Responds only to painful stimuli. Cannot communicate discomfort except by moaning or restlessness. OR Has a sensory impairment that limits the ability to feel pain or discomfort over half of body.	*Slightly limited:* Responds to verbal commands but cannot always communicate discomfort or need to be turned. OR Has some sensory impairment that limits ability to feel pain or discomfort in 1 or 2 extremities.	*No impairment:* Responds to verbal commands. Has no sensory deficit that would limit ability to feel or voice pain or discomfort.
Moisture Degree to which skin is exposed to moisture	*Constantly moist:* Skin is kept moist almost constantly by perspiration, urine, etc. Dampness is detected every time client is moved or turned.	*Very moist:* Skin is often, but not always, moist. Linen must be changed at least once a shift.	*Occasionally moist:* Skin is occasionally moist, requiring an extra linen change approximately once a day.	*Rarely moist:* Skin is usually dry; linen requires changing only at routine intervals. *Continued.*

Copyright 1988 Barbara Braden and Nancy Bergstrom.

*Score client in each of the six subscales. Maximum score is 23, indicating little or no risk. 15-18 = low risk, 13-14 = moderate risk, 10-12 = high risk, and ≤9 = very high risk.

Braden Scale for Predicting Pressure Ulcer Risk*—cont'd

	1 Point	2 Points	3 Points	4 Points
Activity Degree of physical activity	*Bedfast:* Confined to bed.	*Chairfast:* Ability to walk severely limited or nonexistent. Cannot bear own weight and/or must be assisted into chair or wheelchair.	*Walks occasionally:* Walks occasionally during day, but for very short distances, with or without assistance. Spends majority of each shift in bed or chair.	*Walks frequently:* Walks outside the room at least twice a day and inside room at least once every 2 hours during waking hours.
Mobility Ability to change and control body position	*Completely immobile:* Does not make even slight changes in body or extremity position without assistance.	*Very limited:* Makes occasional slight changes in body or extremity position but unable to make frequent or significant changes independently.	*Slightly limited:* Makes frequent though slight changes in body or extremity position independently.	*No limitations:* Makes major and frequent changes in position without assistance.
Nutrition Usual food intake pattern	*Very poor:* Never eats a complete meal. Rarely eats more than one third of any food offered. Eats 2 servings or less of protein (meat or dairy products) per day. Takes fluids poorly. Does not	*Probably inadequate:* Rarely eats a complete meal and generally eats only about half of any food offered. Protein intake includes only 3 servings of meat or dairy products per day. Occasionally	*Adequate:* Eats over half of most meals. Eats a total of 4 servings of protein (meat, dairy products) each day. Occasionally will refuse a meal, but will usually take a supplement if offered.	*Excellent:* Eats most of every meal. Never refuses a meal. Usually eats a total of 4 or more servings of meat and dairy products. Occasionally eats between meals. Does not require supplements.

Friction and shear	take a liquid dietary supplement. OR Is NPO and/or maintained on clear liquids or IVs for more than 5 days. *Problem:* Requires moderate to maximal assistance in moving. Complete lifting without sliding against sheets is impossible. Frequently slides down in bed or chair, requiring frequent repositioning with maximal assistance. Spasticity, contractions, or agitation leads to almost constant friction.	will take a dietary supplement. OR Receives less than optimal amount of liquid diet or tube feeding. *Potential problem:* Moves feebly or requires minimal assistance. During a move skin probably slides to some extent against sheets, chair, restraints, or other devices. Maintains relatively good position in chair or bed most of the time but occasionally slides down.	OR Is on a tube-feeding or TPN regimen that probably meets most nutritional needs. *No apparent problem:* Moves in bed and in chair independently and has sufficient muscle strength to sit up completely during move. Maintains good position in bed or chair at all times.

*Score client in each of the six subscales. Maximum score is 23, indicating little or no risk. 15-18 = low risk, 13-14 = moderate risk, 10-12 = high risk, and ≤9 = very high risk.

Notes

Screening for Common Orthopedic Problems in Infancy and Childhood

Deformity	Screening
Congenital hip dislocation (CHD) Complete or partial displacement of femoral head out of the acetabulum.	Barlow's maneuver (for dislocation of femoral head): flex hip to 90 degrees; grasp symphysis in front and sacrum in back with one hand; with other hand, apply lateral pressure to medial thigh with thumb and longitudinal pressure to knee with palm; abduct flexed hip. A positive sign is sensation of abnormal movement. Reverse hands for examining other hip (Figure 3).

Figure 3

From Stanhope M, Lancaster J: *Community health nursing: promoting health of aggregates, families, and individuals,* ed 4, St. Louis, 1996, Mosby.

Continued.

Screening for Common Orthopedic Problems in Infancy and Childhood—cont'd

Deformity	Screening
Congenital hip dislocation (CHD)—cont'd Complete or partial displacement of femoral head out of the acetabulum—cont'd.	Ortolani's maneuver (for reduction of femur): abduct hip to 80 degrees, lifting proximal femur anteriorly with fingers placed on lateral thigh. A positive sign is sensation of a jerk or snap with reduction into socket (Figure 4). Limited full abduction of hips: with child flat on back, abduct hips one at a time, then together. Figure 5 illustrates degrees of hip abduction. Apparent shortening of femur: 1. Allis' sign: with child lying on back, pelvis flat, knees flexed and feet planted firmly, observe knees. If the knee projects further anteriorly, femur is longer; if one knee is higher, the tibia is longer. 2. With child on back, both legs are extended out with pressure on knees. Heels are matched and observed for equal or unequal length. 3. Trendelenburg sign: with child standing on one leg, observe pelvis. When child stands on abnormal leg, the pelvis drops on normal side (Figure 6).
Metatarsus adductus (varus) Adduction or turning in of forefoot with high longitudinal arch and wide space between first and second toes. Commonly associated with tibial torsion.	Test foot for flexibility and elicit tonic foot reflexes. Rigidity is indicated by eversion or inversion when foot does not move beyond neutral position or does not respond to toe grasping or by dorsiflexing. Signs of metatarsus adductus are illustrated in Figure 7.

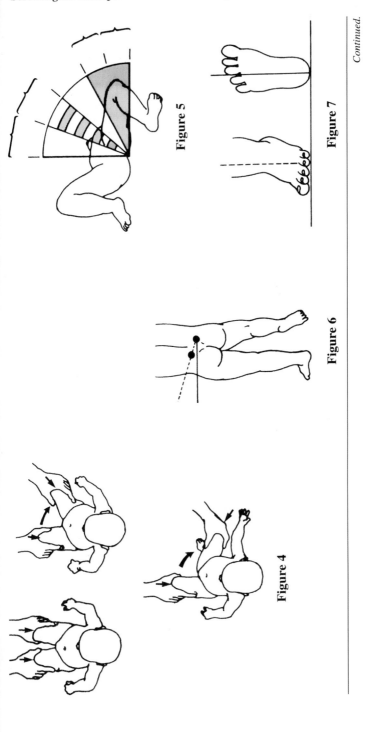

Figure 5

Figure 7

Figure 6

Figure 4

Continued.

Screening for Common Orthopedic Problems in Infancy and Childhood—cont'd

Deformity	Screening
Pes planus (flat feet) When child is weight bearing, longitudinal arch of foot appears flat on floor. 1. Pseudo flat feet: very common until ages 2-3; created by plantar fat pad. Feet are flexible, exhibit hypermobility of joint, and have a low arch. 2. Rigid flat feet: uncommon; created by tightness of heel cord or tarsal coalition (a cartilaginous fibrous or bony connection between bones).	1. Observe feet in weighted and unweighted positions. 2. Stand child on toes. Arch disappears with weight bearing in flexible flat foot and reappears when on toes (Figure 8). 3. Elicit dorsal and plantar flexion to rule out tight heel cord. 4. Elicit eversion and inversion flexion to rule out tarsal coalition. Same as for preceding No. 1 (pseudo flat feet).
Genu valgum (knock-knees) A deviant axis of thighs and calves of more than 10-15 degrees (normal from ages 2-6).	1. Observe axis of thighs and calves with child standing. Normally axis is parallel with 10-15 degrees deviance (Figure 9). 2. Observe space between the knees from front to back. Normal spacing is 1½ inches. 3. Observe space between ankles from front and back. Normal spacing between medial malleoli at heel is 2 inches.

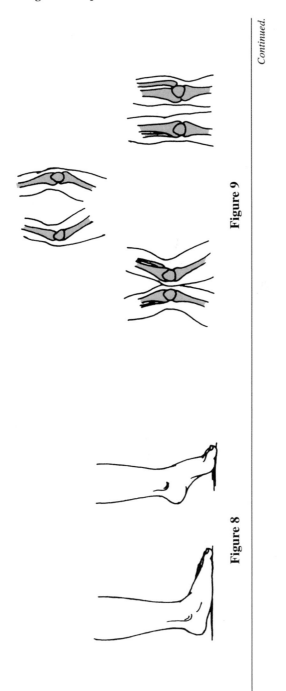

Figure 8

Figure 9

Continued.

Screening for Common Orthopedic Problems in Infancy and Childhood—cont'd

Deformity	Screening
Genu varum (bowlegs) Deviant axis of thighs and calves. 1. Physiological: normal until ages 2-3; occurs with internal tibial torsion and genu valgum. 2. Pathological.	Same as for genu valgum.
Internal tibial torsion Twisting or torsion of tibia usually accompanied by metatarsus adductus.	1. Examine legs for range of motion, flexibility of ankle and elicit tonic foot reflexes. 2. Holding knee firmly with foot in neutral position, observe medial and lateral malleoli. The normal angle between them is approximately 15-20 degrees (Figure 10). 3. Have child sit on examining table and draw a circle over patellar and external malleoli. With patella facing forward only anterior edge of malleolar circle should be seen (Figure 11).
Scoliosis S-shaped lateral curvature of spine with rotation of vertical bodies.	Screening is implemented as follows: 1. Ask the child to bend forward in a 50% flexing position with shoulders drooping forward, arms and head dangling. Observe the spine from above the head and inspect for any lateral curvature or prominent projection of the rib cage on one side (Figure 12).

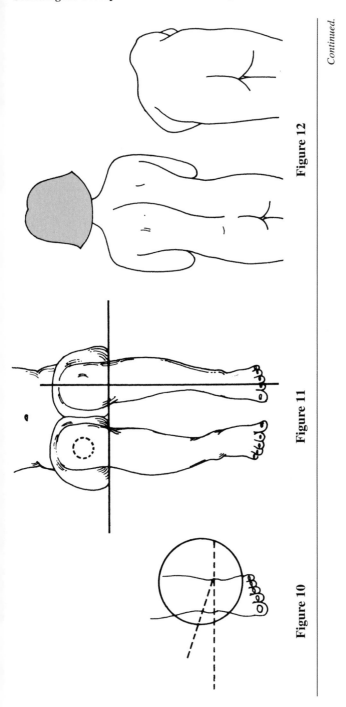

Figure 10

Figure 11

Figure 12

Continued.

Screening for Common Orthopedic Problems in Infancy and Childhood—cont'd

Deformity	Screening

Scoliosis—cont'd
S-shaped lateral curvature of spine with rotation of vertical bodies—cont'd.
	2. While the child is standing erect with weight equal on both feet, observe for:
	    Differences in levels of shoulders, scapula, and hips.
	    Differences in the size of the spaces between the arms and the trunk.
	    Prominence of either scapula or hip.
	    A curve in the vertebral spinous process alignment.
	3. Ask the child to walk and make observations discussed in No. 2 and observe for the presence of a waddle, limp, or tilt.

Criteria for Grading and Recording Muscle Strength

Functional level	Lovett scale	Grade	Percent of normal
No evidence of contractility	Zero (0)	0	0
Evidence of slight contractility	Trace (T)	1	10
Complete range of motion with gravity eliminated	Poor (P)	2	25
Complete range of motion with gravity	Fair (F)	3	50
Complete range of motion against gravity with some resistance	Good (G)	4	75
Complete range of motion against gravity with full resistance	Normal (N)	5	100

From Barkauskas VH et al.: *Health and physical assessment,* ed 2, St. Louis, 1998, Mosby.

Signs and Symptoms of Depression

Depression is a normal response to illness, once the illness has been accepted. The person may describe feelings of sadness or unhappiness. Some common signs of depressed behavior include the following:

1. Decreased interaction with others
2. Lack of interest in activities or environment
3. Voiced concern about illness and amount of care required
4. Expressed wish for or concerns about dying
5. Dependent behavior
6. Decreased activity
7. Complaints of fatigue or inability to sleep
8. Crying spells
9. Change in appetite

Any expressions about suicide should be taken seriously, and the person should be referred for counseling.

Approaches useful when working with a person exhibiting depressed behavior include the following:

1. Approach the client in a serious mood.
2. Convey by action and communication an understanding of what the person must be feeling.
3. Help the person express feelings.
4. Convey acceptance of the right to feel sad.
5. Listen to the person so that the anger can be turned outward.

From Phipps WJ et al.: *Medical surgical nursing: concepts and clinical practices,* ed 6, St. Louis, 1999, Mosby.

Special Musculoskeletal Assessment Techniques

Examination or test	Site	Normal findings	Abnormal findings
Joint range of movements	Any or all joints	Specific range of motion (ROM); no soreness or pain; no edema or elevated temperature in or around joints	Limitation of range of movements in one or more spheres; pain, soreness, muscle weakness, edema, elevated temperature in or around joint or joints
Straight leg raising (Lasegue)	Legs (one at a time)	No pain or soreness in back, buttocks when leg is raised while fully extended at knee; client lies on back	Pain, soreness, or radiation of pain from low back to buttocks; may spread down leg to toes
McMurray	Knee	No excessive or palpable pop or click in knee noted when ankle is grasped to turn knee medially and laterally, and while moving knee backward and forward from full flexion to extension	Click or pop felt or heard; pain or local tenderness is positive for meniscal damage or tears
Febere-Patrick	Knee and hip	Knee can be flexed and brought to almost horizontal position to body with heel resting on opposite knee	Knee cannot be brought to horizontal position; limitation may be in hip, knee, or back (usually hip disease prevents knee rotation to horizontal position)
Drawer: anterior and posterior	Knee	Knee has slight forward or backward movement while flexed on tibia and fibula	Knee has more movement forward or backward (direction indicates tear of either anterior or posterior cruciate ligaments)

Trendelenburg	Pelvis and gluteus muscles	With weight on one leg, pelvis on opposite side will be slightly elevated (observed posteriorly)	With weight on one leg, pelvis will drop (due to weakness or pain in hip joint or its muscles) on opposite side
Thomas	Hip, knee, and lumbar spine	With client on back, hip and knee are flexed to abdomen without flexion simultaneously occurring in lumbar spine	When client flexes knee and hip to abdomen, lumbar spine will flex if there is a pathological condition of the hip, and opposite leg will rise from table
Phalen	Wrists	No tingling of fingers with wrists maximally flexed against each other and held for 1 minute	Tingling felt in the thumb, the index finger, and the middle and lateral half of the ring finger
Tinel	Carpal tunnel of wrist	No tingling into thumb, index, and middle fingers when median nerve is tapped at the wrist	Tingling felt as above for Phalen test
Burdzinski	Back and neck	With client lying on back, no pain is felt in neck or back when head is passively flexed to chest	Pain in back and neck felt with passive flexion of head; knees and hips involuntarily flex to relieve pain (sign of meningeal irritation)
Kernig	Back and leg	No back or leg pain felt when leg is extended (client lies on back with hip and knee flexed)	Pain is felt in lower back, neck, or head when leg is extended from flexed position (sign of meningeal irritation)

From Thompson J et al.: *Mosby's clinical nursing*, ed 4, St. Louis, 1997, Mosby.
These tests are examples of those most commonly done. The reader is referred to Seidel et al.: *Mosby's guide to physical examination*, ed 4, St. Louis, 1999, Mosby, or to Thompson J, Wilson SF: *Health assessment for nursing practice*, St. Louis, 1996, Mosby, for additional special assessments.

Effects of Alcohol on Organ Systems

Body system	Effects	Late effects
Central nervous system	Depression leading to loss of memory and ability to concentrate Lessening of inhibitory functions Self-control and judgment lessened	Unprovoked seizures Wernicke-Korsakoff's syndrome Brain atrophy Sleep disturbances Neuronal damage Neuropathies
Cardiovascular system	Increased pulse rate Vasomotor depression and vasodilation of cutaneous vessels with hypotension Hypertension	Cardiomyopathy (irreversible) Hyperlipidemia Hyperuricemia Coronary artery disease
Skeletal muscles	Lessening awareness of fatigue Reduced muscular capacity for work	Skeletal myopathy
Immunological system	Increased susceptibility to infection	Infections and communicable diseases
Gastrointestinal system	Stimulation of gastric secretions and gastric acid production Irritation of GI mucosa Constipation or diarrhea Vomiting	Pancreatitis Gastritis Nutritional and vitamin deficiencies Cancer of mouth and esophagus Skin syndrome Wernicke-Korsakoff's syndrome

Hepatic system	Few liver changes in acute ingestion	Cirrhosis of the liver
		Cellular damage
		Cell necrosis
		Vitamin depletion (especially B complex vitamins)
		Cell fibrosis
		Liver failure
		Interferes with clotting factors
Renal system	Diuretic effect from inhibition of antidiuretic hormone	
Pancreas	Epigastric pain: vomiting and rigidity of abdominal muscles	Pancreatitis
Hematological system		Anemia
		Thrombocytopenia
		Bone marrow depression
		Prolonged clotting time

From Phipps WJ et al.: *Medical-surgical nursing: concepts and clinical practice*, ed 6, St. Louis, 1999, Mosby.

Levels of Intensity of Hallucinations

Level	Characteristics	Observable client behaviors
Stage I: Comforting **Moderate level of anxiety** Hallucination is generally of a pleasant nature.	The hallucinator experiences intense emotions such as anxiety, loneliness, guilt, and fear, and tries to focus on comforting thoughts to relieve anxiety. The individual recognizes that thoughts and sensory experiences are within conscious control if the anxiety is managed. **Nonpsychotic**	Grinning or laughter that seems inappropriate Moving lips without making any sounds Rapid eye movements Slowed verbal responses as if preoccupied Silent and preoccupied
Stage II: Condemning **Severe level of anxiety** Hallucination generally becomes repulsive.	Sensory experience of any of the identified senses is repulsive and frightening. The hallucinator begins to feel a loss of control and may attempt to distance self from the perceived source. Individual may feel embarrassed by the sensory experience and withdraw from others. **Nonpsychotic**	Increased autonomic nervous system signs of anxiety such as increased heart rate, respiration, and blood pressure Attention span begins to narrow Preoccupied with sensory experience and may lose ability to differentiate hallucination from reality
Stage III: Controlling **Severe level of anxiety** Sensory experiences become omnipotent.	Hallucinator gives up trying to combat the experience and gives in to it. Content of hallucination may become appealing. Individual may experience loneliness if sensory experience ends. **Psychotic**	Directions given by the hallucination will be followed, rather than objected to Difficulty relating to others Attention span of only a few seconds or minutes Physical symptoms of severe anxiety, such as perspiring, tremors, inability to follow directions
Stage IV: Conquering **Panic level of anxiety** Generally becomes elaborate and interwoven with delusions.	Sensory experiences may become threatening if individual does not follow commands. Hallucinations may last for hours or days if there is no therapeutic intervention. **Psychotic**	Terror-stricken behaviors such as panic Strong potential for suicide or homicide Physical activity that reflects content of hallucination, such as violence, agitation, withdrawal, or catatonia Unable to respond to complex directions Unable to respond to more than one person

From Stuart GW, Sundeen SJ: *Principles and practice of psychiatric nursing*, ed 6, St. Louis, 1998, Mosby.

Diagnostic Criteria for Attention-Deficit Hyperactivity Disorder (ADHD)

NOTE: Consider a criterion met only if the behavior is considerably more frequent than that of most people of the same mental age.

1. A disturbance of at least 6 months during which at least six of the criteria for either *inattentive* behavior or *hyperactivity-impulsivity* behavior are met.*
2. Some inattentive or hyperactive-impulsive symptoms that caused impairment were present before age 7 years.
3. Some impairment for the symptoms is present in two or more settings (e.g., at school and at home).
4. Clear evidence of clinically significant impairment exists in social or academic functioning.
5. The symptoms do not occur exclusively during the course of a pervasive developmental disorder, schizophrenia, or other psychotic disorder and are not better accounted for by another mental disorder (e.g., mood disorder, anxiety disorder, dissociative disorder, or a personality disorder).

Modified from American Psychiatric Association: *Diagnostic and statistical manual of mental disorders,* ed 4, Washington, DC, 1994, The Association.

*Refer to *Diagnostic and statistical manual of mental disorders,* ed 4, for the specific criteria.

Notes

Classification of Hearing Loss Based on Symptom Severity

Hearing level (DB)	Effect
Slight—<30 (hard of hearing)	Has difficulty hearing faint or distant speech
	Usually is unaware of hearing difficulty
	Likely to achieve in school but may have problems
	No speech defects
Mild—30-55 (hard of hearing)	Understands conversational speech at 3-5 feet but has difficulty if speech is faint or if not facing speaker
	May have speech difficulties
Moderate—55-70 (hard of hearing)	Unable to understand conversational speech unless loud
	Considerable difficulty with group or classroom discussion
	Requires special speech training
Profound—70-90 (deaf)	May hear a loud voice if nearby
	May be able to identify loud environmental noises
	Can distinguish vowels but not most consonants
	Requires speech training
Extreme—90 (deaf)	May hear only loud sounds
	Requires extensive speech training

From Wong DL: *Whaley and Wong's nursing care of infants and children,* ed 6, St. Louis, 1999, Mosby.

Risk Criteria for Sensorineural Hearing Impairment in Young Children

Neonates (birth to 28 days)

1. Family history of congenital or delayed-onset childhood sensorineural impairment
2. Congenital infection known or suspected to be associated with sensorineural hearing impairment, such as toxoplasmosis, syphilis, rubella, cytomegalovirus, and herpes
3. Craniofacial anomalies, including morphological abnormalities of the pinna and ear canal, absent philtrum, and low hairline
4. Birth weight less than 1500 g (<3.3 pounds)

From American Speech-Language Hearing Association: Joint Committee on Infant Hearing 1990 position statement, *ASHA* 33(suppl 5):3-6, 1991.

5. Hyperbilirubinemia at a level exceeding indication for exchange transfusion
6. Ototoxic medications including but not limited to the aminoglycosides used for more than 5 days (e.g., gentamicin, tobramycin, kanamycin, streptomycin), and loop diuretics used in combination with aminoglycosides
7. Bacterial meningitis
8. Severe depression at birth, which may include infants with Apgar scores of 0 to 3 at 5 minutes and those who fail to initiate spontaneous respiration by 10 minutes or those with hypotonia persisting to 2 hours of age
9. Prolonged mechanical ventilation for a duration equal to or greater than 10 days (e.g., persistent pulmonary hypertension)
10. Stigmata or other findings associated with a syndrome known to include sensorineural hearing loss (e.g., Waardenburg or Usher syndrome)

Risk criteria: infants (29 days to 2 years)

1. Parent/caregiver concern regarding hearing, speech, language, and/or developmental delay
2. Bacterial meningitis
3. Neonatal risk factors that may be associated with progressive sensorineural hearing loss (e.g., cytomegalovirus, prolonged mechanical ventilation, and inherited disorders)
4. Head trauma, especially with either longitudinal or transverse fracture of the temporal bone
5. Stigmata or other findings associated with syndromes known to include sensorineural hearing loss (e.g., Waardenburg or Usher syndrome)
6. Ototoxic medications including but not limited to the aminoglycosides used for more than 5 days (e.g., gentamicin, tobramycin, kanamycin, streptomycin) and loop diuretics used in combination with aminoglycosides
7. Children with neurodegenerative disorders such as neurofibromatosis, myoclonic epilepsy, Werdnig-Hoffmann disease, Tay-Sachs disease, Niemann-Pick disease, any metachromatic leukodystrophy, or any infantile demyelinating neuropathy
8. Childhood infectious diseases known to be associated with sensorineural hearing loss (e.g., mumps, measles)

Hearing Screening: Tuning Fork Tests

A tuning fork test checks for lateralization of sound. Vibrating tuning fork transmits sound through bone directly to inner ear structures, bypassing external and middle ear.

TEST AND STEPS	RATIONALE
Weber's test Hold fork at its base and tap it lightly against heel of palm. Place base of vibrating fork on midline vertex of client's head or middle of forehead (Figure 13). Ask client if sound is heard equally in both ears or better in one ear.	Client with normal hearing hears sound equally in both ears or in midline of head. In conduction deafness, sound is heard in impaired ear. In unilateral sensorineural hearing loss, sound is heard only in normal ear.

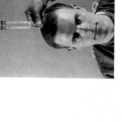

Figure 13 Weber's test

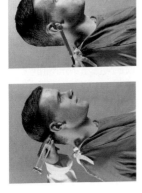

Figure 14 Rinne test

Rinne test

Place stem of vibrating tuning fork against client's mastoid process (Figure 14). Begin counting interval with your watch. Ask client to tell you when sound is no longer heard; note number of seconds. Quickly place still vibrating tines 1-2 cm (1/2-1 inch) from ear canal, and ask client to tell you when sound is no longer heard. (See Figure 14.) Continue counting the time the sound is heard by air conduction. Compare number of seconds for bone conduction versus air conduction.

Air-conducted sound should be heard twice as long as bone-conducted sound. In conduction deafness, bone-conducted sound can be heard longer. In sensorineural loss, sound is not as loud and is heard longer through air.

Modified from Perry A, Potter P: *Clinical nursing skills and techniques*, ed 4, St. Louis, 1998, Mosby.

Clinical Manifestations for Detecting Hearing Impairment

Infants

Lack of startle or blink reflex to a loud sound

Failure to be awakened by loud environmental noises

Failure to localize a source of sound by 6 months of age

Absence of babble or inflections in voice by age 7 months

General indifference to sound

Lack of response to the spoken word; failure to follow verbal directions

Response to loud noises as opposed to the voice

Children

Use of gestures rather than verbalization to express desires, especially after age 15 months

Failure to develop intelligible speech by age 24 months

Monotone quality, unintelligible speech, lessened laughter

Vocal play, head banging, or foot stamping for vibratory sensation

Yelling or screeching to express pleasure, annoyance (tantrums), or need

Asking to have statements repeated or answering them incorrectly

Responding more to facial expression and gestures than to verbal explanation

Avoidance of social interaction; often puzzled and unhappy in such situations; prefer to play alone

Inquiring, sometimes confused facial expression

Suspicious alertness, sometimes interpreted as paranoia, alternating with cooperation

Frequently stubborn because of lack of comprehension

Irritable at not making themselves understood

Shy, timid, and withdrawn

Often appear "dreamy," "in a world of their own," or markedly inattentive

---

From Wong D: *Whaley and Wong's nursing care of infants and children,* ed 6, St. Louis, 1999, Mosby.

Notes:

Vital Signs Along the Age Continuum

Age	Temperature	Sex	Pulse	Respiratory rate	Blood pressure (upper limits)
Newborn	99.1	Male	120	35	110/75
	99.1	Female	120	35	110/75
1 year	99.1	Male	120	30	110/75
	98.8	Female	120	30	110/75
2 years	99.0	Male	110	25	110/75
	98.8	Female	110	25	110/75
4 years	98.6	Male	100	23	110/75
	98.5	Female	100	23	110/75
6 years	98.4	Male	100	21	120/80
	98.5	Female	100	21	120/80
8 years	98.3	Male	90	20	120/80
	98.3	Female	90	20	120/80

10 years	Male	98.0	90	19	125/85
	Female	98.1	90	19	125/85
12 years	Male	97.8	85	19	125/85
	Female	97.9	90	19	125/85
14 years	Male	97.6	80	18	135/90
	Female	97.9	85	18	135/90
16 years	Male	97.3	75	17	135/90
	Female	97.8	80	17	135/90
18 years	Male	97.2	70	16-18	135/90
	Female	97.9	75	16-18	135/90
Adults		97.3	60-90	12-20	
Older adults		More sensitive to temperature	Slows with age	No variation	

Data from Yaladian I, Porter D: *Physical growth and development*, Boston, 1977, Little, Brown; Thompson JM et al.: *Clinical nursing*, St. Louis, 1986, Mosby; U.S. Department of Health and Human Services: *The 1984 report of the Joint National Committee on Detection, Evaluation, and Treatment of High Blood Pressure*, NIH Pub No 84-1088, Bethesda, Md, 1984.

TOOLS AND MEASUREMENTS

PAIN MEASUREMENT

The following scales show various ways to help quantify the amount of pain a client feels. Different approaches to quantification will be appropriate with different clients. Factors such as age and intellectual ability should be considered when choosing a scale.

Notes

Typical Areas of Referred Pain

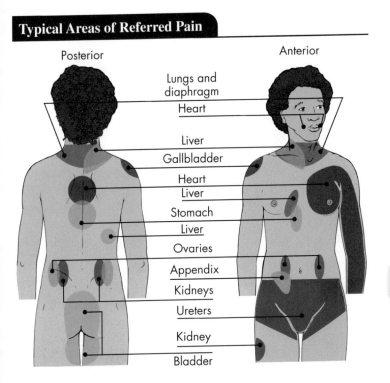

Posterior

Anterior

Lungs and diaphragm
Heart
Liver
Gallbladder
Heart
Liver
Stomach
Liver
Ovaries
Appendix
Kidneys
Ureters
Kidney
Bladder

From Lewis SM et al.: *Medical-surgical nursing: assessment and management of clinical problems,* ed 4, St. Louis, 1996, Mosby.

Notes

Initial Pain Assessment Tool

Client's Name _____ Age _____ Date _____
Room _____
Diagnosis _____ Physician _____
Nurse _____

1. LOCATION: Client or nurse mark drawing.

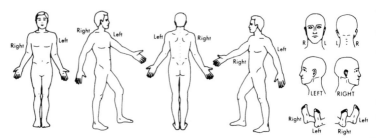

2. INTENSITY: Client rates the pain. Scale used _____
    Present: _____
    Worst pain gets: _____
    Best pain gets: _____
    Acceptable level of pain: _____
3. QUALITY: (Use client's own words, e.g., prick, ache, burn, throb, pull, sharp.) _____
   _____

4. ONSET, DURATION, VARIATIONS, RHYTHMS: _____
   _____

5. MANNER OF EXPRESSING PAIN: _____
   _____
   _____

6. WHAT RELIEVES THE PAIN? _____
   _____
   _____

7. WHAT CAUSES OR INCREASES THE PAIN? _____
8. EFFECTS OF PAIN: (Note decreased function, decreased quality of life.)
    Accompanying symptoms (e.g., nausea) _____
    Sleep _____
    Appetite _____
    Physical activity _____
    Relationship with others (e.g., irritability) _____
    Emotions (e.g., anger, suicidal, crying) _____
    Concentration _____
    Other _____
9. OTHER COMMENTS: _____
   _____

10. PLAN: _____
    _____

_____

From McCaffery M, Pasero C: *Pain: clinical manual,* ed 2, St. Louis, 1999, Mosby.

What Does Your Pain Feel Like?

Some of the words below describe your *present* pain. Circle *ONLY* those words that best describe it. Leave out any category that is not suitable. Use only a single word in each appropriate category—the one that applies best.

Sensory domain
Temporal
Flickering
Quivering
Pulsing
Throbbing
Beating
Pounding

Spatial
Jumping
Flashing
Shooting

Punctuated pressure
Pricking
Boring
Drilling
Stabbing
Lancinating

Incisive pressure
Sharp
Cutting
Lacerating

Constrictive pressure
Pinching
Pressing

Gnawing
Cramping
Crushing

Traction pressure
Tugging
Pulling
Wrenching

Thermal
Hot
Burning
Scalding
Searing

Brightness
Tingling
Itchy
Smarting
Stinging

Dullness
Dull
Sore
Hurting
Aching
Heavy

Miscellaneous
Tender
Taut
Rasping
Splitting

Affective domain
Tension
Tiring
Exhausting

Autonomic
Sickening
Suffocating

Fear
Fearful
Frightful
Terrifying

Punishment
Punishing
Grueling
Cruel
Vicious
Killing

Evaluative/ cognitive domain
Annoying
Miserable
Unbearable
Troublesome
Intense

Miscellaneous
Spreading
Radiating
Penetrating
Piercing
Tight
Numb
Drawing
Squeezing
Tearing
Cool
Cold
Freezing
Nagging
Nauseating
Agonizing
Dreadful
Torturing

From Barker E: *Neuroscience nursing,* St. Louis, 1994, Mosby.

How Intense Is Your Pain?

People agree that the following five words represent pain of increasing intensity. They are as follows:

CATEGORY SCALE Representing pain intensity:

1	2	3	4	5
Mild	Discomforting	Distressing	Horrible	Excruciating

PATTERN OF PAIN As it changes with time:

1	2	3
Continuous	Rhythmic	Brief
Steady	Periodic	Momentary
Constant	Intermittent	Transient

Brief Pain Inventory (Short Form)

Date:_____/_____/_____   Time:_____

Name: _____ _____ _____
                Last   First   Middle Initial

1. Throughout our lives, most of us have had pain from time to time
   (such as minor headaches, sprains, and toothaches). Have you had
   pain other than these everyday kinds of pain today?
   1. Yes   2. No

2. On the diagram, shade in the areas where you feel pain. Put an X
   on the area that hurts the most.

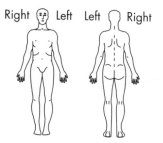

Right 😕 Left   Left   Right

3. Please rate your pain by circling the one number that best describes your pain at its **worst** in the past 24 hours.
   0   1   2   3   4   5   6   7   8   9   10
   No   Pain as bad as
   pain   you can imagine

4. Please rate your pain by circling the one number that best describes your pain at its **least** in the past 24 hours.
   0   1   2   3   4   5   6   7   8   9   10
   No   Pain as bad as
   pain   you can imagine

5. Please rate your pain by circling the one number that best describes your pain on the **average.**
   0   1   2   3   4   5   6   7   8   9   10
   No   Pain as bad as
   pain   you can imagine

6. Please rate your pain by circling the one number that tells how
   much pain you have **right now.**
   0   1   2   3   4   5   6   7   8   9   10
   No   Pain as bad as
   pain   you can imagine

_____

From Pain Research Group, Department of Neurology, University of Wisconsin-Madison.

7. What treatments or medications are you receiving for your pain?

---

8. In the past 24 hours, how much **relief** have pain treatments or medications provided? Please circle the one percentage that most shows how much relief you have received.

0%   10%   20%   30%   40%   50%   60%   70%   80%   90%   100%
No   Complete
relief   relief

9. Circle the one number that describes how, during the past 24 hours, **pain has interfered** with your:

A. General activity

0   1   2   3   4   5   6   7   8   9   10
Does not   Completely
interfere   interferes

B. Mood

0   1   2   3   4   5   6   7   8   9   10
Does not   Completely
interfere   interferes

C. Walking ability

0   1   2   3   4   5   6   7   8   9   10
Does not   Completely
interfere   interferes

D. Normal work (includes both work outside the home and housework)

0   1   2   3   4   5   6   7   8   9   10
Does not   Completely
interfere   interferes

E. Relations with other people

0   1   2   3   4   5   6   7   8   9   10
Does not   Completely
interfere   interferes

F. Sleep

0   1   2   3   4   5   6   7   8   9   10
Does not   Completely
interfere   interferes

G. Enjoyment of life

0   1   2   3   4   5   6   7   8   9   10
Does not   Completely
interfere   interferes

Pain Intensity Scales

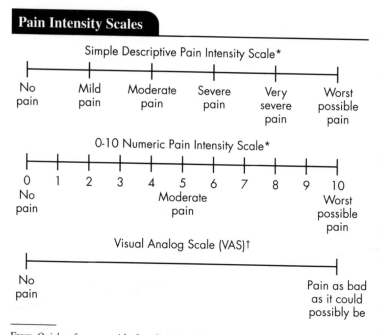

From *Quick reference guide for clinicians #9: Management of cancer pain: adults,*
DHHS-AHCPR 94-0593, 1994.

*If used as a graphic rating scale, a 10-cm baseline is recommended.
†A 10-cm baseline is recommended for VAS scales.

Notes

Wong-Baker FACES Pain Rating Scale

Explain to child that each face is for a person who feels happy because there is no pain (hurt) or sad because there is some or a lot of pain. Face 0 is very happy because there is no hurt. Face 1 hurts just a little bit. Face 2 hurts a little more. Face 3 hurts even more. Face 4 hurts a whole lot, but Face 5 hurts as much as you can imagine, although you don't have to be crying to feel this bad. Ask child to choose face that best describes own pain. May be used with children as young as 3 years.

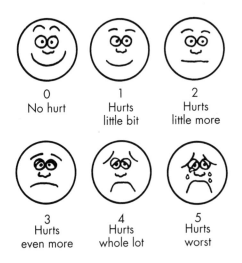

0	1	2
No hurt	Hurts little bit	Hurts little more

3	4	5
Hurts even more	Hurts whole lot	Hurts worst

From Wong D: *Whaley and Wong's nursing care of infants and children,* ed 6, St. Louis, 1999, Mosby.

Notes

OTHER MEASUREMENTS

Lesion Size Measurement

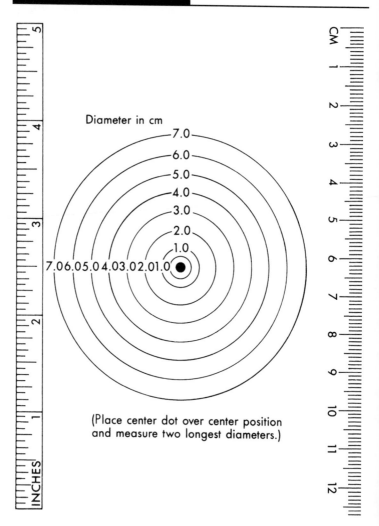

Redrawn from ConvaTec, a Bristol-Meyers Squibb Company, Princeton, NJ.

Guidelines for Referral Regarding Communication Impairment

Age	Assessment findings
2 years	Failure to speak any meaningful words spontaneously
	Consistent use of gestures rather than vocalizations
	Difficulty in following verbal directions
	Failure to respond consistently to sound
3 years	Speech is largely unintelligible
	Failure to use sentences of three or more words
	Frequent omission of initial consonants
	Use of vowels rather than consonants
5 years	Stutters, stammers, or has any other type of dysfluency
	Sentence structure noticeably impaired
	Substitutes easily produced sounds for more difficult ones
	Omits word endings (plurals, tenses of verbs, and so on)
School age	Poor voice quality (monotonous, loud, or barely audible)
	Vocal pitch inappropriate for age
	Any distortions, omissions, or substitutions of sounds after age 7 years
	Connected speech characterized by use of unusual confusions or reversals
General	Any child with signs that suggest a hearing impairment
	Any child who is embarrassed or disturbed by own speech
	Parents who are excessively concerned or who pressure the child to speak at a level above that appropriate for the child's age

From Wong DL: *Clinical manual of pediatric nursing,* ed 4, St. Louis, 1996, Mosby.

Glasgow Coma Scale

A reliable guide to the quick determination of the level of neurological status in an individual who may or may not be able to participate in more advanced testing is the Glasgow Coma Scale (GCS). This scale measures three faculties: eye opening, best motor response, and best verbal response. Numbers are assigned to each of the responses in the three categories. The lowest possible score is 3; 15 is the highest. A GCS of less than 7 indicates a coma state. Serial scores have value in trending client status. To score, the client's best response is elicited in each category and the points added.

Category	Response	Score (points)
Eye opening	Eyes open spontaneously	4
	Eyes open in response to voice	3
	Eyes open in response to pain	2
	No eye opening response	1
Best verbal	Oriented (e.g., to person, place, time)	5
	Confused, speaks but is disoriented	4
	Inappropriate, but comprehensible words	3
	Incomprehensible sounds but no words are spoken	2
	None	1
Best motor	Obeys command to move	6
	Localizes painful stimulus	5
	Withdraws from painful stimulus	4
	Flexion, abnormal decorticate posturing	3
	Extension, abnormal decerebrate posturing	2
	No movement or posturing	1
TOTAL POINTS POSSIBLE		**3-15**

Rancho Los Amigos Scale of Cognitive Levels and Expected Behaviors

The Rancho Los Amigos scale of cognitive functioning was developed as a behavioral rating scale to aid in assessment and treatment of the head-injured person. It represents the progression of recovery of cognitive abilities as demonstrated through behavioral change. The tool is used to assess the client and to give some structure to interventions.

For purposes of client management, eight levels of cognitive functioning are grouped in the following four basic recovery phases and intervention strategies:

Level	Recovery phase	Approach
II, III	Decreased response	Stimulation
IV	Agitated response	Structure
V, VI	Confused response	Structure
VII, VIII	Automatic response	Community

From Malkmus D et al.: *Rehabilitation of the head-injured adult—comprehensive cognitive management,* Downey, Calif, 1980, Professional Staff Association of Rancho Los Amigos Hospital.

Levels of Cognitive Functioning

I. NO RESPONSE

Client is completely unresponsive to any stimuli.

II. GENERALIZED RESPONSE

Client reacts inconsistently and nonpurposefully to stimuli in nonspecific manner.

III. LOCALIZED RESPONSE

Client reacts specifically but inconsistently to stimuli.

IV. CONFUSED—AGITATED

Client is in heightened state of activity with severely decreased ability to process information.

V. CONFUSED—INAPPROPRIATE

Client appears alert and is able to respond to simple commands fairly consistently.

VI. CONFUSED—APPROPRIATE

Client shows goal-directed behavior but depends on external input for direction.

VII. AUTOMATIC—APPROPRIATE

Client appears appropriate and oriented within hospital and home setting, goes through daily routine automatically, with minimal to absent confusion and has shallow recall of actions.

VIII. PURPOSEFUL—APPROPRIATE

Client is alert and oriented, is able to recall and integrate past and recent events, and is aware of and responsive to culture.

Normal Values of Cellular Blood Components*

Complete blood cell count

Red blood cells (RBC)	4.25-6.1 × 10/ml (males)
	3.6-5.4 × 10/ml (females)
White blood cells (WBC)	5000-10,000/mm^3
Hemoglobin (Hgb)	13-18 g/dl (males)
	12-16 g/dl (females)
Hematocrit (Hct)	45-54% (males)
	37-47% (females)

Coagulation

Platelet	150,000-350,000/ml
Prothrombin time (PT)	10-14 sec
Partial thromboplastin time (PTT)	30-45 sec
Thrombin time (TT)	Control ± 5 sec
Fibrinogen split products (FSP)	Negative reaction at >1:4 dilution
Iron/ferritin (Fe) (deficiency)	0-20 ng/ml
Reticulocyte count	0.5-1.5% of red blood cells

From Peterson V: *Just the facts: a pocket guide to basic nursing,* ed 2, St. Louis, 1999, Mosby.
*Averages may vary per facility.

Normal Values of Cellular Blood Components*—cont'd

Blood chemistry

Sodium (Na)	135-145 mEq/L
Potassium (K)	3.5-4.5 mEq/L
Chloride (Cl)	98-106 mEq/L
Carbon dioxide (CO_2)	24-32 mEq/L
Blood urea nitrogen (BUN)	7-25 mg/dl
Creatinine (Cr)	0.7-1.3 mg/dl (males)
	0.6-1.2 mg/dl (females)
Glucose	70-110 mg/dl
Calcium (Ca)	8.5-10.5 mg/dl
Magnesium (Mg)	1.3-2.1 mg/dl
Phosphorus	3.0-4.5 mg/dl
Osmolality	275-295 mOsm/kg
Bilirubin	
Direct	0-0.2 mg/dl
Total	0.2-1.0 mg/dl
Indirect is total minus direct	
Amylase	50-150 U/L
Lipase	0-110 U/L
Anion gap	8-16 mEq/L

Urine electrolytes

Sodium (Na)	40-220 mEq/L
Potassium (K)	25-125 mEq/L
Chloride (Cl)	110-250 mEq/L

Arterial blood gases

Acid-base balance (pH) Measures hydrogen concentration (7.35-7.45)

Oxygenation (Pao_2) Measures partial pressure of dissolved oxygen in the blood (80-100 mm Hg)

Saturation (So_2) Measures percentage of oxygen to hemoglobin (95-98%)

Ventilation ($Paco_2$) Measures partial pressure of carbon dioxide (38-45 mm Hg)

---

*Averages may vary per facility.

Diagnostic Tests for Phenylketonuria

Test	Method	Use
Urine tests		
Diaper test	10% ferric chloride dropped on freshly wet diaper; green spot (positive); probable PKU	Inexpensive: useful in screening large groups of infants but not of value until infant is at least 4-6 weeks of age
Phenistix test	Prepared test stick pressed against wet diaper or dipped in urine; green color reaction: probable PKU	Simple; more accurate than diaper test; useful in screening large groups of infants but not of value until after infant is 6 weeks of age
Serum phenylalanine tests		
Guthrie inhibition assay methods	Drops of blood placed on filter paper; laboratory uses bacterial growth inhibition test; phenylalanine level above 8 mg/dl blood: diagnostic of PKU	Effective in newborn period; used also to monitor PKU diet; blood easily obtained by heel or finger puncture; inexpensive; used for wide-scale screening
LaDu-Michael method	5 ml of blood; serum separated and tested for phenylalanine; level above 8 mg/dl blood: PKU; in persons with PKU, phenylalanine level above 8-12 mg/dl blood: loss of dietary control	Useful diagnostic tool and to monitor PKU diet; requires blood drawn from person; laboratory method difficult (test not available in many laboratories)
McCarnan and Robins fluorometric method	5 ml of blood; serum separated and tested for phenylalanine; level above 8 mg: PKU or loss of dietary control	Diagnostic and diet monitoring tool; laboratory procedure simpler than LaDu-Michael method; test not available in many laboratories

Modified from Williams SR: *Nutrition and diet therapy,* ed 8, St. Louis, 1997, Mosby.

Notes

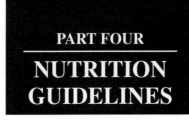

Good nutrition is integral to a healthy life for everyone. Nutrition balance is the goal for all ages, and the nurse should assist clients in a practical and informed way. The following instruments will aid the nurse in gathering appropriate data from across the life span.

GUIDELINES FOR CHILDREN

Diet History for Children

What are the family's usual mealtimes?
Do family members eat together or at separate times?
Who does the family grocery shopping and meal preparation?
How much money is spent to buy food each week?
How are most foods prepared—baked, broiled, fried, other?
How often does the family or your child eat out?
    What kinds of restaurants do you go to?
    What kinds of food does your child typically eat at restaurants?
Does your child eat breakfast regularly?
Where does your child eat lunch?
What are your child's favorite foods, beverages, and snacks?
    What are the average amounts eaten per day?
    What foods are artificially sweetened?
    What are your child's snacking habits?
    When are sweet foods usually eaten?
    What are your child's toothbrushing habits?
What special cultural practices are followed?
    What ethnic foods are eaten?
What foods and beverages does your child dislike?
How would you describe your child's usual appetite (hearty eater, picky eater)?

From Wong D, Whaley L: *Clinical manual of pediatric nursing,* ed 4, St. Louis, 1996, Mosby.

What are your child's feeding habits (breast, bottle, cup, spoon, eats by self, needs assistance, any special devices)?

Does your child take vitamins or other supplements; do they contain iron or fluoride?

Are there any known or suspected food allergies; is your child on a special diet?

Has your child lost or gained weight recently?

Are there any feeding problems (excessive fussiness, spitting up, colic, difficulty sucking or swallowing) or any dental problems or appliances, such as braces, that affect eating?

What types of exercise does your child do regularly?

Is there a family history of cancer, diabetes, heart disease, high blood pressure, or obesity?

Additional questions for parents of infants

What was the infant's birth weight; when did it double, triple?

Was the infant premature?

Are you breast-feeding or have you breast-fed your infant? For how long?

If you use a formula, what is the brand?

How long has the infant been taking it?

How many ounces does the infant drink a day?

Are you giving the infant cow's milk (whole, low fat, skimmed)?

When did you start?

How many ounces does the infant drink a day?

Do you give your infant extra fluids (water, juice)?

If your infant takes a bottle to bed at nap or nighttime, what is in the bottle?

At what age did you start cereal, vegetables, meat or other protein sources, fruit/juice, finger food, table food?

Do you make your own baby food or use commercial foods such as infant cereal?

Does the infant take a vitamin/mineral supplement? If so, what type?

Has the infant shown an allergic reaction to any foods? If so, list the foods and describe the reaction.

Does the infant spit up frequently, have unusually loose stools, or have hard, dry stools? If so, how often?

How often do you feed your infant?

How would you describe your infant's appetite?

Clinical Assessment of Nutritional Status in Children

Evidence of adequate nutrition	Evidence of deficient or excess nutrition	Deficiency/excess*
General growth		
Within 5th and 95th percentiles for height, weight, and head circumference	Below 5th or above 95th percentiles for growth	Protein, calories, fats, and other essential nutrients, especially vitamin A, pyridoxine, niacin, calcium, iodine, manganese, zinc
Steady gain with expected growth spurts during infancy and adolescence	Absence of or delayed growth spurts; poor weight gain	
Sexual development appropriate for age	Delayed sexual development	Excess vitamin A, D
Skin		
Smooth, slightly dry to touch	Hardening and scaling	Vitamin A
Elastic and firm	Seborrheic dermatitis	Excess niacin
Absence of lesions	Dry, rough, petechiae	Riboflavin
Color appropriate to genetic background	Delayed wound healing	Vitamin C
	Scaly dermatitis on exposed surfaces	Riboflavin, vitamin C, zinc
	Wrinkled, flabby	Niacin
	Crusted lesions around orifices, especially nares	Protein and calories
		Zinc
	Pruritus	Excess vitamin A, riboflavin, niacin
	Poor turgor	Water, sodium
	Edema	Protein, thiamin
		Excess sodium

From Wong D, Whaley L: *Clinical manual of pediatric nursing*, ed 4, St. Louis, 1996, Mosby.
*Nutrients listed are deficient unless specified as excess.

Continued.

Clinical Assessment of Nutritional Status in Children—cont'd

Evidence of adequate nutrition	Evidence of deficient or excess nutrition	Deficiency/excess*
Skin—cont'd		
	Yellow tinge (jaundice)	Vitamin B_{12}
		Excess vitamin A, niacin
	Depigmentation	Protein, calories
	Pallor (anemia)	Pyridoxine, folic acid, vitamin B_{12}, C, E (in premature infants), iron
		Excess vitamin C, zinc
	Paresthesia	Excess riboflavin
Hair		
Lustrous, silky, strong, elastic	Stringy, friable, dull, dry, thin	Protein, calories
	Alopecia	Protein, calories, zinc
	Depigmentation	Protein, calories, copper
	Raised areas around hair follicles	Vitamin C
Head		
Even molding, occipital prominence, symmetrical facial features	Softening of cranial bones, prominence of frontal bones, skull flat and depressed toward middle	Vitamin D
Fused sutures after 18 months	Delayed fusion of sutures	Vitamin D
	Hard tender lumps in occiput	Excess vitamin A
	Headache	Excess thiamin

Neck		
Thyroid not visible, palpable in midline	Thyroid enlarged; may be grossly visible	Iodine
Eyes		
Clear, bright	Hardening and scaling of cornea and conjunctiva	Vitamin A
Conjunctiva—pink, glossy	Burning, itching, photophobia, cataracts, corneal vascularization	Riboflavin
Good night vision	Night blindness	
Ears		
Tympanic membrane—pliable	Calcified (hearing loss)	Excess vitamin D
Nose		
Smooth, intact nasal angle	Irritation and cracks at nasal angle	Riboflavin
		Excess vitamin A
Mouth		
Lips—smooth, moist, darker color than skin	Fissures and inflammation at corners	Riboflavin
		Excess vitamin A
Gums—firm, coral pink color, stippled	Spongy, friable, swollen, bluish-red or black color, bleed easily	Vitamin C
Mucous membranes—bright pink, smooth, moist	Stomatitis	Niacin
Tongue—rough texture, no lesions, taste sensation	Glossitis	Niacin, riboflavin, folic acid
	Diminished taste sensation	Zinc

Continued.

Clinical Assessment of Nutritional Status in Children—cont'd

Evidence of adequate nutrition	Evidence of deficient or excess nutrition	Deficiency/excess*
Mouth—cont'd		
Teeth—uniform white color, smooth, intact	Brown mottling, pits, fissures	Excess fluoride
	Defective enamel	Vitamin A, C, D, calcium, phosphorus
	Caries	Excess carbohydrates
Chest		
In infants, shape is almost circular	Depressed lower portion of rib cage	Vitamin D
In children, lateral diameter increases in proportion to anteroposterior diameter	Sharp protrusion of sternum	
Smooth costochondral junctions	Enlarged costochondral junctions	Vitamin C, D
Breast development—normal for age	Delayed development	See General growth on p. 307, especially zinc
Cardiovascular system		
Pulse and blood pressure (BP) within normal limits	Palpitations	Thiamin
	Rapid pulse	Potassium
		Excess thiamin
	Arrhythmias	Magnesium, potassium
		Excess niacin, potassium
	Increased BP	Excess sodium
	Decreased BP	Thiamin
		Excess niacin

Abdomen

In young children, cylindrical and prominent	Distended, flabby, poor musculature	Protein, calories
	Prominent, large	Excess calories
	Potbelly, constipation	Vitamin D
Older children, flat	Diarrhea	Niacin
		Excess vitamin C
Normal bowel habits	Constipation	Excess calcium, potassium

Musculoskeletal system

Muscles—firm, well-developed, equal strength bilaterally	Flabby, weak, generalized wasting	Protein, calories
	Weakness, pain, cramps	Thiamin, sodium, chloride, potassium, phosphorus, magnesium
		Excess thiamin
	Muscle twitching, tremors	Magnesium
	Muscular paralysis	Excess potassium
Spine—cervical and lumbar curves (double S curve)	Kyphosis, lordosis, scoliosis	Vitamin D
Extremities—symmetrical; legs straight with minimum bowing	Bowing of extremities, knock-knees	Vitamin D, calcium, phosphorus
	Epiphyseal enlargement	Vitamin A, D
	Bleeding into joints and muscles, joint swelling, pain	Vitamin C

Clinical Assessment of Nutritional Status in Children—cont'd

Evidence of adequate nutrition	Evidence of deficient or excess nutrition	Deficiency/excess*
Musculoskeletal system—cont'd		
Joints—flexible, full range of motion, no pain or stiffness	Thickening of cortex of long bones with pain and fragility, hard tender lumps in extremities	Excess vitamin A
	Osteoporosis of long bones	Calcium Excess vitamin D
Neurological system		
Behavior—alert, responsive, emotionally stable	Listless, irritable, lethargic, apathetic (sometimes apprehensive, anxious, drowsy, mentally slow, confused)	Thiamin, niacin, pyridoxine, vitamin C, potassium, magnesium, iron, protein, calories
		Excess vitamin A, D, thiamin, folic acid, calcium
	Masklike facial expression, blurred speech, involuntary laughing	Excess manganese
Absence of tetany, convulsions	Convulsions	Thiamin, pyridoxine, vitamin D, calcium, magnesium
		Excess phosphorus (in relation to calcium)
Intact peripheral nervous system	Peripheral nervous system toxicity (unsteady gait, numb feet and hands, fine motor clumsiness)	Excess pyridoxine
Intact reflexes	Diminished or absent tendon reflexes	Thiamin, vitamin E

A Diet History Questionnaire for Infants Through Teenagers

Questionnaire I—infants (birth to 1 year)

Date _____ Age _____

Name _____ Birth date _____

Please answer the following questions by checking the appropriate box or filling in the blank. Answer only those questions that apply to you or your child. All information is confidential.

1. Is the baby breast-fed?   Yes _____ No _____
   If yes, does he or she also receive milk or formula?
   Yes _____ No _____
   If yes, what kind? _____

2. Does the baby receive formula? Yes _____ No _____
   If yes: Ready-to-feed   _____
            Concentrated liquid _____
            Powdered   _____
            Evaporated milk   _____
            Other   _____
   How is formula prepared? _____
   Is the formula iron fortified? _____
   Yes _____ No _____
   Do not know _____

3. Does the baby drink milk?   Yes _____ No _____
   If yes: Whole milk _____
            2% milk   _____
            Skim milk   _____
            Other _____

4. Does the baby drink any fluids other than milk or formula?
   Yes _____ No _____
   If yes, what? _____

5. How many times does the baby eat each day, including milk or formula feedings? _____

6. Does the baby usually take a bottle to bed?
   Yes _____ No _____
   If yes, what is usually in the bottle? _____

7. If the baby drinks milk or formula, what is the usual amount in a day?
   Less than 16 oz (2 cups)   _____
   16 to 32 oz   _____
   More than 32 oz (1 quart) _____

From Bureau of Maternal and Child Health/Nutrition: *Diet history questionnaire,* Washington, DC, 1978. The Bureau.

8. Does the baby take vitamin or iron drops?
Yes _____ No _____
If yes, how often? _____ What kind? _____

9. Is the baby on a special diet now?   Yes _____ No _____
If yes: Allergy   _____
         Weight reduction _____
         Other _____
         Who recommended the diet? _____

10. Does the baby eat clay, paint chips, dirt, paper, or anything else
that is not considered food?
Yes _____ No _____
If yes, what? _____ How often? _____

11. Do you think the baby has a feeding problem?
Yes _____ No _____
If yes, describe _____

12. Who usually feeds the baby? _____
Does the person have the use of:
    Working stove   _____
    Refrigerator   _____
    Piped water   _____

13. Does the family participate in:
    Food stamp program   Yes _____ No _____
    WIC program   Yes _____ No _____
    Day care food program   Yes _____ No _____

14. Please check which, if any, of the following foods the baby eats
and how often.

	Less than once a week	Not daily but at least once a week	Every day or nearly every day
Cheese, yogurt, ice cream, pudding	_____	_____	_____
Milk or formula	_____	_____	_____
Eggs	_____	_____	_____
Dried beans, peas, peanut butter, nuts	_____	_____	_____
Meat, fish, poultry, wild game	_____	_____	_____
Bread, rice, grits, cereal, tortillas, noodles, spaghetti	_____	_____	_____
Fruits or fruit juices	_____	_____	_____
Vegetables (including potatoes)	_____	_____	_____
Candy, desserts, sweets	_____	_____	_____

15. If the baby eats fruits or drinks fruit juices every day or nearly every day, which ones does he or she eat or drink most often (not more than three)?

_____   _____   _____

16. If the baby eats vegetables every day or nearly every day, which ones does he or she eat most often (not more than three)?

_____   _____   _____

17. Does the baby eat:
   Sticky or sweet foods   Yes _____   No _____
   Salty foods   Yes _____   No _____
   If yes, what are the foods? _____

   _____
   Is salt added to the baby's food?   Yes _____   No _____
18. Below list the foods and beverages the baby has had during the last 24 hours.

Time	Food eaten	Amount	How is this food prepared?

Questionnaire II—preschool and young school-age child (guardian responds)

Date _____   Age _____
Name _____   Birth date _____

   Please answer the following questions by checking the appropriate box or filling in the blank. Answer only those questions that apply to you or your child. All information is confidential.

1. Does the child drink milk?   Yes _____   No _____
   If yes: Whole milk   _____
            2% milk   _____
            Skim milk   _____
            Other _____
   If yes: Less than 8 oz (1 cup)   _____
            8 to 32 oz   _____
            More than 32 oz (1 quart)_____

2. Does the child drink anything from a bottle?
Yes _____   No _____
If yes: Milk _____
         Other _____
Does the child take a bottle to bed?   Yes _____   No _____
If yes, what is usually in the bottle?

_____

3. How many times a day does the child usually eat, including snacks? _____
Does the child eat anything after he or she has gone to bed?
Yes _____   No _____
If yes, what? _____

4. Does the child take vitamins or iron?
Yes _____   No _____
If yes, how often? _____
What kind? _____

5. Is the child on a special diet now?   Yes _____   No _____
If yes: Allergy   _____
         Weight reduction _____
         Other _____
Who recommended the diet? _____

6. Does the child eat clay, paint chips, dirt, paper, or anything else not usually considered food?
Yes _____   No _____
If yes, what? _____ How often? _____

7. How would you describe the child's appetite?
         Good   _____
         Fair   _____
         Poor   _____
         Other (specify) _____

8. Who usually feeds the child? _____
Does this person have use of:
         Working stove _____
         Refrigerator   _____
         Piped water   _____

9. Does the family participate in:
         Food stamp program   Yes _____   No _____
         WIC program   Yes _____   No _____
Does the child participate in:
         School breakfast   Yes _____   No _____
         School lunch   Yes _____   No _____
         Day care food program   Yes _____   No _____
         Summer food program   Yes _____   No _____

10. Please check which, if any, of the following foods the child eats and how often.

	Less than once a week	Not daily but at least once a week	Every day or nearly every day
Cheese, yogurt, ice cream, pudding	_____	_____	_____
Milk	_____	_____	_____
Eggs	_____	_____	_____
Dried beans, peas, peanut butter, nuts	_____	_____	_____
Meat, fish, poultry, wild game	_____	_____	_____
Bread, rice, grits, cereal, tortillas, noodles, spaghetti	_____	_____	_____
Fruits or fruit juices	_____	_____	_____
Vegetables (including potatoes)	_____	_____	_____
Candy, desserts, sweets	_____	_____	_____

11. If the child eats fruits or drinks fruit juices every day or nearly every day, which ones does he or she eat or drink most often (not more than three)?

_____   _____   _____

12. If the child eats vegetables every day or nearly every day, which ones does he or she eat most often (not more than three)?

_____   _____   _____

13. Does the child usually eat between meals? Yes _____ No _____
If yes, name the two or three snacks (including bedtime snacks) that the child has most often.

_____   _____   _____

14. Does the child eat:
   Sticky or sweet foods   Yes _____ No _____
   Salty foods   Yes _____ No _____
   If yes, what are the foods? _____
   _____
   Is salt added to the child's food? Yes _____ No _____

15. Below list the foods and beverages the child has had in the last 24 hours.

Time	Food eaten	Amount	How is this food prepared?

Questionnaire III—school-age child and teenager

Date _____ Age _____

Name _____ Birth date _____

   Please answer the following questions by checking the appropriate box or filling in the blank. Answer only those questions that apply to you or your child. All information is confidential.

1. Do you drink milk?   Yes _____ No _____
   If yes: Whole milk   _____
             2% milk   _____
             Skim milk   _____
             Other _____
   How often? _____
   Are there other beverages you often drink?
   Yes _____   No _____
   If yes, what? _____

2. How many times a day do you eat, including snacks?
   _____

3. Do you take vitamins or iron?   Yes _____ No _____
   If yes, how often? _____ What kind? _____

4. Are you on a special diet?   Yes _____ No _____
   If yes: Allergy   _____
            Weight reduction   _____
            Other _____
   Who recommended the diet? _____

5. Do you eat clay, paint chips, dirt, paper, or anything else not usually considered food?   Yes _____ No _____
   If yes, what? _____ How often? _____

6. Does anyone in your household participate in:
             Food stamp program   Yes _____ No _____
             WIC program   Yes _____ No _____
   Do you participate in:
             School breakfast   Yes _____ No _____
             School lunch   Yes _____ No _____
             Summer food program   Yes _____ No _____

7. Who usually prepares your meals? _____
   Does this person have use of:
             Working stove _____
             Refrigerator _____
             Piped water   _____

8. Do you eat any:
             Sticky or sweet foods   Yes _____ No _____
             Salty foods   Yes _____ No _____
   Do you add salt to your food?   Yes _____ No _____

9. Please check which of the following foods you eat and how often.

	Less than once a week	Not daily but at least once a week	Every day or nearly every day
Cheese, yogurt, ice cream, pudding	_____	_____	_____
Milk	_____	_____	_____
Eggs	_____	_____	_____
Dried beans, peas, peanut butter, nuts	_____	_____	_____
Meat, fish, poultry, wild game	_____	_____	_____
Bread, rice, grits, cereal, tortillas, noodles, spaghetti	_____	_____	_____
Fruits or fruit juices	_____	_____	_____
Vegetables (including potatoes)	_____	_____	_____
Candy, desserts, sweets	_____	_____	_____

10. If you eat fruits or drink fruit juices every day or nearly every day, which ones do you eat or drink most often (not more than three)?

_____   _____   _____

11. If you eat vegetables every day or nearly every day, which ones do you eat most often (not more than three)?

_____   _____   _____

12. Do you usually eat anything between meals?
Yes _____ No _____
If yes, name the two or three snacks (including bedtime snacks) that you have most often.

_____   _____   _____

13. Below list the foods and beverages you have had in the last 24 hours.

Time	Food eaten	Amount	How is this food prepared?

Guidelines for Feeding During the First Year

Age/type of feeding	Specific recommendations
Birth to 6 months	
Breast-feeding	Most desirable complete diet for first half of year
	Requires supplements of fluoride (0.25 mg), regardless of the fluoride content of the local water supply, and iron by 6 months of age
	Requires supplements of vitamin D (400 units) if mother's diet is inadequate or if infant is not exposed to sufficient sunlight
Formula	Iron-fortified commercial formula is a complete food for the first half of the year*
	Requires fluoride supplements (0.25 mg) when the concentration of fluoride in the drinking water is below 0.3 parts per million (ppm)
	Evaporated milk formula requires supplements of vitamin C, iron, and fluoride (in accordance with the fluoride content of the local water supply)
6 to 12 months	
Solid foods	May begin to add solids by 5-6 months of age; earlier introduction tends to contribute to overfeeding
	First foods are strained, pureed, or finely mashed
	"Finger foods," such as teething crackers, raw fruit, or vegetables, can be introduced by 6-7 months
	Chopped table food or commercially prepared junior foods can be started by 9-12 months
	With the exception of cereal, the order of introducing foods is variable; a recommended sequence is weekly introduction of other foods, beginning with fruit, then vegetables, and then meat
	Breast-fed infants require more high-protein foods than formula-fed children
	As the quantity of solids increases, the amount of formula should be limited to approximately 900 ml (30 oz) daily

Method of introduction

Introduce solids when infant is hungry

Begin spoon feeding by pushing food to back of tongue because of infant's natural tendency to thrust tongue forward

Use small spoon with straight handle; begin with 1 or 2 teaspoons of food; gradually increase to 2-3 tablespoons per feeding

Introduce one food at a time, usually at intervals of 4-7 days; identify food allergies

As the amount of solid food increases, decrease the quantity of milk to prevent overfeeding

Never introduce foods by mixing them with the formula in the bottle

Cereal

Introduce commercially prepared iron-fortified infant cereals and administer daily until 18 months

Rice cereal is usually introduced first because of its low allergenic potential

Can discontinue supplemental iron once cereal is given

Fruits and vegetables

Applesauce, bananas, and pears are usually well tolerated

Avoid fruits and vegetables marketed in cans that are not specifically designed for infants because of variable and sometimes high lead content and addition of salt, sugar, or preservatives

Offer fruit juice only from a cup, not a bottle, to reduce the development of "nursing bottle caries"

Meat, fish, and poultry

Avoid fatty meats

Prepare by baking, broiling, steaming, or poaching

Include organ meats such as liver, which has a high iron, vitamin A, and vitamin B complex content

If soup is given, be sure all ingredients are familiar to child's diet

Avoid commercial meat/vegetable combinations because protein is low

Eggs and cheese

Serve egg yolk hard-boiled and mashed, soft cooked, or poached

Introduce egg white in small quantities (1 tsp) toward end of first year to detect an allergy

Use cheese as a substitute for meat and as "finger food"

From Wong D, Whaley L: *Clinical manual of pediatric nursing*, ed 4, St. Louis, 1996, Mosby.

*The Academy of Pediatrics recommends breast-feeding or commercial formula-feeding for up to 12 months of age. After 1 year whole cow's milk can be given.

This section may be photocopied and distributed to families.

Guidelines for Formula-Feeding

Age	Average quantity taken in individual feedings	Average number of feedings per 24 hours
Birth to 3 weeks	2-3 oz	6-10
2 weeks to 2 months	5 oz	5-8
2 to 3 months	5-7 oz	5-6

Modified from Bobak IM, Lowdermilk DL, Jensen MD: *Maternity nursing,* ed 4, St. Louis, 1995, Mosby.

Notes

Normal and Special Infant Formulas*

Formula (manufacturer)	Protein source	Carbohydrate source	Fat sources	Indications for use	Comments (nutritional considerations)
Human and cow's milk formulas					
Human breast milk	Mature human milk; whey/casein ratio: 60:40	Lactose	Mature human milk	For all full-term infants except those with galactosemia; may be used with low–birth-weight infants	Recommended sole form of feeding for first 5-6 months; nutritionally complete except for fluoride
Evaporated cow's milk formulas	Milk protein; whey/casein ratio: 18:82	Lactose, sucrose	Butterfat	For full-term infants with no special nutritional requirements; use of undiluted cow's milk after 12 months	Supplement with iron and vitamin C; A and D if not fortified; fluoride if fluoridated water is not used for formula preparation
Commercial infant formulas					
Enfamil (Mead Johnson)	Nonfat cow's milk, demineralized whey; whey/casein ratio: 60:40	Lactose	Palm olein, soy, coconut, HOSun† oils	For full-term and premature infants with no special nutritional requirements	Available fortified with iron, 12 mg/L Also available in 24 cal/oz

Continued.

From Wong D: *Whaley and Wong's nursing care of infants and children*, ed 6, St. Louis, 1999, Mosby.
*All formulas provide 20 kcal/oz except as noted in product information from the formula manufacturers. For the most current information, consult product labels or package enclosures.
†HOSun, high-oleic sunflower.

Normal and Special Infant Formulas*—cont'd

Formula (manufacturer)	Protein source	Carbohydrate source	Fat sources	Indications for use	Comments (nutritional considerations)
Commercial infant formulas—cont'd					
Improved Similac (Ross)	Nonfat cow's milk; whey/casein ratio: 48:52	Lactose	Soy, coconut oils, and high-oleic safflower oil	For full-term and premature infants with no special nutritional requirements	Available fortified with iron, 1.8 mg/100 cal, nucleotides, 72 mg/L Also available in 24 cal/oz with iron
Baby Formula (Gerber)	Nonfat cow's milk; whey/casein ratio: 18:82	Lactose	Palm olein, soy, coconut, HOSun oils	For full-term and premature infants with no special nutritional requirements	Available fortified with iron, 12 mg/L
Good Start H.A. (Carnation)	Hydrolyzed whey	Lactose, maltodextrin	Palm olein, soy, safflower, coconut oils	For full-term infants	Manufacturer's claim regarding hypoaller-genicity has been withdrawn
Good Nature (Carnation)	Nonfat cow's milk	Corn syrup solids	Palm, corn, oleic oils	For feeding older infants	Contains more protein and calcium than "starter" formulas

Product	Protein source	Carbohydrate source	Fat source	Indications	Comments
Similac Natural Care Human Milk Fortifier (Ross)	Nonfat cow's milk; whey protein concentrate	Hydrolyzed corn starch, lactose	MCT,‡ coconut, soy oils	For low–birth-weight infants; fed mixed with human milk or fed alternately with human milk; improves vitamin/mineral content of human milk	Protein, 2.7 g/100 cal osmolality; 300 mOsm/kg water, 24 cal/oz
Similac NeoCare with Iron	Nonfat cow's milk, whey/casein ratio: 50:50	Corn syrup and lactose	MCT oils	Preterm infants, 22 cal/oz	Protein, 2.6 g/100 cal Phosphorus, 62 mg/100 cal Calcium, 105 mg/100 cal
Enfamil Human Milk Fortifier (Mead Johnson)	Whey protein concentrate, casein	Corn syrup solids	Trace	For low–birth-weight infants; fed mixed with human milk; increases protein, calories, calcium, phosphorus, and other nutrients	Used only as human milk fortifier, not as separate formula; one packet of powder supplies 3.5 kcal/ml and less than 0.1 g/dl fat
For milk protein–sensitive infants ("milk allergy"), lactose intolerance					
Prosobee (Mead Johnson)	Soy protein isolate	Corn syrup solids	Palm, soy, coconut, HOSun oils	With milk protein allergy, lactose intolerance, lactase deficiency, galactosemia	Hypoallergenic, zero band antigen; lactose- and sucrose-free

Continued.

*All formulas provide 20 kcal/oz except as noted in product information from the formula manufacturers. For the most current information, consult product labels or package enclosures.

‡MCT, medium-chain triglycerides.

Normal and Special Infant Formulas*—cont'd

For milk protein–sensitive infants ("milk allergy"), lactose intolerance—cont'd

Formula (manufacturer)	Protein source	Carbohydrate source	Fat sources	Indications for use	Comments (nutritional considerations)
Isomil (Ross)	Soy protein isolate	Corn syrup, sucrose	Soy, coconut oils	With milk protein allergy, lactose intolerance, lactase deficiency, galactosemia	Hypoallergenic; lactose-free
Isomil SF (Ross)	Soy protein isolate	Hydrolyzed corn starch	Soy, coconut oils	For use during diarrhea	Lessens amount and duration of watery stools; contains fiber
Lactofree (Mead Johnson)	Milk protein isolate	Corn syrup solids	Palm olein, soy, HOSun oils	With lactose intolerance, lactase deficiency, galactosemia	Lactose-free
Soyalac (Loma Linda)	Soybean solids	Sucrose, corn syrup	Soy oil	With milk protein allergy, lactose intolerance, lactase deficiency, galactosemia	Lactose-free
I-Soyalac (Loma Linda)	Soy protein isolate	Sucrose tapioca dextrin	Soy oil	With milk protein allergy, lactose intolerance, lactase deficiency, galactosemia	Lactose- and corn-free

For infants with malabsorption syndromes, milk allergy (hydrolysate formulas)

	Protein source	Carbohydrate source	Fat source	Indication	Comments
RCF (Ross Carbohydrate Free) (Ross)	Soy protein isolate		Soy, coconut oils	With carbohydrate intolerance	Carbohydrate is added according to amount infant will tolerate
Portagen (Mead Johnson)	Sodium caseinate	Corn syrup solids, sucrose, lactose	MCT (coconut source), corn oil	For impaired fat absorption secondary to pancreatic insufficiency, bile acid deficiency, intestinal resection, lymphatic anomalies	Nutritionally complete
Nutramigen (Mead Johnson)	Casein hydrolysate, L-amino acids§	Corn syrup solids, modified corn starch	Corn, soy oils	For infants and children sensitive to food proteins; use in galactosemic patients	Nutritionally complete; hypoallergenic formula; lactose- and sucrose-free
Pregestimil (Mead Johnson)	Casein hydrolysate, L-amino acids	Corn syrup solids, modified tapioca starch	MCT, soy, HOSun oils	Disaccharidase deficiencies, malabsorption syndromes, cystic fibrosis, intestinal resection	Nutritionally complete; easily digestible protein, carbohydrate, and fat; lactose- and sucrose-free
Alimentum (Ross)	Casein hydrolysate, L-amino acids	Sucrose, modified tapioca starch	MCT, oleic, soy oils	For infants and children sensitive to food proteins or with cystic fibrosis	Nutritionally complete; hypoallergenic formula; lactose-free

*All formulas provide 20 kcal/oz except as noted in product information. For the most current information, consult product labels or package enclosures.

§L-Amino acids include L-cystine, L-tyrosine, and L-tryptophan, which are reduced in hydrolyzed, charcoal-treated casein.

Continued.

Normal and Special Infant Formulas*—cont'd

Formula (manufacturer)	Protein source	Carbohydrate source	Fat sources	Indications for use	Comments (nutritional considerations)
Specialty formulas					
Lonalac (Mead Johnson)	Casein	Lactose	Coconut	For children with congestive heart failure, who require reduced sodium intake	For long-term management, additional sodium must be given; supplement with vitamins C and D and iron; Na = 1 mEq/L
Similac PM 60/40 (Ross)	Whey protein concentrate, sodium caseinate (60:40 ratio)	Lactose	Coconut, corn oils	For newborns predisposed to hypocalcemia and infants with impaired renal, digestive, and cardiovascular functions	Low calcium, potassium, and phosphorus; relatively low solute load; Na = 7 mEq/L; available in powder only
Diet modifiers					
Polycose (Ross)		Glucose polymers (corn syrup solids)		Used to increase calorie intake, as in failure-to-thrive infants	Carbohydrate only; a powdered or liquid calorie supplement; powder, 23 kcal/tbsp

Moducal (Mead Johnson)		Hydrolyzed corn starch	Used to increase carbohydrate intake	Carbohydrate only; a powdered calorie supplement: 30 kcal/tbsp
Casec (Mead Johnson)	Calcium caseinate		Used to increase protein intake	Protein only; negligible fat and no carbohydrate
MCT Oil (Mead Johnson)			90% MCT (coconut source)	Supplement in fat malabsorption conditions	Fat only; 8.3 kcal/g; 115 kcal/tbsp
For infants with phenylketonuria[II]				
Lofenalac (Mead Johnson)	Casein hydrolysate, L-amino acids	Corn syrup solids, modified tapioca starch	Corn oil	For infants and children	111 mg phenylalanine per quart of formula (20 cal/oz); must be supplemented with other foods to provide minimal phenylalanine
Phenyl-free (Mead Johnson)	L-Amino acids	Sucrose, corn syrup solids, modified tapioca starch	Corn, coconut oils	For children over 1 year of age	Phenylalanine-free; permits increased supplementation with normal foods

*All formulas provide 20 kcal/oz except as noted in product information from the formula manufacturers. For the most current information, consult product labels or package enclosures.

[II]Ross Laboratories and Mead Johnson manufacture several specialty formulas for metabolic disorders for infants.

Continued.

Normal and Special Infant Formulas*—cont'd

Formula (manufacturer)	Protein source	Carbohydrate source	Fat sources	Indications for use	Comments (nutritional considerations)
For infants with phenylketonuria[II]—cont'd					
Phenex-1 (Ross)	L-Amino acids	Hydrolyzed corn starch	Soy, coconut, palm oils	For infants	Phenylalanine-free; fortified with L-tyrosine, L-glutamine, L-carnitine, and taurine; contains vitamins, minerals, and trace elements
Phenex-2 (Ross)	L-Amino acids	Hydrolyzed corn starch	Soy, coconut, palm oils	For children and adults	Phenylalanine-free; fortified with L-tyrosine, L-glutamine, L-carnitine, and taurine; contains vitamins, minerals, and trace elements
Pro-Phree (Ross)	None	Hydrolyzed corn starch	Soy, coconut, palm oils	For infants and toddlers requiring reduced protein intake	Must be supplemented with protein; has vitamins, minerals, and trace elements

*All formulas provide 20 kcal/oz except as noted in product information from the formula manufacturers. For the most current information, consult product labels or package enclosures.

[II]Ross Laboratories and Mead Johnson manufacture several specialty formulas for metabolic disorders for infants.

Nutrition Guidelines for Diabetes in Pediatrics

Description

Diabetes during the pediatric years requires a balance of insulin, diet, and exercise. The major goal of nutrition therapy in insulin dependent diabetes mellitus is to ensure a pattern of growth and maturation that simulates the pattern of healthy children without diabetes.

Indications

The nutrition guidelines outlined under an adult diabetic diet for consistent carbohydrate intake should also be used for children with diabetes mellitus.

How to determine diet

Consistent carbohydrate
Specify Level I, II, III
Specify number of snacks (0, 1, 2, 3)

Nutritional adequacy

This diet is planned to meet nutrient requirements in accordance with the Recommended Dietary Allowances. Individual food choice and intake will determine actual nutritional adequacy.

Modified from *Diet manual,* Lexington, Ky, 1997, Department of Dietetics and Nutrition, University of Kentucky Hospital Chandler Medical Center.

Nutrition Guidelines for Children With Hypoglycemia

Treat hypoglycemia with one of the following: sugar, fruit juice with sugar, candy, jelly, honey, Monogel, or sweetened beverages. Follow with a small snack to stabilize blood glucose. An extra snack should be eaten before and after strenuous exercise to prevent hypoglycemia.

Meal pattern

Breakfast
Juice, unsweetened
Cereal
Toast
Margarine
Milk, low fat
Sugar substitute

Lunch
Soup
Sandwich
Fruit, fresh or unsweetened
Milk, low fat

All between-meal feedings
Meat or substitute
Bread or substitute
Milk, low fat

Supper
Meat or substitute
Potato or substitute
Vegetable or salad
Bread
Fruit, fresh or unsweetened
Margarine
Milk, low fat

From *Diet manual,* Lexington, Ky, 1997, Department of Dietetics and Nutrition, University of Kentucky Hospital Chandler Medical Center.

Nutrition Guidelines for Children With Cystic Fibrosis

Description
Maintenance of nutritional status is of primary importance in clients with cystic fibrosis. Inadequate growth occurs in the majority of clients with cystic fibrosis because of increased energy needs imposed by malabsorption, chronic pulmonary disease, and infection.

Indications
These guidelines should be considered in the individual with cystic fibrosis.

How to determine diet
High-calorie, high-protein diet with between-meal feedings.

General guidelines
1. The diet should be individualized based on nutritional status, growth velocity, and degree of malabsorption.
2. Pancreatic enzymes are necessary to improve absorption of dietary fat.
3. Fat should be included in the diet to increase calorie intake, but the amount is determined by individual tolerance. Indications for fat restriction include excessive steatorrhea in spite of pancreatic enzyme supplementation, prolapse of the rectum, and abdominal distention.
4. Cystic fibrosis clients presenting with acute pancreatitis should follow nutritional guidelines for pancreatitis.
5. Additional dietary fiber is encouraged. Snacks may include peanuts, or fruits with peanut butter.

Nutritional adequacy
This diet is planned to meet nutrient requirements in accordance with the Recommended Dietary Allowances. Individual food choice and intake will determine actual nutritional adequacy. A multivitamin supplement at double the normal dosage is routinely recommended. In the presence of malabsorption, additional vitamin supplementation may be indicated.

From *Diet manual,* Lexington, Ky, 1997, Department of Dietetics and Nutrition, University of Kentucky Hospital Chandler Medical Center.

Calorie requirements

An intake of one and one half to two times the normal requirement is recommended.

Infants: 150-200 kcal/kg/day
Older children (1-9 years): 130-180 kcal/kg/day
Males ($\geq$10 years): 100-130 kcal/kg/day
Females ($\geq$10 years): 80-110 kcal/kg/day

Protein requirements

An intake of two to two and one half times the normal requirement is recommended.

Infants: 4 g/kg/day
Older children (1-9 years): 3 g/kg/day
Young adults ($\geq$10 years): 2.5-3 g/kg/day

Nutrition Guidelines for Children With Phenylketonuria

Description

Phenylketonuria (PKU) is one of a group of inherited disorders of phenylalanine metabolism, some of which are associated with mental retardation. Each newborn in the state of Kentucky is screened for PKU, and those with elevated serum phenylalanine levels are referred for confirmation of diagnosis. The only known treatment for PKU is dietary restriction of phenylalanine. Diet therapy should be instituted before the third week of life to prevent permanent brain damage.

Indications

These nutrition guidelines should be implemented for the individual with phenylketonuria.

How to determine diet

Consult the dietician before ordering a diet restricted in phenylalanine.

General guidelines

1. Phenylalanine is found in large amounts in all protein-rich foods, such as commercial infant formula, meat, milk, eggs, and cheese. These foods are eliminated from the diet.

Modified from *Diet manual,* Lexington, Ky, 1997, Department of Dietetics and Nutrition, University of Kentucky Hospital Chandler Medical Center.

2. Limited amounts of starches, vegetables, and fruits are allowed.
3. Lofenalac and Phenyl-Free are two specially prepared commercial formulas from which the majority of phenylalanine has been removed. These products are the basis of the diet and provide for nitrogen and amino acid requirements.
4. The low-phenylalanine diet should be continued throughout life. Recent studies indicate that deterioration in intellectual function occurs in children with PKU who have discontinued the phenylalanine-restricted diet. Adults who discontinue the phenylalanine-restricted diet experience short-term memory deficits. Continuation of the diet is even more critical for women with PKU during their childbearing years to prevent problems such as mental retardation, microcephaly, and birth defects in their offspring.

Nutritional adequacy

This diet is planned to meet nutrient requirements in accordance with the Recommended Dietary Allowances. Individual food choice and intake will determine actual nutritional adequacy. Regular monitoring and adjustments in the meal plan are necessary.

Recommended Nutrient and Energy Intake for Phenylketonuria

Age	Phenylalanine mg/kg	Protein	Calories
<3 months	40-70	2.5 g/kg	120 kcal/kg
3-6 months	25-50	2.5 g/kg	115 kcal/kg
6-9 months	25-40	2.25 g/kg	110 kcal/kg
9-12 months	20-35	2.25 g/kg	105 kcal/kg
1-4 years	15-30	25 g	1300 kcal
4-7 years	12-25	35 g	1700 kcal
7-11 years	10-20	45 g	2400 kcal
Females			
11-15 years	10-20	50 g	2200 kcal
15-19 years	8-20	50 g	2100 kcal
19-23 years	8-15	46 g	2100 kcal
>23 years	8-15	46 g	1800 kcal
Males			
11-15 years	10-20	50 g	2700 kcal
15-19 years	10-20	60 g	2800 kcal
>19 years	8-15	60 g	2700 kcal

From *Diet manual,* Lexington, Ky, 1997, Department of Dietetics and Nutrition, University of Kentucky Hospital Chandler Medical Center.

"BRAT" Diet

Description
The "BRAT" diet is low in residue and high in carbohydrate.

Indications
The "BRAT" diet is used for short periods of time for children with diarrhea. It has not been shown to be clinically effective in controlled studies.

How to determine diet
"BRAT" diet.

General guidelines
1. Allowed foods are served often and in small amounts. Only one or two items per meal may be given to small children.
2. Other foods may be gradually added until a general diet is tolerated.
3. Milk and milk products should be the last foods to be resumed.

Nutritional adequacy
This diet is inadequate in all nutrients and should be used only for a limited period of time.

Meal pattern
Breakfast
Banana, ½
Rice cereal or Cream of Wheat
Toast, white
Jelly
Fruit-flavored beverage

Between-meal feedings
Applesauce
Crackers, saltines
Fruit ice
Popsicle

From *Diet manual,* Lexington, Ky, 1997, Department of Dietetics and Nutrition, University of Kentucky Hospital Chandler Medical Center.

Lunch/supper

Broth

Toast, white, or rice

Banana, ½

Gelatin or Popsicle

Jelly

Fruit-flavored beverage

Sample Menus for Pregnant Adolescents

	Day 1	Day 2
Breakfast	1 cup unsweetened, ready-to-eat cereal with 1 cup 2% milk ¾ cup orange juice	2 pancakes, 1 medium waffle, or 1 slice French toast 2 Tbsp syrup 1 cup 2% milk
Snack	1 blueberry muffin 1 cup 2% milk	2 graham crackers 1 6-oz can apple juice
Lunch	1 cheeseburger (fast food) 1 banana Carrot sticks 1 cup 2% milk	3 slices pizza 1 apple Small salad 1 Tbsp dressing 1 cup 2% milk
Snack	1 apple 3 Tbsp peanut butter Caffeine-free soda*	½ cup cottage cheese dip Raw vegetables Caffeine-free soda*
Dinner	1 cup spaghetti with meat sauce Salad 2 Tbsp dressing 1 roll ½ cup chocolate pudding 1 glass water[†]	3 oz baked chicken 1 cup rice 1 cup green beans 1 roll 1 ice cream sandwich 1 glass water[†]
Snack	1 slice angel food cake ½ cup fresh or frozen fruit, no sugar added Calories = 2525[‡]	3 cups popcorn 1 glass ginger ale Calories = 2568[‡]

*Sample diets should include foods that patients normally eat and, therefore, provide teaching opportunities about better choices (example: caffeinated beverage vs. caffeine-free drink).

†Encourage adequate water consumption daily—6 to 8 glasses.

‡Calorie calculations are based on the maximum allowance for growth; however, the best indication that a pregnant adolescent is eating sufficient calories is to monitor weight gain throughout pregnancy. If inadequate or excess weight gain occurs, consultation with a registered dietician is recommended.

Nutrition counseling for pregnant adolescents

The purpose of nutrition counseling is to increase the adolescent's knowledge of nutrients and ability to plan, select, and prepare optimally nutritive foods for herself and her family. The nutritional needs of the mature (15 years and older) pregnant adolescent approach those of pregnant adults. Additional amounts of vitamins, minerals, and calories are needed to meet the growth needs of the pregnant adolescent and her fetus and to correct deficiencies resulting from inadequate intake of nutrients before, during, and after pregnancy. Iron supplements are needed to provide for the growing muscle mass and blood volume increase in the pregnant adolescent. Most adolescent females consume at least one snack per day, with a range of one to seven. Snacks contribute more than "empty calories." Nutrients found in many of the snacks eaten by adolescent females contribute approximately half the RDA of riboflavin, vitamin C, and thiamin. Pregnant adolescents should be encouraged to eat nutritious snacks such as peanut butter crackers, cheese, fruit, and juice.

As an integral part of health care programs for pregnant adolescents, the nutrition consultant must be skillful in establishing rapport and developing a relationship that promotes effective patient counseling in the nutritional aspects of reproduction. Counseling should include setting a weight gain goal together with the pregnant adolescent, preferably at the initial prenatal examination, and explaining why weight gain is important. Additional strategies include building on cultural practices; categorizing nutrition practices as beneficial, neutral, or harmful; and reinforcing those practices that are positive and promoting change only in those that are harmful. Counseling should extend to the postpartum period to ensure a significant and lasting effect on the future of the parents and child.

From Wong D, Perry S: *Maternal-child nursing care,* St. Louis, 1998, Mosby.

Very young teens (younger than 15 years old) should gain at the upper end of recommended ranges. Weight gain should be plotted at each prenatal visit to detect erratic changes. Erratic weight gain suggests fluid retention. If the adolescent has an inadequate diet, vitamin and mineral supplements are recommended. Supplements should be taken between meals and at bedtime for best absorption. Those with a recent weight loss and a body mass index (BMI) less than 19.8 should be evaluated for an eating disorder.

Notes

GUIDELINES FOR ADULTS

Clinical Signs of Nutritional Status

Features	Good	Poor
General appearance	Alert, responsive	Listless, apathetic, cachexic
Hair	Shiny, lustrous, healthy scalp	Stringy, dull, brittle, depigmented
Neck glands	No enlargement	Thyroid enlarged
Skin, face, neck	Smooth, slightly moist, good color, reddish pink mucous membranes	Greasy, discolored, scaly
Eyes	Bright, clear, no fatigue circles	Dryness, signs of infection, increased vascularity, glassiness, thickened conjunctivae
Lips	Good color, moist	Dry, scaly, swollen, angular lesions (stomatitis)
Tongue	Good pink color, surface papillae present, no lesions	Papillary atrophy, smooth appearance, swollen, red, beefy (glossitis)
Gums	Good pink color, no swelling or bleeding, firm	Marginal redness or swelling, receding, spongy
Teeth	Straight, no crowding, well-shaped jaw, clean, no discoloration	Unfilled cavities, absent teeth, worn surface, mottled, malpositioned

Skin, general	Smooth, slightly moist, good color	Rough, dry, scaly, pale, pigmented, irritated; petechiae, bruises
Abdomen	Flat	Swollen
Legs, feet	No tenderness, weakness, swelling, good color	Edema, tender calf, tingling, weakness
Skeleton	No malformations	Bowlegs, knock-knees, chest deformity at diaphragm, beaded ribs, prominent scapulas
Weight	Normal for height, age, body build	Overweight or underweight
Posture	Erect, arms and legs straight, abdomen in, chest out	Sagging shoulders, sunken chest, humped back
Muscles	Well-developed, firm	Flaccid, poor tone, undeveloped, tender
Nervous control	Good attention span for age, does not cry easily, not irritable or restless	Inattentive, irritable
Gastrointestinal function	Good appetite and digestion, normal, regular elimination	Anorexia, indigestion, constipation or diarrhea
General vitality	Endurance, energetic, sleeps well at night, vigorous	Easily fatigued, no energy, falls asleep in school, looks tired, apathetic

From Williams S: *Nutrition and diet therapy*, ed 8, St. Louis, 1997, Mosby.

Nutritional Screening Tool

Section I. Assess factors that may indicate need for medical social worker assessment/follow-up.

Psychosocial Factors: Circle the specific findings in each line, e.g., if in item #4, there is no water but the refrigeration is adequate, circle "water" only

	"✓" if any negative findings in an item
1) Lives alone and is physically or mentally dependent for meal preparation	
2) Homebound with no one to assist with shopping	
3) Limited financial resources for the purchase of food	
4) Inadequate means for food storage and/or preparation, i.e., water, refrigeration	
5) Illness-related psychiatric condition, i.e., depression, anxiety, confusion	
6) Caregivers present but unwilling and/or unable to provide nutrition assistance	
TOTAL: each "✓" should be added to arrive at total	

Risk   2-3   Moderate nutritional risk due to psychosocial and/or environmental problems
Scale   4-6   High nutritional risk due to psychosocial and/or environmental problems
Plan   [Indicate by ✓]
☐   Medical social worker referral indicated: problems have potential to have an impact on the client's rate of recovery and/or response to medical treatment. Notify client's physician.
☐   No additional referral at this time. Skilled nurse to continue to assess.
☐   Other [Specify]

Section II. Assess factors that may indicate need for nutritional follow-up by skilled nurse and/or registered dietician.

Medical Factors: Circle the specific findings in each line, e.g., if in item #1, the problems are anorexia and dysphasia, circle both

	"✓" if any negative findings in an item
1) Anorexia, dysphasia, or problems with teeth, mouth, gums	

2) Wound that will not heal, despite medical treatment regimen	
3) Presence of nausea, vomiting, diarrhea, or constipation	
4) Unexplained weight loss or gain of 10 pounds in past 6 months	
5) Transitional diet, e.g., tube feeding to oral intake; hyperalimentation to oral	
6) Complicated and restricted therapeutic diet ordered: no prior instruction and/or does not understand instructions, e.g., diabetic diet, renal diet	
7) Multiple medications with potential for food interactions	
8) Presence of uncontrolled pain	
9) Terminal client: special considerations for comfort during end stage of life	
10) On hyperalimentation and/or tube feedings	
11) Other physical findings: e.g., dry skin, decreased elasticity, sunken eyes, coarse hair, bleeding/sore gums, disruption of tissue on oral cavity, appears emaciated, appears obese. Other:	
TOTAL: each "✓" should be added to arrive at total	

Risk   3-6   Moderate nutritional risk due to medical factors
Scale   7-11   High nutritional risk due to multiple medical factors
           [Indicate by ✓]

Plan
☐   Registered dietitian referral indicated: follow-up required the skills of a nutritional specialist.
☐   No additional referral at this time. Skilled nurse to develop nutrition care plan and continue to assess response to expected outcome.
☐   Other [Specify, e.g., ESRD client refer to Dialysis Center]

Client Name _____   PT # _____

RN _____   Visit Date _____

From *Home Care Nurse News*, Dec 1996.

Mini Nutritional Assessment (MNA)

ID# _____

Last Name _____ First Name _____ M.I. _____

Sex _____ Date _____ Age _____

Weight, kg _____ Height, cm _____ Knee Height, cm _____

Complete the form by writing the numbers in the boxes. Add the numbers in the boxes and compare the total assessment with the Malnutrition Indicator Score.

Anthropometric Assessment

	Points

1. Body Mass Index (BMI) (weight in kg)/(height in m)^2
   a. BMI <19   = 0 points
   b. BMI 19 to <21 = 1 point
   c. BMI 21 to <23 = 2 points
   d. BMI ≥23   = 3 points
	☐

2. Mid-arm circumference (MAC) in cm
   a. MAC <21   = 0.0 points
   b. MAC 21 ≤22 = 0.5 points
   c. MAC >22   = 1.0 points
	☐.☐

3. Calf circumference (CC) in cm a. CC <31 = 0 points b. CC ≥31 = 1 point	☐

4. Weight loss during last 3 months
   a. weight loss greater than 3 kg (6.6 lbs) = 0 points
   b. does not know   = 1 point
   c. weight loss between 1 and 3 kg
      (2.2 and 6.6 lbs)   = 2 points
   d. no weight loss   = 3 points
	☐

General Assessment

5. Lives independently (not in a nursing home or hospital) a. no = 0 points b. yes = 1 point	☐
6. Takes more than 3 prescription drugs per day a. yes = 0 points b. no = 1 point	☐
7. Has suffered psychological stress or acute disease in the past 3 months a. yes = 0 points b. no = 2 points	☐

8. Mobility
   a. bed or chair bound   = 0 points
   b. able to get out of bed/chair but does
     not go out   = 1 point
   c. goes out   = 2 points
	☐

9. Neuropsychological problems
   a. severe dementia or depression = 0 points
   b. mild dementia   = 1 point
   c. no psychological problems = 2 points
	☐

10. Pressure sores or skin ulcers a. yes = 0 points b. no = 1 point	☐

Modified from Nestec Ltd (Nestle Research Center)/Clintec Nutrition Company.
Ref. Gurgot Y. Vellus B and Gerry PJ. 1994. Mini Nutritional Assessment: A practical assessment tool for grading the nutritional state of elderly clients. *Facts and Research in Gerontology:* Supplement #2: 15-59.
© 1994 Nestec Ltd (Nestlé Research Center)/Clintec Nutrition Company

Continued.

Dietary Assessment

	Points
11. How many full meals does the client eat daily? a. 1 meal = 0 points b. 2 meals = 1 point c. 3 meals = 2 points	☐
12. Selected consumption markers for protein intake • At least one serving of dairy products (milk, cheese, yogurt) per day? yes ☐ no ☐ • Two or more servings of legumes or eggs per week? yes ☐ no ☐ • Meat, fish, or poultry every day? yes ☐ no ☐ a. If 0 or 1 yes = 0.0 points b. If 2 yes = 0.5 points c. If 3 yes = 1.0 points	☐.☐
13. Consumes two or more servings of fruits or vegetables per day? a. no = 0 points b. yes = 1 point	☐
14. Has food intake declined over the past three months due to loss of appetite, digestive problems, chewing or swallowing difficulties? a. severe loss of appetite = 0 points b. moderate loss of appetite = 1 point c. no loss of appetite = 2 points	☐
15. How much fluid (water, juice, coffee, tea, milk, . . .) is consumed per day? (1 cup = 8 oz.) a. less than 3 cups = 0.0 points b. 3 to 5 cups = 0.5 points c. more than 5 cups = 1.0 points	☐.☐
16. Mode of feeding a. unable to eat without assistance = 0 points b. self-fed with some difficulty = 1 point c. self-fed without any problem = 2 points	☐

Self Assessment

	Points
17. Do they view themselves as having nutritional problems? a. major malnutrition = 0 points b. do not know or moderate malnutrition = 1 point c. no nutritional problem = 2 points	☐
18. In comparison with other people of the same age, how do they consider their health status? a. not as good = 0.0 points b. does not know = 0.5 points c. as good = 1.0 points d. better = 2.0 points	☐.☐

Assessment Total (max. 30 points):   ☐☐.☐

Malnutrition Indicator Score		
≥24 points	well-nourished	☐
17 to 23.5 points	at risk of malnutrition	☐
<17 points	malnourished	☐

Nutritional Strategies for Two Types of Diabetes

Dietary strategy	IDDM (nonobese)	NIDDM (usually obese)
Decrease energy intake (kcalories)	No	Yes
Increase frequency and number of feedings	Yes	Usually no
Have regular daily intake of kcalories, carbohydrates, protein, and fat	Very important	Not important if average caloric intake remains in low range
Plan consistent daily ratio of protein, carbohydrates, and fat for each feeding	Desirable	Not necessary
Use extra or planned ahead food to treat or prevent hypoglycemia	Very important	Not necessary
Plan regular times for meals/snacks	Very important	Not important
Use extra food for unusual exercise	Yes	Usually not necessary
During illness, use small, frequent feedings of carbohydrates to prevent starvation ketosis	Important	Usually not necessary because of resistance to ketosis

From Williams S: *Nutrition and diet therapy*, ed 8, St. Louis, 1997, Mosby.

Calorie Controlled Diet

Description
The Calorie Controlled Diet is a modification of the regular diet used to reduce food intake below the level needed for maintenance of present weight.

Indications
The Calorie Controlled diet is used to promote weight loss.

How to determine diet
Calorie Controlled Diet
Specify calorie level

General guidelines
1. Decrease calorie intake by 500-1000 calories per day to promote a weight loss of 1-2 pounds per week.
2. It is recommended that men and women not be placed on calorie levels below 1200-1500 and 1000-1200 calories per day, respectively.
3. The Exchange List for Meal Planning is used in meal planning.

Nutritional adequacy
This diet is planned to meet nutrient requirements in accordance with the Recommended Dietary Allowances. Individual food choice and intake will determine actual nutritional adequacy. Generally, diets providing 1200 calories or more are adequate.

Calorie requirements for various activity levels

| | Activity level | | |
	Sedentary	Moderate	Marked
Maintenance	30 Kcal/kg	35 Kcal/kg	40 Kcal/kg
Weight Reduction	20-25 Kcal/kg	30 Kcal/kg	35 Kcal/kg

From *Diet manual,* Lexington, Ky, 1997, Department of Dietetics and Nutrition, University of Kentucky Hospital Chandler Medical Center.

Meal pattern—1200 calories

BREAKFAST

Fruit	1 exchange
Meat or substitute	1 exchange
Bread or Starch	1 exchange
Fat	1 exchange
Milk, skim	1 exchange

LUNCH

Meat or substitute	2 exchanges
Vegetable, free	1 serving
Bread or Starch	2 exchanges
Fruit	1 exchange
Fat	1 exchange
Milk, skim	1 exchange

SUPPER

Meat or substitute	2 exchanges
Vegetable	2 exchanges
Bread or Starch	1 exchange
Fruit	1 exchange
Fat	1 exchange

Food pattern

Refer to the Exchange Lists for Meal Planning.

Nutrition Guidelines for Diabetes

Description

Guidelines for diabetes are based on recommendations by the American Diabetes Association and the American Dietetic Association. The diet for diabetes provides consistency in carbohydrate intake from day to day at breakfast, at lunch, at supper, and at snacks.

Indications

The Nutrition Guidelines for Diabetes are used for Type I, Type II, and secondary diabetes.

Modified from *Diet manual,* Lexington, Ky, 1997, Department of Dietetics and Nutrition, University of Kentucky Hospital Chandler Medical Center.

How to determine diet

Consistent Carbohydrate
Specify level I, II, III (See calorie section)
Specify number of snacks (0, 1, 2, 3)

General guidelines

1. Overall recommendations for macronutrients and other components of the diet are the same for Type I and Type II diabetes whether treated with insulin, with oral agents, or by diet alone.
2. A decrease in calories is recommended when diabetes is associated with obesity.

Nutritional adequacy

This diet is planned to meet nutrient requirements in accordance with the Recommended Dietary Allowances. Individual food choice and intake will determine actual nutritional adequacy.

Macronutrients and dietary components

Calories   Calories should be provided for weight loss, weight gain, or maintenance, as appropriate. Even a modest reduction in weight in the obese/overweight person can improve glycemic control.

Level I provides approximately 1200 calories.
Level II provides approximately 1800 calories.
Level III provides approximately 2400 calories.

Carbohydrate   Composes approximately 50% of total calorie intake. Carbohydrate content at breakfast, at lunch, at supper, and at snacks is consistent from day to day. Emphasis is on complex, unrefined carbohydrate, which results in an increase in fiber intake. Sucrose and other refined sugars are incorporated as a portion of the total carbohydrate content.

Protein   Composes approximately 20% of total calorie intake. Derived from both animal and vegetable sources.

Fat   Composes approximately 30% of total calorie intake. Due to the increased incidence of atherosclerotic disease among individuals with diabetes, saturated fat is limited. Cholesterol is also limited to 300 milligrams or less per day.

Fiber	Provided by a wide variety of food sources, including fruits, vegetables, legumes, and whole grain breads and cereals.
Sweeteners	Artificial sweeteners are routinely provided.

Aspartame, saccharin, and acesulfame K are considered safe for use. The calorie contribution to total calories is negligible.

Women with diabetes who are pregnant are encouraged to reduce intake of artificial sweeteners; however, they are not expressly prohibited.

Meal Distribution and Frequency	Unless a specific meal pattern distribution is ordered (e.g. three meals and three snacks), three meals are provided. Children and adolescents with diabetes should receive additional feedings. One, two, or three snacks may be ordered.
Pregnancy	Meal pattern should be planned to provide three meals and between meal feedings for insulin-requiring individuals. Additional milk and calcium sources are included to meet increased calcium requirements. Level I provides inadequate calories and is not recommended.

Meal pattern

Breakfast

Fruit (fresh or juice pack)
    or unsweetened juice
Cereal
Egg
Toast
Margarine
Milk, low-fat
Beverage, sugar-free
Diet jelly
Sugar substitute/salt/pepper

Lunch/Supper

Meat or substitute
Potato or substitute
Vegetable or salad
Fruit (fresh or juice pack)
Bread
Margarine
Milk, low-fat
Beverage, sugar-free
Sugar substitute/salt/pepper

All between meal feedings

Meat or substitute
Bread or substitute

Nutrition Strategies

Strategy	Type II diet controlled	Type II oral agents	Type I/Type II Type II/insulin
Calories	Decrease, if overweight	Decrease, if overweight	Decrease, if overweight
Regular meal times	Not crucial	Important	Important
Consistency of day-to-day intake	Not critical, but can be beneficial	Not critical, but can be beneficial	Important
Increased number and frequency of feedings	Not usually necessary	Not usually necessary	Important
Extra food for exercise	Not usually necessary	Not usually necessary	Important
Modification of amount and type of fat	Important	Important	Important
Use of food to treat hypoglycemia	Not usually necessary	Important	Important

Nutrition Guidelines for Diabetes During Pregnancy

Description
This diet is based on the Exchange List for Meal Planning with modification in the frequency of meals and an increase in calcium-containing foods to meet nutritional needs during pregnancy.

Indications
The Nutrition Guidelines for Diabetes During Pregnancy are used for gestational diabetes and preexisting diabetes and pregnancy.

How to determine diet
Diabetic Diet for Pregnancy
Specify calorie level

Modified from *Diet manual,* Lexington, Ky, 1997, Department of Dietetics and Nutrition, University of Kentucky Hospital Chandler Medical Center.

General guidelines

1. Calorie intake should be sufficient to achieve desired weight gain without promoting ketonuria.
2. The diet should consist of approximately 45% carbohydrate, 15-20% protein, and 35-40% fat as a percentage of total calories.
3. Emphasis is on complex, unrefined carbohydrate sources, which results in an increase in fiber intake.
4. The meal pattern provides three meals and three between meal feedings. The bedtime feeding should contain a protein source.
5. Additional milk or calcium sources are included to meet increased calcium requirements.
6. Reduced intake of artificial sweeteners is encouraged; however, they are not expressly prohibited. Aspartame is preferred over saccharin.
7. Supplementation with a prenatal vitamin is recommended since food intake may not supply adequate levels of nutrients such as folic acid and iron. Additional iron supplementation may be recommended. Individuals should be counseled about food sources of nutrients with particular attention to folic acid and iron.

Nutritional adequacy

This diet is planned to meet nutrient requirements in accordance with the Recommended Dietary Allowances. Iron and folic acid intake may be inadequate without supplementation. Individual food choice and intake will determine actual nutritional adequacy.

Calorie requirements for diabetes during pregnancy

1st Trimester	30-32 Kcal/kg ideal body weight
2nd/3rd Trimester	38 Kcal/kg ideal body weight
>120% IBW	24 Kcal/kg present body weight

Meal pattern

Breakfast
Meat or substitute
Bread
Cereal
Milk, 1/2 cup
Margarine

Lunch/supper
Meat or substitute
Vegetable
Potato
Bread or substitute,
    1-2 servings
Fruit
Milk, 1 cup
Margarine

Mid-morning
Bread or substitute, 1-2 servings

Mid-afternoon
Bread or substitute, 1-2 servings
Milk or yogurt, 1 cup

Bedtime
Meat or substitute, 1 oz
Bread or substitute, 1-2 servings
Milk, 1 cup

Food pattern
Refer to the Exchange Lists for Meal Planning.

High Carbohydrate, High Fiber Diet

Macronutrients and dietary components

Fiber	Approximately 40 grams of plant fiber per day. Recent research has demonstrated that when plant fiber is ingested with carbohydrate, the resultant rise in blood glucose and insulin concentrations is lower than when carbohydrate is ingested without fiber. Diets high in plant fiber are usually accompanied by reductions in serum cholesterol and triglyceride levels. It is especially important to include foods rich in soluble fiber, such as oat products and dried beans.
Sweeteners	Artificial sweeteners are routinely provided.
Meal Distribution and Frequency	Unless a specific meal pattern distribution is ordered (e.g. three meals and three snacks), three meals and a bedtime feeding are provided.

Modified from *Diet manual,* Lexington, Ky, 1997, Department of Dietetics and Nutrition, University of Kentucky Hospital Chandler Medical Center.
From HCF Nutrition Research Foundation, Lexington, Ky.

Food values for high carbohydrate, high fiber exchange lists

Exchange list	Pro (g)	Fat (g)	Cho (g)	Fiber (g)	Kcal
Starches	2	0	15	2	70
Garden Vegetables	1	0	5	2	25
Fruits	0	0	15	2.5	60
Cereals	3	0	20	4	90
Beans	7	0	17	4	90
Milk	8	0.5	12	5	95
Protein	8	2	0	0	85
Fats	0	5	0	0	50
					45

Pro — Protein   g — grams
Fat — Fat   Kcal — calories
Cho — Carbohydrate

High carbohydrate, high fiber exchange lists

STARCHES

Breads and flour

Bagel, whole grain	½ bagel
Bread crumbs, whole grain	¾ cup
Bread, pita	½ pocket
Bread, pumpernickel, rye	1 slice (1 oz)
Bread, whole grain	1 slice (1 oz)
Cornmeal, dry	2½ Tbsp
English muffin, whole grain	½ muffin
Flour, oat, wheat, rye, buckwheat	2½ Tbsp
Oat bran muffin	½ muffin
Roll, rye or wheat	1 small (1 oz)
Tortilla, corn or flour	1 small (1 oz)

Grains

Barley, dry	1½ Tbsp
Bulgur, dry	1½ Tbsp
Pasta, cooked	½ cup
Rice, cooked	⅓ cup

Starchy vegetables

Corn	½ cup or 4-inch ear
Parsnips, cooked	½ cup
Peas, green	½ cup
Potato, with peel	1 small (2½ oz)
Pumpkin	1 cup
Squash, winter, cooked	¾ cup
Sweet potato, cooked	⅓ cup or ½ small
Yam, cooked	⅓ cup or ½ small

Crackers/snacks

Crispbreads	2 slices
Flatbreads	4 slices
Graham crackers, 2½ inch square	2
Melba toast (lower in fiber)	4 slices
Popcorn, popped, no oil	3 cups
Rice cakes	2
Rye crackers	6 small squares
Soda crackers (lower in fiber)	6 squares

GARDEN VEGETABLES

Artichoke, cooked	½ medium
Asparagus, cooked	½ cup or 4 spears
Bamboo shoots, cooked	1 cup
Beans, green, raw or cooked	½ cup
Beet greens, cooked	½ cup
Beets, cooked	½ cup
Broccoli, raw	1 cup
Broccoli, cooked	½ cup
Brussel sprouts, cooked	½ cup
Cabbage, Chinese, cooked	1 cup
Cabbage, raw or cooked	½ cup
Carrots, raw or cooked	½ cup
Cauliflower, raw	1 cup
Cauliflower, cooked	½ cup
Celery, cooked	1 cup
Chard, Swiss, cooked	½ cup
Collard greens, cooked	½ cup
Eggplant, raw	1 cup
Eggplant, cooked	½ cup
Kale, cooked	½ cup
Kohlrabi, cooked	½ cup
Leeks, raw or cooked	½ cup
Mung bean sprouts, raw	1 cup
Mushrooms, cooked or canned	½ cup
Mustard greens, cooked	1 cup
Okra, raw or cooked	½ cup
Onions, raw or cooked	½ cup
Rutabaga, cooked	½ cup
Sauerkraut, canned	½ cup
Snow peas, raw or cooked	½ cup
Spinach, cooked	½ cup
Squash, summer, raw	1 cup
Squash, summer, cooked	½ cup

Tomatoes, raw	1 cup or 1 medium
Tomatoes, cooked	½ cup
Turnip greens, cooked	½ cup
Turnips, raw or cooked	½ cup
Water chestnuts, raw	½ cup
Zucchini, raw	1 cup
Zucchini, cooked	½ cup

These selections are lower in fiber:

Carrot juice	¼ cup
Tomato juice	½ cup
Tomato paste	2 Tbsp
Vegetable juice	½ cup

FRUITS

Apple, raw, small	1 apple
Apple slices	1 cup
Applesauce, unsweetened	½ cup
Apricots, fresh	3 apricots
Apricots, canned, water-pack	8 halves
Apricots, canned, juice-pack	4 halves
Banana, 9 inch long	½ banana
Blackberries	¾ cup
Blueberries	¾ cup
Boysenberries	¾ cup
Cantaloupe	⅓ melon
Cantaloupe, cubed	1 cup
Casaba melon	⅛ melon
Casaba melon, cubed	1 cup
Cherries, sweet	12 cherries
Cranberries	1¼ cup
Dates	2½ dates
Figs, large	1 fig
Fruit cocktail, water-pack	¾ cup
Fruit cocktail, juice-pack	½ cup
Fruit salad, water-pack	¾ cup
Fruit salad, juice-pack	½ cup
Grapefruit	½ grapefruit
Grapefruit sections	¾ cup
Grapes	15 grapes
Honeydew melon	⅛ melon
Honeydew melon, cubed	1 cup
Kiwi, large	1 kiwi
Mango	½ mango
Melon balls	1 cup
Nectarine	1 nectarine
Orange	1 orange

Orange sections	¾ cup
Papaya	½ papaya or 1 cup
Peach, medium	1 peach
Peaches, canned, water-pack	1 cup
Peaches, canned, juice-pack	½ cup
Pear	½ pear
Pears, canned, water-pack	3 halves
Pears, canned, juice-pack	½ cup
Pineapple	¾ cup
Pineapple, canned, water-pack	¾ cup
Pineapple, canned, juice-pack	½ cup
Plums, medium	2 plums
Pomegranate	½ pomegranate
Prunes	3 prunes
Raisins	2 Tbsp
Raspberries	1 cup
Rhubarb	2 cups
Strawberries	1¼ cup
Tangelo, medium	1 tangelo
Tangerine	2 tangerines
Watermelon	1¼ cup

These selections are lower in fiber:

Apple juice	½ cup
Grape juice	⅓ cup
Grapefruit juice	½ cup
Orange juice	½ cup
Pineapple juice	½ cup
Prune juice	⅓ cup

CEREALS

All-Bran*	⅓ cup
All-Bran with extra fiber*	⅓ cup
100% Bran*	⅓ cup
Bran Chex*	⅔ cup
Bran Flakes*	⅔ cup
Fiber One*	½ cup
Grapenuts	¼ cup
Grapenuts Flakes	¾ cup
Grits, cooked	¾ cup
Grits, dry	3 Tbsp
Most	⅔ cup
Nutri-Grain	¾ cup
Oat Bran*, cooked	¾ cup
Oat Bran*, dry	⅓ cup

*These cereals provide over 5 g of fiber per serving.

CEREALS—CONT'D

Oat Flakes	⅔ cup
Oatmeal, cooked	¾ cup
Oatmeal, dry	⅓ cup
Raisin Squares	½ cup
Ralston, cooked	¾ cup
Ralston, dry	2½ Tbsp
Shredded Wheat	1 biscuit
Shredded Wheat, spoon size	⅔ cup
Toasted Wheat and Raisins	1 cup
Total	1 cup
Wheat Chex	⅔ cup
Wheaties	1 cup

Cereals that are lower in fiber may be chosen occasionally. These include Corn Chex, Corn Flakes, Cream of Rice, Cream of Wheat, Rice Chex, Product 19, Puffed Rice, Rice Krispies, and Special K. Choose cereals that contain less than 2 g of fat and 5 g of sugar per serving.

BEANS

Black-eyed peas (cowpeas)	½ cup
Butter beans	½ cup
Chick peas (garbanzo beans)	⅓ cup
Kidney beans	½ cup
Lentils	½ cup
Lima beans	½ cup
Other beans and peas	½ cup
Peas, split	½ cup
Pinto beans	½ cup
Soybeans	½ cup plus 1 fat exchange
White beans	½ cup

MILK

Buttermilk, lowfat	1 cup
Dry milk, nonfat	5 Tbsp
Milk, ½%	1 cup
Milk, 1%	1 cup plus ½ fat exchange
Milk, 2%	1 cup plus 1 fat exchange
Skim milk	1 cup
Skim milk, evaporated	½ cup
Yogurt, plain, nonfat	5 oz

*These cereals provide over 5 g of fiber per serving.

PROTEIN

Amounts listed are for raw meat, fish, and poultry.

Fish	Abalone, bass, cod, flounder, grouper, halibut, mackerel, monkfish, orange roughy, pompano, sole, snapper, and other varieties of whitefish	2 oz
	Crab, lobster, scallops, shrimp, clams	2 oz
	Herring, in tomato sauce	1 oz
	Salmon	1 oz
	Swordfish	1½ oz
	Tuna, fresh or frozen	1 oz
	Tuna, canned in water	¼ cup
Cheese	Cottage, dry curd	½ cup
	Cottage, 1% fat	¼ cup
	Low calorie, less than 50 calories/oz	1 oz
	Mozzarella, part-skim	½ oz
	Parmesan	2 Tbsp
Eggs	Egg substitute, less than 200 calories/cup	¼ cup
	Egg whites	3 whites
Poultry	Chicken, without skin	1 oz
	Turkey, without skin	1 oz
Meats	Beef—round, flank, sirloin, tenderloin	1 oz
	Lamb	1 oz
	Pork (lean)—chops, tenderloin; fresh, canned, boiled, or cured ham	1 oz
	Veal (lean)—chops, roast	1 oz
Other	Tofu	2½ oz

FATS

Avocado, medium	⅛ avocado
Margarine	1 tsp
Margarine, reduced-calorie	1 Tbsp
Mayonnaise	1 tsp
Mayonnaise, reduced-calorie	1 Tbsp
Nuts	
Almonds	6 whole (¼ oz)
Cashews	4 whole (¼ oz)
Chopped	1 Tbsp (¼ oz)
Peanuts	10 large (¼ oz)
	20 small
Pecans	5 halves (¼ oz)
Pistachios	15 whole (¼ oz)
Walnuts	5 halves (¼ oz)

FATS—CONT'D

Oil—corn, cottonseed, olive, safflower, soybean, sunflower	1 tsp
Olives, black	8 small
Olives, green	6 medium
Peanut butter	1½ tsp
Salad dressing, mayonnaise type	2 tsp
Salad dressing, mayonnaise type, reduced-calorie	1 Tbsp
Seeds	
Pumpkin	2 tsp (⅓ oz)
Soybean kernels	1½ Tbsp (⅓ oz)
Squash	2 tsp (⅓ oz)
Sunflower	1 Tbsp (¼ oz)

FREE VEGETABLES

Each serving is equal to ½ cup raw. If more than 2 cups of free vegetables are eaten per day, count each additional serving as ½ garden vegetable exchange.

Alfalfa sprouts	Lettuce
Cabbage	Parsley
Cabbage, Chinese	Mushrooms
Cabbage, red	Radishes
Celery	Romaine
Cucumbers	Spinach
Endive	Swiss Chard
Escarole	Watercress
Hot peppers	

FREE FOODS

Artificial sweetener	Lemon and lemon juice
Bouillon, low-fat	Lime and lime juice
Broth, low-fat	Mineral water
Butter flavorings	Mustard
Carbonated water	Nonstick pan spray
Club soda	Pickles, dill
Coffee and tea	Salad dressing, with less than
Gelatin, sugar-free	10 calories/Tbsp
Herbs and spices	Sugar-free beverages
Horseradish	Vinegar

No–Concentrated Sweets Diet

Description
Liberalized carbohydrate intake and portions may be appropriate for individuals with diabetes who cannot fully implement the standard diabetic diet. Decreased calorie intake as a result of anorexia may also necessitate a liberalization of diet.

Indications
This diet may be used for individuals with diabetes who do not require insulin or who cannot fully understand or implement the diabetic diet. It may also be used for individuals with diabetes who have a decreased appetite.

How to determine diet
No Concentrated Sweets Diet

General guidelines
1. This diet is adapted from the basic meal pattern.
2. Foods containing simple sugar are omitted.
3. Moderate fat intake is encouraged with an emphasis on reducing saturated fat.

Nutritional adequacy
This diet is planned to meet nutrient requirements in accordance with the Recommended Dietary Allowances. Individual food choice and intake will determine actual nutritional adequacy.

Meal pattern

Breakfast	Lunch/supper
Fruit or juice	Meat or substitute
Cereal	Potato or substitute
Egg	Vegetable or salad
Toast	Fruit
Milk	Bread
Margarine	Margarine
Beverage, sugar-free	Milk (supper)
Diet jelly	Beverage, sugar-free
Sugar substitute/salt/pepper	Sugar substitute/salt/pepper

Modified from *Diet manual,* Lexington, Ky, 1997, Department of Dietetics and Nutrition, University of Kentucky Hospital Chandler Medical Center.

Food pattern

FOOD GROUP	FOODS ALLOWED	FOODS OMITTED
Milk	All except chocolate Yogurt, plain	Chocolate milk Sweetened condensed milk
Eggs	Prepared any style	None
Meat and Substitutes	All meats, poultry, and fish Peanut butter Cheese	None
Fruits and Vegetables	Fresh, frozen, or prepared without sugar, honey, or syrup	Any sweetened with sugar, honey, or syrup Corn, cream style
Breads and Cereals	Whole grain or enriched breads and cereals Pasta Rice Hominy and grits Biscuits and cornbread Crackers	Doughnuts and sweet rolls Presweetened cereals Cereals that contain sugar-coated fruit pieces
Fats and Oils	Margarine and butter Oil and shortening Mayonnaise and salad dressings Gravy Sour cream	None

Desserts and Sweets	Gelatin, sugar-free
	Pudding, sugar-free
	On occasion
	  Ice cream and sherbet
	  Gelatin and custard
	  Cake, without frosting
	  Cookies, without frosting
		In excess amounts and frequency
		Pies, marshmallows, candy
		Cake with frosting

Beverages	Coffee and tea Sugar-free beverages Sugar-free, fruit-flavored beverages	Sweetened soft drinks and fruit-flavored beverages Other sweetened beverages Alcoholic beverages, unless approved by physician
Miscellaneous	Herbs and spices Sugar substitute Salt and pepper Pickles, dill	Sugar Syrup, honey, and molasses Jam, jelly, and preserves Pickles and relish, sweet

Nutrition Guidelines for Reactive Hypoglycemia

Description
A diet that is modified in carbohydrate and meal frequency may improve symptoms of reactive hypoglycemia.

Indications
The nutrition guidelines are used for reactive hypoglycemia.

How to describe diet
Hypoglycemia Diet
Specify number of feedings

General guidelines
1. Simple carbohydrates, concentrated sweets, and fruit are limited because of the potential for rapid glucose absorption and subsequent blood glucose rise.
2. Adequate protein, fat, and fiber are encouraged in combination with carbohydrate-rich foods in an attempt to blunt blood glucose response.
3. Three meals, and if needed, one, two, or three snacks, are provided.
4. The diet should be adapted to individual tolerance.
5. This diet is adapted from the basic meal pattern general guidelines, limiting fruit to 0-2 servings per day.

Nutritional adequacy
This diet is planned to meet nutrient requirements in accordance with the Recommended Dietary Allowances. Individual food choice and intake will determine actual nutritional adequacy.

Meal pattern

Breakfast	Lunch/supper
Fruit (fresh or juice pack) or unsweetened juice 0-1 serving	Meat or substitute
Cereal	Potato or substitute
Egg	Vegetable or salad
Toast	Fruit (fresh or juice pack) 0-1 serving
Milk, low-fat	Bread
Margarine	Milk, low-fat
Beverage, sugar-free	Margarine
Sugar substitute/salt/pepper	Beverage, sugar-free
Diet jelly	Sugar substitute/salt/pepper

Modified from *Diet manual,* Lexington, Ky, 1997, Department of Dietetics and Nutrition, University of Kentucky Hospital Chandler Medical Center.

Food pattern

FOOD GROUP	FOODS ALLOWED	FOODS OMITTED
Milk	All except chocolate	Chocolate milk
	Yogurt, plain or sugar-free	Sweetened condensed milk
Eggs	Prepared any style	None
Meat and Substitutes	All meats, poultry, and fish	None
	Peanut butter	
	Cheese	
Fruits and Vegetables	Fresh, frozen, or prepared without sugar, honey, or syrup	Any sweetened with sugar, honey, or syrup
		Corn, cream style
Breads and Cereals	Whole grain or enriched breads and cereals	Doughnuts and sweet rolls
	Pasta	Presweetened cereals
	Rice	Cereals that contain sugar-coated fruit pieces
	Hominy and grits	
	Biscuits and cornbread	
	Crackers	
Fats and Oils	Margarine and butter	None
	Oil and shortening	
	Mayonnaise and salad dressings	
	Gravy	
	Sour cream	
Desserts and Sweets	Gelatin, sugar-free	In excess amounts and frequency
	Pudding, sugar-free	Pies, marshmallows, candy
	Other sugar-free desserts	Cake, custard, cookies, ice cream, sherbet, or other sugar-sweetened desserts
Beverages	Coffee and tea	Sweetened soft drinks and fruit-flavored beverages
	Sugar-free beverages	Other sweetened beverages
	Sugar-free, fruit-flavored beverages	Alcoholic beverages, unless approved by physician
Miscellaneous	Herbs and spices	Sugar
	Sugar substitute	Syrup, honey, and molasses
	Salt and pepper	Jam, jelly, and preserves
	Pickles, dill	Pickles and relish, sweet

Nutrition Guidelines for Pregnancy and Lactation

Description
Additional nutrients in the form of food and vitamins are required during pregnancy and lactation.

Indications
The diet for pregnancy and lactation provides adequate nutrition to support maternal weight gain and lactation and in the adolescent to support continued growth and development.

How to determine diet
Regular diet for pregnancy/lactation; regular diet for pregnancy/lactation (adolescent).

General guidelines
1. Calorie intake should be sufficient to achieve recommended weight gain during pregnancy. Intentional weight loss is contraindicated.
2. If milk and milk products are not consumed, calcium supplementation may be indicated.
3. Between-meal feedings are offered three times per day at midmorning, midafternoon, and bedtime to increase calorie intake.
4. A sodium restriction is not indicated during pregnancy.

Minimum recommended daily food intake during pregnancy and lactation

Food group	Adult	Adolescent
Milk and dairy products	4 servings	5 servings
Meat or protein substitute	2-3 servings	3 servings
Fruits and vegetables	5 servings	5 servings
	Include a vitamin C source daily	
	Include a vitamin A source at least three times per week	
Breads and cereals	6 servings	6 servings
Fluids, other than milk	6-8 cups	6-8 cups

Modified from *Diet manual,* Lexington, Ky, 1997, Department of Dietetics and Nutrition, University of Kentucky Hospital Chandler Medical Center.

Nutritional adequacy

The diet is planned to meet nutrient requirements in accordance with the Recommended Dietary Allowances. Individual food choice and intake will determine actual nutritional adequacy. Supplementation with a prenatal vitamin is recommended because food intake may not supply adequate levels of folic acid and iron.

Meal pattern

Breakfast
Fruit or juice
Cereal
Egg or substitute
Bread
Margarine
Milk
Jelly
Sugar/salt/pepper

Midmorning
Fruit

Lunch/supper
Meat or substitute
Starch or substitute
Vegetable or salad
Margarine
Fruit or dessert
Bread
Milk
Sugar/salt/pepper

Midafternoon
Bread or starch
Milk

Bedtime
Meat or substitute
Bread or starch

Calorie requirements during pregnancy

Normal weight	13-16 kcal/lb or 29-35 kcal/kg
Underweight	17 kcal/lb or 37 kcal/kg
Overweight	11 kcal/lb or 24 kcal/kg
Adolescents	18-21 kcal/lb or 40-46 kcal/kg

Use current pregnancy weight to assess calorie needs; in morbid obesity, adjusted weight should be used.

Protein requirements during pregnancy and lactation

Pregnancy 18+ years	60 g/day
Lactation	
First 6 months	65 g/day
Second 6 months	62 g/day

Recommended weight gain during pregnancy

Normal weight	25-35 lb
Underweight	28-40 lb
Overweight	15-35 lb
Obese	15 lb
Twins	44 lb
Adolescents	35 lb

Exchange Lists for Meal Planning

STARCH LIST

Melba toast	4 slices
Oyster crackers	24
Popcorn (popped, no fat added or low-fat microwave)	3 cups
Pretzels	¾ oz
Rice cakes, 4-inch across	2
Saltine-type crackers	6
Snack chips, fat-free (tortilla, potato)	15-20 (¾ oz)
Whole-wheat crackers, no fat added	2-5 slices (¾ oz)

The Exchange Lists are the basis of a meal planning system designed by a committee of the American Diabetes Association and the American Dietetic Association. While designed primarily for people with diabetes and others who must follow special diets, the Exchange Lists are based on principles of good nutrition that apply to everyone. © 1995 American Diabetes Association, Inc., the American Dietetic Association.

Starchy foods prepared with fat
Count as 1 starch exchange, plus 1 fat exchange.

Biscuit, 2½-inch across	1
Chow mein noodles	½ cup
Corn bread, 2-inch cube	1 (2 oz)
Crackers, round butter type	6
French fried potatoes	16-25 (3 oz)
Granola	¼ cup
Muffin, small	1 (1½ oz)
Pancake, 4-inch across	2
Popcorn, microwave	3 cups
Sandwich crackers, cheese or peanut butter filling	3
Stuffing, bread (prepared)	⅓ cup
Taco shell, 6-inch across	2
Waffle, 4½-inch square	1
Whole-wheat crackers, fat added	4-6 (1 oz)

FRUIT LIST
Fruit

Apple, unpeeled, small	1 (4 oz)
Apples, dried	4 rings
Applesauce, unsweetened	½ cup
Apricots, fresh	4 whole (5½ oz)
Apricots, dried	8 halves
Apricots, canned	½ cup
Banana, small	1 (4 oz)
Blackberries	¾ cup
Blueberries	¾ cup
Cantaloupe, small	⅓ melon (11 oz)
Cantaloupe, cubes	1 cup
Cherries, sweet, fresh	12 cherries (3 oz)
Cherries, sweet, canned	½ cup
Dates	3
Figs, fresh	1½ large or 2 medium (3½ oz)
Figs, dried	1½
Fruit cocktail	½ cup
Grapefruit, large	½ grapefruit (11 oz)
Grapefruit sections, canned	¾ cup
Grapes, small	17 grapes (3 oz)
Honeydew melon	1 slice (10 oz)

Honeydew melon, cubes	1 cup
Kiwi	1 (3½ oz)
Mandarin oranges, canned	¾ cup
Mango, small	½ fruit (5½ oz) or
	½ cup
Nectarine, small	1 (5 oz)
Orange, small	1 (6½ oz)
Papaya	½ fruit (8 oz) or
	1 cup cubes
Peach, medium, fresh	1 (6 oz)
Peaches, canned	½ cup
Pear, large, fresh	½ (4 oz)
Pears, canned	½ canned
Pineapple, fresh	¾ cup
Pineapple, canned	½ cup
Plums, small	2 (5 oz)
Plums, canned	½ cup
Prunes, dried	3
Raspberries, raw	1 cup
Strawberries, whole	1 ¼ cup
Tangerine, small	2 (8 oz)
Watermelon	1 slice (13½ oz)
Watermelon, cubes	1¼ cup

Fruit juice

Apple juice/cider	½ cup
Cranberry juice cocktail	⅓ cup
Cranberry juice cocktail, reduced-calorie	1 cup
Fruit juice blends, 100% juice	⅓ cup
Grape juice	⅓ cup
Grapefruit juice	½ cup
Orange juice	½ cup
Pineapple juice	½ cup
Prune juice	⅓ cup

MILK LIST

One exchange is equal to any one of the following items.

Skim and very low-fat milk

Buttermilk, nonfat or low-fat	1 cup
Dry milk, nonfat	⅓ cup
Evaporated skim milk	½ cup
Milk, ½%	1 cup
Milk, 1%	1 cup
Skim milk	1 cup

Yogurt, nonfat or low-fat fruit-
  flavored sweetened with aspartame
  or with a nonnutritive sweetener
	1 cup

Yogurt, plain, nonfat	¾ cup

Lowfat milk

Milk, 2%	1 cup
Sweet acidophilus milk	1 cup
Yogurt, plain, lowfat	¾ cup

Whole milk

Evaporated whole milk	½ cup
Goat's milk	1 cup
Kefir	1 cup
Whole milk	1 cup

OTHER CARBOHYDRATES LIST

One exchange equals 15 grams carbohydrate or 1 starch, or 1 fruit, or 1 milk.

	Amount	Exchanges
Angel food cake, unfrosted	¹⁄₁₂th cake	2 CHO
Brownie, small, unfrosted	2-inch square	1 CHO, 1 FAT
Cake, unfrosted	2-inch square	1 CHO, 1 FAT
Cake, frosted	2-inch square	2 CHO, 1 FAT
Cookie, fat-free	2 small	1 CHO
Cookie or sandwich cookie with creme filling	2 small	1 CHO, 1 FAT
Cranberry sauce, jellied	¼ cup	2 CHO
Cupcake, frosted	1 small	2 CHO, 1 FAT
Doughnut, plain cake	1 medium	1½ CHO, 2 FAT
Doughnut, glazed	3¾-inch across	2 CHO, 2 FAT
Fruit juice bars, 100% juice	1 bar	1 CHO

Fruit snacks, chewy	1 roll	1 CHO
Fruit spreads, 100% fruit	1 Tbsp	1 CHO
Gelatin, regular	½ cup	1 CHO
Gingersnaps	3	1 CHO
Granola bar	1 bar	1 CHO, 1 FAT
Granola bar, fat-free	1 bar	2 CHO
Hummus	⅓ cup	1 CHO, 1 FAT
Ice cream	½ cup	1 CHO, 2 FAT
Ice cream, fat-free, no sugar added	½ cup	1 CHO
Ice cream, light	½ cup	1 CHO, 1 FAT
Jam or jelly, regular	2 Tbsp	1 CHO
Milk, chocolate, whole	1 cup	2 CHO, 1 FAT
Pie, fruit, 2 crusts	⅙ pie	3 CHO, 2 FAT
Pie, pumpkin or custard	⅛ pie	1 CHO, 2 FAT
Potato chips	12-18 (1 oz)	1 CHO, 2 FAT
Pudding, regular (made with low-fat milk)	½ cup	2 CHO
Pudding, sugar-free (made with low-fat milk)	½ cup	1 CHO
Salad dressing, fat-free	¼ cup	1 CHO
Sherbet, sorbet	½ cup	2 CHO
Spaghetti/pasta sauce, canned	½ cup	1 CHO, 1 FAT
Sweet roll or Danish	1 (1½ oz)	2½ CHO, 2 FAT
Syrup, light	2 Tbsp	1 CHO
Syrup, regular	1 Tbsp	1 CHO
Syrup, regular	¼ cup	4 CHO
Tortilla chips	6-12 (1 oz)	1 CHO, 2 FAT
Vanilla wafers	5	1 CHO, 1 FAT
Yogurt, frozen, fat-free, no sugar added	½ cup	1 CHO
Yogurt, frozen, low-fat, fat-free	⅓ cup	1 CHO, 0-1 FAT
Yogurt, low-fat with fruit	1 cup	3 CHO, 0-1 FAT

CHO—Carbohydrate Exchange
FAT—Fat Exchange

VEGETABLE LIST

One exchange is equal to ½ cup of cooked vegetables or vegetable juice and 1 cup of raw vegetables.

Artichoke
Artichoke hearts
Asparagus
Bean sprouts
Beans (green, wax, Italian)
Beets
Broccoli
Brussels sprouts
Cabbage
Carrots
Cauliflower
Celery
Cucumber
Eggplant
Green onions or scallions
Greens (collard, kale, mustard, turnip)
Mushrooms

Okra
Onions
Pea pods
Radishes
Peppers (all varieties)
Salad greens (endive, escarole, lettuce, romaine, spinach)
Sauerkraut
Spinach
Summer squash
Tomato
Tomatoes, canned
Tomato sauce
Tomato/vegetable juice
Turnips
Water chestnuts
Watercress
Zucchini

MEAT LIST

One meat exchange is equal to any one of the following items.

Very lean meat and substitutes list

Poultry	Chicken or turkey (white meat, no skin), Cornish hen (no skin)	1 oz
Fish	Fresh or frozen cod, flounder, haddock, halibut, trout; tuna (fresh or canned in water)	1 oz
Shellfish	Clams, crab, lobster, scallops, shrimp, imitation shellfish	1 oz
Game	Duck or pheasant (no skin), venison, buffalo, ostrich	1 oz
Cheese	With 1 gram or less fat per oz	
	Nonfat or low-fat cottage cheese	¼ cup
	Fat-free cheese	1 oz

Other	Processed sandwich meats with 1 g or less fat per oz, such as deli thin, shaved meats, chipped beef, ham, turkey	1 oz
	Egg whites	2
	Egg substitutes, plain	¼ cup
	Hot dogs, 1 gram or less fat per oz	1 oz
	Kidney (high in cholesterol)	1 oz
	Sausage, 1 gram or less fat per oz	1 oz

Count as one very lean meat and one starch exchange.

| Dried beans, peas, lentils (cooked) | ½ cup |

Lean meat and substitutes

Beef	USDA Select or Choice grades of lean beef trimmed of fat, such as round, sirloin, and flank steak; tenderloin; roast (rib, chuck, rump); steak (T-bone) porterhouse, cubed, ground round	1 oz
Pork	Lean pork, such as fresh ham; canned, cured or boiled ham; Canadian bacon; tenderloin, center loin chop	1 oz
Lamb	Roast, chop, leg	1 oz
Veal	Lean chop, roast	1 oz
Poultry	Chicken, turkey (dark meat, no skin), chicken white meat (with skin), domestic duck or goose (well-drained of fat, no skin)	1 oz
Fish	Herring (uncreamed or smoked)	1 oz
	Oysters	6 medium
	Salmon (fresh or canned), catfish	1 oz
	Sardines, canned	2 medium
	Tuna (canned in oil, drained)	1 oz
Game	Goose (no skin), rabbit	1 oz
Cheese	4.5%-fat cottage cheese	¼ cup
	Grated parmesan	2 Tbsp
	Cheese, 3 grams or less fat per oz	1 oz
Other	Hot dogs, 3 grams or less fat per oz	1½ oz
	Processed sandwich meat, 3 grams or less fat per oz, such as turkey pastrami or kielbasa	1 oz
	Liver, heart (high in cholesterol)	1 oz

MEAT LIST—CONT'D

Medium-fat meat and substitutes

Beef	Most beef products fall into this category (ground beef, meatloaf, corned beef, short ribs, prime grades or meat trimmed of fat, such as prime rib)	1 oz
Pork	Top loin, chop, Boston butt, cutlet	1 oz
Lamb	Rib roast, ground	1 oz
Veal	Cutlet (ground or cubed, unbreaded)	1 oz
Poultry	Chicken dark meat (with skin), ground turkey or ground chicken, fried chicken (with skin)	1 oz
Fish	Any fried fish product	1 oz
Cheese	With 5 g or less fat per oz	
	Feta	1 oz
	Mozzarella	1 oz
	Ricotta (2 oz)	¼ cup
Other	Egg (high in cholesterol, limit to 3 per week)	1
	Sausage, 5 g or less fat per oz	1 oz
	Soy milk	1 cup
	Tempeh	¼ cup
	Tofu (4 oz)	½ cup

High-fat meat and substitutes

Pork	Spareribs; ground pork, pork sausage	1 oz
Cheese	All regular cheese, such as American, cheddar, Monterey Jack, Swiss	1 oz
Other	Processed sandwich meats with 8 g or less per oz, such as bologna, pimento loaf, salami	1 oz
	Sausage, such as bratwurst, Italian, knockwurst, Polish, smoked	1 oz
	Hot dog (turkey or chicken)	1 (10/lb)
	Bacon	3 slices

Count as one high-fat meat plus one fat exchange.

Hot dog (beef, pork, or combination)	1 (10/lb)
Peanut butter	1 Tbsp

FAT LIST

Monounsaturated fats

Avocado, medium	⅛ avocado (1 oz)
Nuts	
almonds, cashews	6 nuts
mixed (50% peanuts)	6 nuts
peanuts	10 nuts
pecans	4 halves
Oil (canola, olive, peanut)	1 tsp
Olives: ripe (black)	8 large
green, stuffed	10 large
Peanut butter, smooth or crunchy	2 tsp
Sesame seeds	1 Tbsp
Tahini paste	2 tsp

Polyunsaturated fats

Margarine: stick, tub, or squeeze	1 tsp
lower fat (30%-50% vegetable oil)	1 Tbsp
Mayonnaise: regular	1 tsp
reduced-fat	1 Tbsp
Miracle Whip Salad Dressing: regular	2 tsp
reduced-fat	1 Tbsp
Nuts, walnuts, English	4 halves
Oil (corn, safflower, soybean)	1 tsp
Salad dressing: regular	1 Tbsp
reduced-fat	2 Tbsp
Seeds: pumpkin, sunflower	1 Tbsp

Saturated fats

Bacon, cooked	1 slice (20 slices/lb)
Bacon, grease	1 tsp
Butter: stick	1 tsp
whipped	2 tsp
reduced-fat	1 Tbsp
Chitterlings, boiled	2 Tbsp (½ oz)
Coconut, sweetened, shredded	2 Tbsp
Cream, half and half	2 Tbsp
Cream cheese: regular	1 Tbsp (½ oz)
reduced-fat	2 Tbsp (1 oz)
Fatback or salt pork	1 inch × 1 inch × ¼ inch
Shortening or lard	1 tsp
Sour cream: regular	2 Tbsp
reduced-fat	3 Tbsp

FREE FOODS

The following foods contain less than 20 calories per serving. If no serving size is specified, they may be used in unlimited amounts. If a serving size is specified, servings should be limited to three servings per day.

Drinks
Bouillon, broth, consommé
Bouillon or broth, low-sodium
Carbonated or mineral water
Club soda
Cocoa powder, unsweetened (1 Tbsp)
Coffee
Diet soft drinks, sugar-free
Drink mixes, sugar-free
Tea
Tonic water, sugar-free

Sugar-free/low-sugar foods
Candy, hard, sugar-free (1 candy)
Gelatin dessert, sugar-free
Gelatin, unflavored
Gum, sugar-free
Jam/jelly, low-sugar/light (2 tsp)
Sugar substitutes
Syrup, sugar-free (2 Tbsp)

Fat-free/reduced-fat foods
Cream cheese, fat-free (1 Tbsp)
Creamers, nondairy, liquid (1 Tbsp)
Creamers, nondairy, powdered (2 tsp)
Margarine, fat-free (1 Tbsp)
Margarine, reduced-fat (1 tsp)
Mayonnaise, fat-free (1 Tbsp)
Mayonnaise, reduced-fat (1 tsp)
Miracle Whip, nonfat (1 Tbsp)
Miracle Whip, reduced-fat (1 tsp)
Nonstick cooking spray
Salad dressing, fat-free (1 Tbsp)
Salad dressing, fat-free, Italian (2 Tbsp)
Salsa (1/4 cup)
Sour cream, fat-free, reduced-fat (1 Tbsp)
Whipped topping, regular or light (2 Tbsp)

Condiments
Catsup (1 Tbsp)
Horseradish
Lemon/lime juice
Mustard
Pickles, dill (1½ large)
Soy sauce, regular/light
Taco sauce (1 Tbsp)
Vinegar

Seasonings
Flavoring extracts
Garlic
Herbs, fresh or dried
Pimento
Spices
Tabasco/hot pepper sauce
Wine, used in cooking
Worcestershire sauce

Dietary Strategies for Vomiting

Dietary strategies (appropriate food choices decrease the likelihood of emesis):

- Cold, clear liquids are often the first foods tolerated. Begin with Popsicles, sherbets, sorbets, frozen ices, Jell-O, and beverages; establishment of tolerance before advancing increases the client's willingness to increase intake slowly. Gradual incorporation of soft, smooth foods such as ice cream, milkshakes, puddings, hot cereals, and soups is usually tolerated next, although some clients best tolerate lower-fat options.
- Vitamin tastes from many supplements may increase nausea, but Scandishakes are usually better tolerated because they can be made with a juice base.
- Small, frequent meals reduce distention and reflux.
- Cold or room-temperature foods decrease aroma-related nausea. Nurses should remove the lids to hot foods outside the room to decrease odors for clients.
- Avoid fatty, fried foods that delay stomach emptying if the client observes increased nausea and vomiting with such foods.

Behavioral strategies (simple changes around eating times may decrease nausea):

- Rest after eating, avoiding excessive movement and exercise.
- Keep the head elevated to allow gravity to work against reflux. The stomach empties fastest with client lying on the right side.
- Avoid gagging activities (mouth care, pills) immediately after eating as well as highly textured foods that stimulate gagging.
- Relaxation techniques, including guided imagery, may be beneficial.
- An initial continuous antiemetic dosage plan is best, even after the client seems to have improved. Doses can be weaned gradually to determine whether the client is doing well because of the medication or truly no longer needs it. Prevention is crucial. As-needed dosing of secondary antiemetic medications must be thoroughly explained to clients, or they will be unaware of the need to request them.

From Gates R, Fink R: *Oncology nursing secrets,* Philadelphia, 1997, Hanley & Belfus.

Overcoming Taste Problems

Eliminating problematic tastes

- Practicing good mouth care and rinsing the mouth with a solution of salt, baking soda, and warm water before eating helps to eliminate bad tastes.
- Drink fluids with meals to rinse away bad tastes. Fruit-flavored drinks such as Hi-C, Kool-Aid, or Gatorade are well tolerated; coffee and tea frequently are not.
- Use plastic eating utensils and glass or plastic cooking containers if you notice a metallic taste while eating.
- If red meats seem bitter, substitute chicken, dairy, pork, fish, and eggs as protein sources.
- Minimize odors that can affect taste by drinking fluids cold and with a straw and by choosing cold foods such as cheese, milkshakes, cold cuts, tuna and egg salad.
- Hard candies and fresh fruit eliminate bad tastes in the mouth and leave a more pleasant taste.
- Retry foods; what tastes "off" this week may work next week.
- Eat foods cold or at room temperature.

Enhancing flavors

- Use more strongly seasoned foods, such as Italian, Mexican, curried, or barbequed foods, unless you have mouth sores. These stronger flavors increase the probability you will sense the taste.
- Tart foods help to overcome metallic tastes. Use lemon, citrus or cranberry juices, and lemon drops.
- Marinate food in wine, fruit juice, soy or teriyaki sauce, Italian dressing, or barbeque sauce.
- Sauces and gravies help to spread taste through the mouth and add calories, too.
- Eat meats with something sweet, such as applesauce, jelly, glazes, or cranberry sauce.
- Salt decreases the excessive sweetness of sugary foods.

Dry mouth

- Choose moist foods, adding sauces, gravies, fat, and other lubricants whenever possible. Dry foods such as breads, crackers, or dry meats are not well tolerated alone.

- Use tart substances such as lemon juice, or suck on hard candies (especially sugarless lemon drops) to stimulate maximal production of saliva.
- Drink lots of fluids (juices, broth soups, and fruit-flavored beverages); switch to liquid diet if necessary.
- Sucking on ice chips keeps the mouth lubricated.
- Rinse your mouth frequently with a saline solution.
- Artificial saliva may be helpful, but some clients complain that such products are thick and have a sticky consistency.
- Regular mouth care is essential with decreased saliva to prevent cavities, gum disease, or mouth ulceration.

Smell sensitivity

- Choose cold foods, which lack the volatile compounds that reach the nose.
- Caretakers can reduce smells in meal preparation using fans, covered pans, microwaves, or outdoor grills.
- Friends may cook meals at their homes and bring them over, reducing the smells of preparation for the client.
- Take-out foods from restaurants may help.
- Dietary staff and nurses serving meals can reduce odors in clients' rooms by uncovering the trays in the hallway before entering.

Dietary Modifications for Diarrhea

- Complex carbohydrates (fruits and starches) are particularly well absorbed and beneficial to gut healing. However, highly insoluble fiber, such as bran, should be limited. Diarrhea is a marker of GI damage, and food safety precautions to limit introduction of pathogenic organisms is recommended.
- Avoid gastric irritants such as caffeine, pepper, and alcohol.
- Absorption of lactose may be impaired by the damage to the GI tract. The lactase enzyme is easily lost and leaves the carbohydrate available for breakdown by normal gut flora. Their metabolic byproduct is gas, which creates the bloating and cramping and, ultimately, the diarrhea associated with lactose intolerance. Alternatives to milk products include soy milk, supplements, sorbet, and

From Gates R, Fink R: *Oncology nursing secrets,* Philadelphia, 1997, Hanley & Belfus.

tofutti frozen dessert as well as lactose-free milks. Lactase tablets or drops (available over the counter) may be used if milk products are highly desired.

- Fluid replacement is essential to replace the increased losses in the stool. Nonacidic juices are well tolerated: nectars, fruit-ade drinks, Gatorade. Some clients find that it helps to avoid liquids at meal times and to limit liquids with high sugar content.

Vegetarian Diet

Description
Vegetarian diets are designed to use combinations of vegetable and plant proteins to meet essential protein needs. They are classified according to the extent animal foods are excluded.

Indications
The vegetarian diet is used for clients who choose to restrict animal products in the diet.

How to determine diet
Vegetarian diet; lacto-ovo vegetarian diet, if known; lacto vegetarian diet, if known.

General guidelines
1. Adequate calories are provided to meet energy needs and spare protein to promote efficient protein use.
2. A variety of vegetable and plant proteins are included in each vegetarian diet.
3. A variety of meat substitutes (cheese, peanut butter, nuts, dried beans/peas) are included in each vegetarian diet.
4. The vegetarian, or vegan, diet is not recommended without nutrition counseling. Nutrition counseling should include a discussion of nutrients and their sources.
5. Food preferences will be obtained to determine individual client practices and will be incorporated into the meal pattern.

From *Diet manual,* Lexington, Ky, 1997, Department of Dietetics and Nutrition, University of Kentucky Hospital Chandler Medical Center.

Nutritional adequacy

Individual food choice and intake will determine actual nutritional adequacy. More nutrients are deficient with progressive levels of restriction. Nutrients that may be deficient are high biological value protein, vitamin B_{12}, vitamin D, riboflavin, calcium, iron, and zinc. Specific nutrients are listed by classification of vegetarian diet.

Meal pattern

Breakfast
Fruit or juice
Cereal, cooked
Meat substitute
Bread
Margarine
Jelly
Sugar/salt/pepper

Lunch/supper
Vegetarian soup
Meat substitute
Starch or substitute
Vegetable or salad
Bread
Fruit or juice
Margarine
Sugar/salt/pepper

Classification of vegetarian diets

Classification	Foods allowed	Foods omitted	Limiting nutrients
Lacto-ovo	Fruits, grains, legumes, nuts, seeds, eggs, vegetables, milk/milk products	Animal meat	Iron
Lacto	Fruits, grains, legumes, nuts, seeds, vegetables, milk/milk products	Animal meat Eggs	Iron Vitamin D Calcium Riboflavin
Vegan	Fruits, grains, legumes, nuts, seeds, vegetables	All animal products	HBV protein* Iron Calcium Vitamin D Riboflavin Vitamin B_{12}

*HBV, high biological value.

Protein complement guide

Food group	Limiting essential amino acid	Protein complementation
Eggs	None	Complete protein
Grains	Lysine, isoleucine	Grains and legumes Grains and milk or eggs
Legumes	Methionine, cystine, tryptophan (except when soy protein is included in diet)	Legumes and grains Legumes and seeds or nuts
Milk products	None	Complete protein
Nuts and seeds	Lysine, isoleucine (except when cashews and pumpkin seeds are included in diet)	Nuts, seeds, and legumes
Other vegetables	Cystine, methionine, isoleucine (except spinach)	Vegetable and nuts, seeds, and legumes Vegetable and grain Vegetable and eggs or milk/milk products

Vegetarian Varieties

Nine types of vegetarians are described. They are listed here by degree of exclusion of animal foods and by the foods included in the diet.

- *Zen macrobiotics*—eat only brown rice and herb tea. This is done to achieve a perfect balance of yin and yang, to fend off disease, and to reach a higher spiritual state.
- *Vegans*—rely solely on grains, legumes, vegetables, fruits, nuts, and seeds. They refuse any source of animal protein. Some also reject the use of fortified foods or nutritional supplements.
- *Fruitarians*—eat only fresh and dried fruits, nuts, honey, and sometimes olive oil.
- *Lactovegetarians*—allow milk, cheese, yogurt, and other milk products as the only source of animal protein in their diets.
- *Ovovegetarians*—allow eggs as their only source of animal protein.

From Williams S: *Nutrition and diet therapy,* ed 8, St. Louis, 1997, Mosby.

- *Lactoovovegetarians*—consume milk and milk products as well as eggs but use no other animal products.
- *Pescovegetarians*—permit fish as the only animal product in their diets.
- *Pollovegetarians*—allow poultry as the only animal product in their diets.
- *"Red-meat abstainers"*—eat any animal product except red meat but still consider themselves vegetarians.

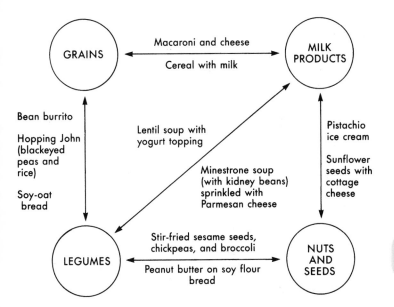

Complementary proteins. The circled items are major types of protein in many vegetarian diets. Items connected by arrows are complementary. Examples of dishes providing complementary proteins are given beside the arrows. *From Lowdermilk DL, Perry SE, Bobak IM: Maternity and women's health care, ed 6, St. Louis, 1997, Mosby.*

Fat in Selected Vegetarian Foods

Food	Fat (g)
Butter, 1 pat	4
Margarine, 1 pat	4
Salad dressing, creamy, 2 tbsp	16
Vegetable oil, 1 tbsp	14
Nuts and seeds, 1 oz	14
Peanut butter, 1 tbsp	8
Tofu, 4 oz	5
Cooked dried beans, 1 cup	1
Eggs, 1 large	6
Skim milk, 1 cup	Trace
Soy milk, 1 cup	7
Whole milk, 1 cup	8
Cheese, 3 oz	27
Ice cream, 1 cup	14
Tofu ice cream, 1 cup	2-17
Fruit, 1 medium	0
Grains, cooked, 1 cup	1
Vegetables, 1 cup	0-1
Crackers, 4	1-4
Cookies, 4	4-12
Bread, 1 slice	1
Chips, 10	7
French fries, 10	8
Olives, 4 medium	2
Avocado, half	15
Coconut, 2 tbsp	3
For comparison:	
Hamburger on bun	20

From the Vegetarian Resource Group, Baltimore.

Use this table and food labels to make choices so the total amount of fat in your diet is low. A low-fat diet does not mean never eating salad dressing again. It does mean taking a minute to think about all the food you can eat in a day and deciding if you would rather use 2 tablespoons of salad dressing or get about the same amount of fat from a tablespoon of peanut butter and 16 crackers.

The vegetarian's protein intake should be assessed especially carefully. Plant proteins tend to be "incomplete," or lacking in one or more amino acids required for growth and maintenance of body tissues. However, combinations of different types of complementary incomplete proteins, in which one protein source will be rich in an amino acid that the other protein source lacks, and vice versa, can provide sufficient amounts of complete protein. The figure on p. 383 demonstrates complementary protein combinations. It is probably not essential that complementary proteins be consumed at the same meal. It is an excellent practice to become accustomed to planning meals around complementary proteins to ensure that the diet is balanced and that all types of protein foods are included.

GENERAL GUIDELINES

Suggested Weights for Adults

Height*	Weight (in pounds)† 19 to 34	35 and over
5'0"	97-128‡	108-138
5'1"	101-132	111-143
5'2"	104-137	115-148
5'3"	107-141	119-152
5'4"	111-146	122-157
5'5"	114-150	126-162
5'6"	118-155	130-167
5'7"	121-160	134-172
5'8"	125-164	138-178
5'9"	129-169	142-183
5'10"	132-174	146-188
5'11"	136-179	151-194
6'0"	140-184	155-199
6'1"	144-189	159-205
6'2"	148-195	165-210
6'3"	152-200	168-216
6'4"	156-205	173-222
6'5"	160-211	177-228
6'6"	164-216	182-234

From *Guidelines for Americans,* U.S. Government Printing Office, 1995.
*Without shoes.
†Without clothes.
‡The higher weights in the ranges generally apply to men, who tend to have larger body frames and more muscle; the lower weights more often apply to women, who have smaller body frames and less muscle. Weights even below the range may be appropriate for some small-boned people.

Determine Your Nutritional Health

The warning signs of poor nutritional health are often overlooked. Use this checklist to find out if you or someone you know is at nutritional risk.

Nutrition checklist

Read the statements below. Circle the number in the yes column for those that apply to you or someone you know. For each yes answer, score the number in the box. Total your nutritional score.

	Yes
I have an illness or condition that made me change the kind and/or amount of food I eat.	2
I eat fewer than two meals per day.	3
I eat few fruits, vegetables, or milk products.	2
I have three or more drinks of beer, liquor, or wine almost every day.	2
I have tooth or mouth problems that make it hard for me to eat.	2
I do not always have enough money to buy the food I need.	4
I eat alone most of the time.	1
I take three or more different prescribed or over-the-counter drugs a day.	1
Without wanting to, I have lost or gained 20 pounds in the last 6 months.	2
I am not always physically able to shop, cook, and/or feed myself.	2
	Total

Total Your Nutritional Score. If it is—

0-2	Good! Recheck your nutritional score in 6 months.
3-5	You are at moderate nutritional risk. See what can be done to improve your eating habits and lifestyle. Your office on aging, senior nutrition program, senior citizens center, or health department can help. Recheck your nutritional score in 3 months.
6 or more	You are at high nutritional risk. Bring this checklist the next time you see your doctor, dietician, or other qualified health or social service professional. Talk with him or her about any problems you may have. Ask for help to improve your nutritional health.

Remember that warning signs suggest risk but do not represent diagnosis of any condition. To learn more about the warning signs of poor nutritional health, see the following text.

From Nutrition Screening Initiative, a project of the American Academy of Family Physicians, the American Dietetic Association, the National Council on the Aging, Inc, and funded in part by Ross Products Division, Abbott Laboratories.

The nutrition checklist is based on the warning signs described below; use the word DETERMINE to remind you of the warning signs.

Disease

Any disease, illness, or chronic condition that causes you to change the way you eat, or makes it hard for you to eat, putting your nutritional health at risk. Four out of five adults with chronic diseases are affected by diet. Confusion or memory loss that keeps getting worse is estimated to affect one out of five older adults. This can make it hard to remember what, when, or if you have eaten. Feeling sad or depressed, which happens to about one in eight older adults, can cause big changes in appetite, digestion, energy level, weight, and well-being.

Eating poorly

Eating too little and eating too much both lead to poor health. Eating the same foods day after day or not eating fruit, vegetables, and milk products daily will also cause poor nutritional health. One in five adults skip meals daily. Only 23% of adults eat the minimum amount of fruit and vegetables needed. One in four older adults drink too much alcohol. Many health problems become worse if you drink more than one or two alcoholic beverages per day.

Tooth loss/mouth pain

A healthy mouth, teeth, and gums are needed to eat. Missing, loose, or rotten teeth, or dentures that do not fit well or cause mouth sores, make it hard to eat.

Economic hardship

As many as 40% of older Americans have incomes of less than $6000 per year. Having less—or choosing to spend less—than $25 to $30 per week for food makes it hard to get the foods you need to stay healthy.

Reduced social contact

One third of all older people live alone. Being with people daily has a positive effect on morale, well-being, and eating.

Multiple medicines

Many older Americans must take medicines for health problems. Almost half of older Americans take multiple medicines daily. Growing old may change the way we respond to drugs. The more medicines you take, the greater the chance for side effects such as increased or decreased appetite, change in taste, constipation, weakness, drowsiness, diarrhea, and nausea. Vitamins or minerals when taken in large doses act like drugs and can cause harm. Alert your doctor to everything you take.

Involuntary weight loss/gain

Losing or gaining a lot of weight when you are not trying to do so is an important warning sign that must not be ignored. Being overweight or underweight also increases your chance of poor health.

Needs assistance in self-care

Although most older people are able to eat, one of every five has trouble walking, shopping, and buying and cooking food, especially as he or she gets older.

Elder years above age 80

Most older people lead full and productive lives. But as age increases, risk of frailty and health problems increase. Checking your nutritional health regularly makes good sense.

Notes

Family Nutritional Assessment Tool

Family members	Age	Educational level	Developmental stage
1.			
2.			
3.			
4.			
5.			
6.			

Family's perception of health status (describe)

Nutritional practices
Who decides on the menu?
Who does the grocery shopping?
Who prepares the meals?
Number of meals consumed per day?
Describe mealtime (who is present, when, where, and atmosphere).
Does mealtime serve a particular function? (For example, are the day's activities planned? Are problems discussed?)
Snacks consumed and frequency
Knows food sources from the basic four food groups
24-hour food recall

Dietary fat
Use of red meat, fish, and poultry (once a week, three times, etc.)
How often do you eat cheese? What kinds do you purchase?
How often do you use cold cuts?
How often do you use fish/chicken? (Describe preparation.)
How often do you use processed foods such as bakery products, frozen dinners?
How much milk or other dairy products do you consume? What types?

Cholesterol and saturated fat
How many eggs does the family eat per week?
What kind of fat do you use in cooking?
What kind of vegetable oil do you use?

Complex carbohydrates and fiber
How often do you eat fruit? How do you eat it (juices, fresh, canned)?
What kind of vegetables do you eat (canned, frozen, fresh)?
What kind of bread do you eat (whole grain, white)?

Sugar consumption
Do you use sugar in cooking? Do you buy candy, pastries, sweetened cereals?

From Bomar P, editor: *Nurses and family health promotion: concepts, assessment and interventions,* ed 2, Philadelphia, 1996, Saunders.

Sodium
How often do you use processed foods (canned or packaged, such as macaroni and cheese)?
Do you add salt to food?

Alcohol consumption
How often do you use alcohol?

Caffeine
How much coffee and tea do you drink per day?

Supplements
Do you take vitamins or mineral supplements? What and how much? Why?

Cultural influences
"Special" foods
Eating habits unique to culture
Family food preferences or restrictions

Economics
Do you receive any supplementary income to purchase food items?

Eating problems
Do you have problems with indigestion, vomiting, nausea, sore mouth?
Do you have any difficulty swallowing liquids or solids or chewing and feeding yourself?

Medications
Are you on any medications? Do they affect your appetite or weight?

Weight
Has weight changed in the last 6 months? How much? Describe events associated with the change.

Elimination pattern
Describe bowel and urinary patterns.

Activity and exercise patterns
Usual daily/weekly activities of family members

Source of nutrition information
Magazines, family member, schools, health food store

Family work patterns
Do family members work outside of the home? Type of work and hours?

Physical assessment

Describe appearance of the family
Height
Weight
Blood pressure
Pulse/respirations
Percent body fat

$$\text{Relative weight} = \frac{\text{Actual weight} \times 100}{\text{Ideal weight}}$$

Example:
160 (actual weight) × 100 = 16,000
16,000 divided by ideal weight of 140 = 114%
The closer relative weight is to 100%, the better.
 120 to 139 mild obesity
 140 to 159 moderate obesity
 160+ severe obesity
Family strengths/weaknesses
Identify nutritional concerns of the family
Barrier to change? Are there reasons why the family cannot change the
 problem area?

Assessment summary

Check problem area or potential problems
 1. Dietary fat
 2. Cholesterol and saturated fat
 3. Complex carbohydrates and fiber
 4. Sugar
 5. Sodium
 6. Alcohol
 7. Caffeine
 8. Supplements
 9. Cultural influences
10. Economics
11. Eating problems
12. Medications
13. Weight changes
14. Elimination pattern
15. Activity and exercise
16. Nutrition resources
17. Work patterns
18. Notes of concern

Nursing diagnosis
Plan and intervention
Evaluation

Nutritional History Guidelines for Home Care Clients

Client name _____   Marital status _____
Age _____   Family or significant
Gender _____   others _____

Primary medical diagnosis   _____

_____   _____

Height _____   _____
Weight _____   Recent weight change (note)
                                  amount, time period, and cause)
Frame (small, medium, large)   _____

_____   _____

Allergies (food or drug)   Smoking (packs per day) _____

_____   _____

Medications _____   _____

_____   _____

Describe dosage schedule for medications, that is, are they taken with meals or on an empty stomach?

Food preferences _____

_____

Food intolerances or restrictions _____

_____

Therapeutic diet or nutritional support prescription _____

_____

What does the client or family find to be the easiest and most difficult parts of the therapeutic diet or nutritional support plan?

_____

_____

What, if anything, would the client or family like to change about the therapeutic diet or nutritional support plan?

_____

_____

Usual daily dietary intake (including fluids)

_____

_____

From Sebastian T: Nutrition in home care. In Martinson I, Widmer J, editors: *Home health care nursing,* Philadelphia, 1989, Saunders.   *Continued.*

**Nutritional History Guidelines
for Home Care Clients—cont'd**

Availability of foodstuffs:
　　Who does the shopping? _____
　　Where do you shop? _____
　　Do you have transportation problems with regard to shopping?

　　_____
　　Are you limited by seasonal availability of foods? (Explain) _____

_____
Financial concerns regarding diet _____
Cultural/religious concerns _____
What is the meaning of food to this family (e.g., social or sustenance
only)? _____
Food storage:
　　Refrigeration: _____
　　Hygiene: _____
Food preparation:
　　Electricity, gas: _____
　　Functioning stove, oven: _____
　　Sufficient utensils: _____
　　Who prepares the food? _____
　　Who makes food decisions? _____
Health problems (describe in terms of onset, chronology, quality,
associated factors, aggravating factors, alleviating factors, how the
problem is managed, whether the intervention is effective) _____

_____
_____
_____
_____

　　Indigestion (pre- or post-prandial) _____
　　Dysphagia _____
　　Difficulty chewing _____
　　Diabetes _____
　　Cardiovascular disease _____
　　Hypertension _____
　　Condition of teeth/gums _____
　　Dentures (full, partial) _____

Client Teaching Guidelines for Breastfeeding

How to hold your baby for feedings

- Sit or lie down comfortably with your back supported.
- Make sure your baby has one arm on either side of your breast, as you pull the baby close.
- Use firm pillows or folded blankets under the baby to keep the baby supported during the feeding. As your baby gets older, you probably will not need the extra support.
- Support the baby's back and shoulders firmly. Do not push on the back of the baby's head.
- Once the baby's mouth is open wide, pull your baby quickly onto your breast.

Four common breastfeeding positions

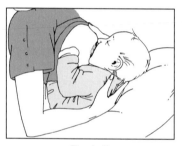

Football

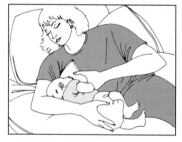

Lying down

- Hold the baby's back and shoulders in the palm of your hand.
- Tuck the baby up under your arm, keeping the baby's ear, shoulder, and hip in a straight line.
- Support the breast. Once the baby's mouth is open wide, pull the baby quickly to you.
- Continue to hold your breast until the baby feeds easily.

- Lie on your side with a pillow at your back, and lay the baby so you are facing each other.
- To start, prop yourself up on your elbow and support your breast with that hand.
- Pull the baby close to you, lining up the baby's mouth with your nipple.
- Once the baby is feeding well, lie back down. Hold your breast with the opposite hand.

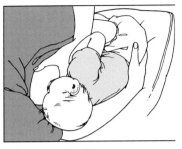

Cradling

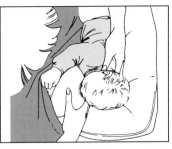

Across the lap

- Cradle the baby in the arm closest to the breast, with the baby's head in the crook of your arm.
- Have your baby's body facing you, tummy to tummy.
- Use your opposite hand to support the breast.

- Lay your baby on firm pillows across your lap.
- Turn the baby facing you.
- Reach across your lap to support the baby's neck and shoulders with the palm of your hand.
- Support your breast from underneath. Once the baby's mouth is open wide, pull your baby quickly onto your breast.

Latching-on

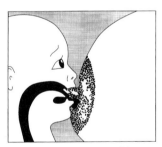

Incorrect tongue position

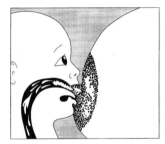

Correct tongue position

- Hold your breast in one hand with your fingers underneath and the thumb on top.
- Have your hand back from the areola (the dark skin around the nipple).
- Line up the baby's lips with your nipple.
- Touch the lips with your nipple until the baby's mouth opens and tongue is down.
- Pull the baby quickly onto the breast.
- If nursing hurts after the first few sucks, take the baby off and start over. Make sure the baby's mouth is open wide and the tongue is down before pulling the baby close.

Breastfeeding is going well when . . .

- Your newborn is feeding about eight times in 24 hours for 30 to 40 minutes at each feeding. Some newborns need to eat more frequently until they learn to breastfeed efficiently. Other babies gain weight well feeding less often.
- At least one breast softens well at each feeding.
- You feel a tug, but not pain, when the baby sucks.
- The baby's arms and shoulders are relaxed during the feeding.
- The baby has bursts of 10 or more sucks and swallows at the beginning of each feeding.
- As your breast softens, the baby slows down to two to three sucks and swallows at a time.
- Your baby is content when you finish breastfeeding.
- By the time the baby is 4 days old, you should see at least six wet diapers and three bowel movements every 24 hours.

Formula Preparation and Feeding

Your newborn baby will be hungry about every 2 1/2 to 3 hours but sometimes may go 3 to 4 hours between feedings. The newborn should not go longer than 4 hours between feedings until a weight gain pattern is established—usually about 2 weeks. Your baby needs to be awake before being fed. If your baby is sleepy, massage the baby's back and chest and talk to him or her.

Your baby's feedings will change a lot in the first week after birth. The first day most babies only drink 1/4 to 1/2 oz (7.5 to 15 ml) of formula at a feeding. By the time they are a week old, most babies drink 1 to 2 oz (30 to 60 ml) at a feeding and then gradually increase their intake as they grow. If you do not use all the formula at a feeding, throw away what is left, because it spoils once it has mixed with the baby's saliva.

You may want to write down how many ounces (milliliters) your baby drinks each day. When you take the baby in for a checkup, the physician or nurse will ask you about how much formula the baby drinks. By a week old, most babies who weigh 7 to 10 lb (3 to 4.5 kg) are drinking about 28 oz (840 ml) in 24 hours. Smaller babies drink a little less. Babies weighing more than 10 lb (4.5 kg) drink about 32 oz (960 ml) each day.

From Lowdermilk D, Perry S, Gobak I: *Maternity and women's health care,* ed 6, St. Louis, 1997, Mosby.

To feed your baby, place the nipple in the baby's mouth on the tongue. It should touch the roof of the mouth to stimulate the baby's sucking reflex. Hold the bottle like a pencil. Keep the bottle tipped so the nipple stays filled with milk and the baby does not suck in air.

Hold your baby close for feedings. This should be a pleasant time for social interaction and cuddling. Some newborns take longer to feed than others. Be patient. It may be necessary to keep the baby awake and encourage continued sucking. Moving the nipple gently in the baby's mouth may stimulate more sucking.

Some newborns swallow air when sucking. Give your baby a chance to burp several times during early feedings. As your baby gets older and you get more experienced, you will know when to stop for burping.

If your baby fusses or cries in between feedings, check the diaper to see if it should be changed and see if the baby needs to be picked up and cuddled. If the baby continues to cry and acts hungry, then he or she needs to be fed. Babies do not get hungry on a schedule.

By placing your baby on the right side after feedings, air bubbles can come up easily. A rolled-up receiving blanket or small towel against the baby's back will keep him or her in the side-lying position. Some babies sleep better on their backs. To decrease the risk of sudden infant death syndrome (SIDS), however, it is important not to put your baby stomach down to sleep.

The stools of a formula-fed newborn are yellow and soft but formed. The baby will probably have a bowel movement during or after each feeding in the first 2 weeks, but this will then gradually decrease to one to two stools each day.

Safety tips
- Babies should be held and never left alone while feeding. Do not prop the bottle. The baby could inhale formula or choke on any that was spit up.
- Know how to use the bulb syringe in case your baby should choke.
- Drinking bottles of formula or juice while falling asleep can cause tooth decay in your children (nursing bottle caries).

Formula preparation
- Wash your hands and clean the bottle, nipple, and can opener carefully before preparing formula.
- If new nipples seem too hard, they can be softened by boiling them for 5 minutes before use.
- Read the label on the container of formula and mix it exactly according to the directions.

- Use tap water to mix concentrated or powdered formula, unless directed otherwise by your baby's physician or nurse.
- Test the size of the nipple hole by holding a prepared bottle upside down. The formula should drip from the nipple. If it runs in a stream, the hole is too big and should not be used. If it has to be shaken for the formula to come out, the hole is too small. You can either buy a new nipple or enlarge the hole by boiling the nipple for 5 minutes with a sewing needle inserted in the hole.
- If a nipple collapses when your baby sucks, loosen the nipple ring a little to let in air.
- Opened cans of ready-to-feed or concentrated formula should be covered and refrigerated. Any unused portions must be discarded after 48 hours.
- Bottles of unopened formula can be stored at room temperature.
- If the formula is refrigerated, warm it by placing the bottle in a pan of hot water. Never use a microwave to warm any food to be given to a baby. Test the temperature of the formula by letting a few drops fall on the inside of your wrist. If the formula feels comfortably warm to you, it is the correct temperature.

Notes

Modifying Behavior to Promote Weight Loss or Maintenance

1. Chew food slowly, and put utensils down between bites.
2. Never shop for food on an empty stomach.
3. Make out a grocery shopping list before starting, and do not add to it as you shop.
4. Leave a small amount of food on your plate after each meal.
5. Fill your plate in the kitchen at the start of the meal; do not put open bowls of food on the table.
6. Eat in only one or two places (e.g., the kitchen and dining room table).
7. Never eat while involved in any other activity, such as watching television.
8. Do not eat while standing.
9. Keep a diary of when and where you eat and under what circumstances (e.g., boredom, frustration, anxiety). Be aware of problem circumstances, and substitute another activity for eating.
10. Keep low-calorie snacks available at all times.
11. Reward yourself for weight loss (e.g., buy new clothes, treat yourself to concert tickets or a trip). Establish a step-wise set of goals with a reward for achieving each goal.
12. If you violate your diet on one occasion, do not use that as an excuse to go off the diet altogether. Acknowledge that setbacks happen, and return to your weight control program.
13. When confronted with an appealing food, remember that this will not be your last chance to have the food. Content yourself with a small portion.

From Moore M: *Nutritional care,* ed 3, St. Louis, 1997, Mosby.

CONTROLLING FAT IN THE DIET

Dietary Principles for Low-fat and Fat-free Diets

Low-fat diet

General description

- This diet contains foods that are low in fat.
- Foods are prepared without the addition of fat.
- Fatty meats, gravies, oils, cream, lard, avocados, and desserts containing eggs, butter, cream, and nuts are avoided.
- Foods should be used in amounts specified and only as tolerated.
- The sample pattern contains approximately 85 g protein, 50 g fat, 220 g carbohydrates, and 1670 kcal.

	ALLOWED	NOT ALLOWED
Beverages	Skim milk, coffee, tea, carbonated beverages, fruit juices	Whole milk, cream, evaporated and condensed milk
Bread and cereals	All kinds	Rich rolls or breads, waffles, pancakes
Desserts	Jell-O, sherbet, water ices, fruit whips made without cream, angel food cake, rice and tapioca puddings made with skim milk	Pastries, pies, rich cakes and cookies, ice cream
Fruits	All fruits, as tolerated	
Eggs	Three allowed per week, cooked any way except fried	Avocados
Fats	Three tsp butter or margarine daily	Fried eggs
Meats and fish	Lean meat such as beef, veal, lamb, liver, lean fish and fowl, baked, broiled, or roasted without added fat	Salad and cooking oils, mayonnaise Fried meats, bacon, ham, pork, goose, duck, fatty fish, fish canned in oil, cold cuts
Cheese	Dry or fat-free cottage cheese	All other cheeses
Potato or substitute	Potatoes, rice, macaroni, noodles, spaghetti, all ~~prepared without added fat~~	Fried potatoes, potato chips

Soups	Bouillon or broth, without fat; soups made with skim milk	Cream soups
Sweets	Jam, jelly, sugar, sugar candies without nuts or chocolate	Chocolate, nuts, peanut butter
Vegetables	All kinds as tolerated	The following should be omitted if they cause distress: broccoli; cauliflower; corn, cucumber, green pepper, radishes, turnips, onions, dried peas, and beans
Miscellaneous	Salt in moderation	Pepper, spices, highly spiced food, olives, pickles, cream sauces, gravies

Suggested menu pattern

Breakfast
Fruit
Cereal
Toast, jelly
1 tsp butter or margarine
Egg 3 times per week
Skim milk, 1 cup
Coffee, sugar

Lunch and dinner
Meat, broiled or baked
Potato
Vegetable
Salad with fat-free dressing
Bread, jelly
1 tsp butter or margarine
Fruit or dessert, as allowed
Skim milk, 1 cup
Coffee, sugar

Fat-free diet

General description

The following additional restrictions are made to the low-fat diet to make it relatively fat free:

1. Meat, eggs, and butter or margarine are omitted.
2. A substitute for meat at the noon and evening meal is 84 g (3 oz) of fat-free cottage cheese.

From Williams S: *Nutritional and diet therapy*, ed 8, St. Louis, 1997, Mosby.

Fat and Cholesterol Content of Selected Foods

Make a habit of reading nutrient labels on foods. They will give information similar to that shown on the food table below, which gives examples of some commonly eaten foods and their fat, cholesterol, and caloric contents.

Food	Serving size	Calories	Fat (g)	Saturated fat (g)	Cholesterol (mg)	Sodium (mg)
Dairy products						
Milk						
Fluid whole	1 cup	150	8.2	5.1	33	120
Skim	1 cup	86	0.4	0.3	4	126
Cheese						
Cheddar	1 oz	114	9.4	6.0	30	176
Cottage—creamed	½ cup	109	4.7	3.0	16	425
Cottage—low fat, 1% fat	½ cup	82	1.2	0.7	5	459
Mozzarella, part skim	1 oz	72	4.5	2.9	16	132
Eggs (whole, raw)	1 med	79	5.6	1.7	213	69
Fats and oils						
Peanut butter (smooth)	2 tsp	63	5.5	0.9	0	52
Butter	1 tsp	36	4.1	2.5	11	41
Tub margarine						
Safflower oil	1 tsp	34	3.8	0.4	0	51
Corn oil	1 tsp	34	3.8	0.7	0	51

Meat, poultry, fish

Food						
Lean beef, average all grades, cooked	1 oz	63	2.9	1.1	25	18
Beef liver, braised	1 oz	46	1.4	0.5	110	30
Lean pork, center loin, fresh, broiled	1 oz	65	3.0	1.0	28	22
Bacon, pan-fried, 4½ slices	1 oz	163	14	5.0	24	452
Frankfurters (beef and pork)	1 oz	91	8.3	3.1	14	318
Chicken, flesh without skin (stewed)						
Light meat	1 oz	45	1.1	0.3	22	18
Dark meat	1 oz	54	2.5	0.7	25	21
Fish						
Flounder, cooked, dry heat	1 oz	33	0.4	0.1	19	30
Salmon, coho, cooked, moist heat	1 oz	52	2.1	0.4	14	17
Tuna, light, canned in water drained solids	1 oz	37	0.1	0.1	—	101
Shellfish						
Lobster, Northern, cooked, moist heat	1 oz	28	0.2	Trace	20	108
Shrimp (cooked)	1 oz	28	0.3	0.1	55	63

Food Tips to Reduce Fat, Saturated Fat, and Cholesterol

- Use fats and oils sparingly in cooking.
- Use small amounts of salad dressings and spreads, such as butter, margarine, and mayonnaise. Try reduced or nonfat substitutes.
- Choose lean cuts of meat and trim visible fat.
- Take skin off poultry before eating the meat.
- Have cooked dry beans and peas instead of meat occasionally.
- Moderate the use of organ meats and egg yolks. An egg a day is okay for people whose serum cholesterol levels are normal.
- Choose skim or low-fat milk and nonfat or low-fat yogurt and cheese most of the time.
- Check labels on foods to see how much fat and saturated fat are in a serving.
- Choose liquid vegetable oils most often because they are lower in saturated fat.
- Choose a diet with plenty of grain products, vegetables, and fruits.
- Eat more vegetables, legumes, fruits, breads, cereals, pasta, and rice. A varied diet that emphasizes these foods supplies important vitamins and minerals, fiber, and complex carbohydrates and is generally lower in fat.
- It is better to get fiber from foods that contain fiber naturally than from supplements. Some of the benefit of a high-fiber diet may come from the food that provides the fiber, not from the fiber alone.

From Edelman C, Mandle C: *Health promotion throughout the lifespan,* ed 4, St. Louis, 1998, Mosby.

Figure Out Your Fat

The recommendation is that no more than 30% of total calories come from fat. Food labels list fat in grams. To find out what *your* total intake of fats in grams should be limited to, multiply your daily calories by 0.30 (30%) and divide by 9 (the number of calories in a gram of fat).

Example: 2200 calories × 0.30 = 660 calories from fat
660 calories ÷ 9 = 73 g of fat

From Grodner M et al.: *Foundations and clinical applications of nutrition,* St. Louis, 1996, Mosby.

EATING DISORDERS

Eating Disorder Definitions

According to the American Psychiatric Association, a person diagnosed as bulimic or anorectic must have all of that disorder's specific symptoms:

Bulimia nervosa

- Recurrent episodes of binge eating (minimum average of two binge-eating episodes a week for at least 3 months)
- A feeling of lack of control over eating during the binges
- Regular use of one or more of the following to prevent weight gain: self-induced vomiting, use of laxatives or diuretics, strict dieting or fasting, or vigorous exercise
- Persistent overconcern with body shape and weight

Anorexia nervosa

- Refusal to maintain weight that is over the lowest weight considered normal for age and height
- Intense fear of gaining weight or becoming fat, even though underweight
- Distorted body image
- In women, three consecutive missed menstrual periods, without pregnancy

From Food and Drug Administration, DHHS pub # 92-1194, HFI-40, 1994, Rockville, Md.

Clinical Manifestations of Bulimia and Anorexia

1. Loss of tooth enamel
2. Tooth decay
3. Infection of the mouth
4. Gastrointestinal bleeding
5. Gastritis or esophagitis

   } associated with vomiting of food and gastric acid

6. Malnutrition
7. Loss of rectal tone
8. Loss of minerals and bone mass
9. Diarrhea

   } associated with purging

10. Amenorrhea
11. Hyperactivity without fatigue
12. Agitated behavior
13. Disorganized thinking
14. Excessive weight loss
15. Sleep disorder
16. Epigastric pain

From Phipps WJ et al: *Medical-surgical nursing: concepts and clinical practice,* ed 5, St. Louis, 1995, Mosby.

Guidelines for Teaching the Client With an Eating Disorder

Educating the client about the eating disorder is important. Elements of the teaching include the following:

1. Disease concept of eating disorders
2. Medical aspects of the disease
3. The need for an adequate and prudent diet
4. The importance of finding healthy ways to cope with life
5. The awareness of an increased tendency to transfer obsessions
6. Signs and symptoms of relapse
7. Importance of aftercare
8. Importance of a stable support system

Expected Outcomes for the Client With an Eating Disorder

Expected outcomes for the client with bulimia or anorexia include but are not limited to the following:

1. Maintains optimal nutrition
2. Maintains adequate hydration
3. Remains free of infection
4. Demonstrates improved activity tolerance
5. Maintains positive body image
6. Verbalizes improved self-esteem
7. Demonstrates improved management of anxiety
8. Demonstrates improved and effective coping mechanisms
9. Admits that bulimia or anorexia is a problem in his or her life
10. Verbalizes a plan to carry out desired health related behavior
11. Verbalizes knowledge of disease and treatment
12. Demonstrates increased ability to cope with interpersonal encounters and social isolation

Evaluation

To evaluate the effectiveness of nursing interventions, compare client behaviors with those stated in the expected client outcomes. Successful achievement of client outcomes for the client with anorexia or bulimia is indicated by the following:

1. Sustains weight gain
2. Has good skin turgor with moist and pink mucous membranes
3. Does not have nosocomial infection
4. Able to be up and about without assistance and able to do own activities of daily living
5. Speaks positively about own body image, and exhibits pleasure at change in appearance
6. Demonstrates improved self-esteem by speaking positively about self
7. Appears less anxious and sits or lies quietly without exhibiting nervousness
8. Demonstrates improved coping mechanisms by being less angry and frustrated and not withdrawing when things do not go as planned

---

From Phipps WJ et al.: Cassmeyer V: *Medical-surgical nursing: concepts and clinical practice,* ed 5, St. Louis, 1995, Mosby.

9. Verbalizes that bulimia or anorexia is a problem that is affecting his or her life and needs to be addressed
10. Discusses how to maintain weight at desired level, participates in moderate exercise, and attends Overeaters Anonymous (OA) meetings regularly
11. Discusses his or her disease, how to care for self, how to avoid complications, and the need for regular follow-up
12. Interacts more comfortably with a variety of persons

Size Acceptance Scale

Assessing size attitudes

This behavior assessment can be used to evaluate your support for the health and well-being of large people. Use the following scale to indicate the frequency of each behavior.

1—never   2—rarely   3—occasionally   4—frequently   5—daily

How often do you:	Never				Daily
1. Make negative comments about your fatness	1	2	3	4	5
2. Make negative comments about someone else's fatness	1	2	3	4	5
3. Directly or indirectly support the assumption that no one should be fat	1	2	3	4	5
4. Disapprove of fatness (in general)	1	2	3	4	5
5. Say or assume that someone is looking good because she or he has lost weight	1	2	3	4	5
6. Say something that presumes that a fat person wants to lose weight	1	2	3	4	5
7. Say something that presumes that fat people should lose weight	1	2	3	4	5
8. Say something that presumes that fat people eat too much	1	2	3	4	5
9. Admire or approve of someone for losing weight	1	2	3	4	5
10. Disapprove of someone for gaining weight	1	2	3	4	5
11. Assume that something is wrong when someone gains weight	1	2	3	4	5
12. Admire weight-loss dieting	1	2	3	4	5
13. Admire rigidly controlled eating	1	2	3	4	5
14. Admire compulsive or excessive exercising	1	2	3	4	5
15. Tease or admonish someone about his/her eating (habits or choices)	1	2	3	4	5
16. Criticize someone's eating to a third person ("so-and-so eats way too much junk")	1	2	3	4	5
17. Discuss food in terms of good/bad	1	2	3	4	5

Continued.

From Kano S: Size acceptance scale, *Obesity and Health,* Jan/Feb 1994, p. 14.

Size Acceptance Scale—cont'd

18. Talk about "being good" and "being bad" in reference to eating behavior	1	2	3	4	5
19. Talk about calories (in the usual dieter's fashion)	1	2	3	4	5
20. Say something that presumes being thin is better (or more attractive) than being fat	1	2	3	4	5
21. Comment that you do not wear a certain style because "it makes you look fat"	1	2	3	4	5
22. Comment that you love certain clothing because "it makes you look thin"	1	2	3	4	5
23. Say something that presumes that fatness is unattractive	1	2	3	4	5
24. Participate in a fat joke by telling one or laughing/smiling at one	1	2	3	4	5
25. Support the diet industry by buying their services and/or products	1	2	3	4	5
26. Undereat and/or exercise obsessively to maintain an unnaturally low weight	1	2	3	4	5
27. Say something that presumes being fat is unhealthy	1	2	3	4	5
28. Say something that presumes being thin is healthy	1	2	3	4	5
29. Encourage someone to let go of guilt	1	2	3	4	5
30. Encourage or admire self-acceptance and self-appreciation/love	1	2	3	4	5
31. Encourage someone to feel good about his/her body as is	1	2	3	4	5
32. Openly admire a fat person's appearance	1	2	3	4	5
33. Openly admire a fat person's character, personality, or actions	1	2	3	4	5
34. Oppose/challenge fattism (intolerance) verbally	1	2	3	4	5
35. Oppose/challenge fattism (intolerance) in writing	1	2	3	4	5
36. Challenge or voice disapproval of a fat joke	1	2	3	4	5
37. Challenge myths about fatness and eating	1	2	3	4	5
38. Compliment ideas, behavior, character, etc. more often than appearance	1	2	3	4	5
39. Support organizations that advance fat acceptance (with your time or money)	1	2	3	4	5

Behaviors 1 to 28 are unhelpful or harmful; look over areas that need improvement and strive to avoid these and similar behaviors in the future. Behaviors 29 to 39 help support size acceptance; reread items you marked "never" (1) or "rarely" (2); make a list of realistic goals for increasing supportive behavior.

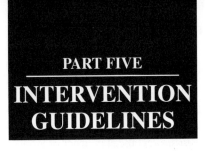

PART FIVE

INTERVENTION GUIDELINES

Often the nurse, in addition to teaching, must carry out clinical procedures in the home. The following guides will help the nurse establish and execute needed care. This list is not considered to be exhaustive but is to be used as a reference for common activities of the nurse.

TECHNIQUES FOR THE NURSE

Hand Washing Technique

1. Use a sink with warm running water, soap, and paper towels.
2. Push wristwatch and long uniform sleeves up above wrists. Remove jewelry, except a plain band, from fingers and arms.
3. Keep fingernails short and filed.
4. Inspect the surface of the hands and fingers for breaks or cuts in the skin and cuticles. Report such lesions when caring for highly susceptible clients.
5. Stand in front of the sink, keeping hands and uniform away from the sink surface. (If hands touch the sink during hand washing, repeat the process.) Use a sink where it is comfortable to reach the faucet.
6. Turn on the water. Turn on hand-operated faucets by covering the faucet with a paper towel.
7. Avoid splashing water against your uniform or clothes.
8. Regulate flow of water so the temperature is warm.
9. Wet hands and lower arms thoroughly under running water. Keep the hands and forearms lower than the elbows during washing.
10. Apply 1 ml of regular or 3 ml of antiseptic liquid soap to the hands, lathering thoroughly. If bar soap is used, hold it throughout the lathering period. Soap granules and leaflet preparations may be used.

Modified from Perry AG, Potter PA: *Clinical nursing skills and techniques,* ed 4, St. Louis, 1998, Mosby.

11. Wash the hands, using plenty of lather and friction for at least 10 to 15 seconds. Interlace the fingers and rub the palms and back of hands with a circular motion at least 5 times each.
12. If areas underlying fingernails are soiled, clean them with fingernails of the other hand and additional soap or a clean orangewood stick. Do not tear or cut the skin under or around the nail.
13. Rinse hands and wrists thoroughly, keeping hands down and elbows up.
14. Repeat steps 10 through 12 but extend the actual period of washing for 1-, 2-, and 3-minute hand washings.
15. Dry the hands thoroughly from the fingers up to the wrists and forearms.
16. Discard paper towel in proper receptacle.
17. To turn off a hand faucet, use a clean, dry paper towel.

Remember to treat the inside of your "black bag" as clean. Always wash hands before removing supplies and equipment from bag or putting clean supplies in the bag. Carry soap and paper towels in outside packets of your bag or at inner top.

Sterilizing Equipment in the Home

Moist-heat sterilization

1. When boiling equipment, have a large pan with handles on both sides and a lid and use wide-mouth jars.
2. It is best to boil equipment about 1 hour before use. It will then be sterile and cool enough to handle.
3. Always boil equipment immersed in water in a covered pan. Start timing after water begins to boil and boil for 10 minutes.
4. If equipment will not be used for a while, keep the lid on the pan until ready for use.

Dry-heat sterilization

1. You can use any metal pan such as a cake or pie pan to sterilize dressings in the oven.
2. Place the clean dressings, wrapped in a clean cloth, into the pie tin and bake in a preheated oven at 350° F for 1 hour. Wrap the cloth so that you will not contaminate the dressings upon unwrapping. Let cool slightly before using.

Modified from Humphrey C: *Home care nursing handbook,* Baltimore, 1994, Aspen.

Solutions

Solutions used as disinfectants

Bleach—undiluted is used for spillage of body fluids, that is, blood, vomitus, and excreta for clients with hepatitis.

Bleach—diluted in a mixture of 1:10 can be used for cleaning contaminated surfaces when caring for clients with AIDS.

Lysol solution should be mixed as directed on bottle. Never use anywhere near food. All items in contact with solution should be rinsed well.

White vinegar in a mixture of 1:3 can be used to disinfect respiratory and tracheostomy equipment. First, wash equipment well with friction and soap and water. Place in vinegar solution and store in a closed container. Allow to air dry before using.

Solutions for wounds and irrigations

Although solutions used for dressing changes and some irrigation procedures can be purchased already prepared and sterilized, client situations often demand that these solutions be made in the home. If high cost, lack of financial resources, long-term use, and lack of transportation are factors in purchasing supplies, the nurse can best ensure that procedures are complied with if clients or their families are taught how to make their own solutions in the home.

Procedures for making and storing solutions in the home are given below in a simple format that can be taught to clients. Once a procedure is established, solutions can be made easily in the home without danger to the client and can result in saving a great deal of money. Things to remember when using solutions in the home are as follows:

- Teach the family cleaning techniques.
- Use a safe container, such as canning jars or mayonnaise jars.
- Label all solutions with name and date prepared.
- Keep solutions out of reach of small children and pets.

Sterile water. A new container of sterile water should be made *daily*. Once the solution is made, the jar should be stored in a cool place.

Equipment: Large pan with a lid, small-mouth glass jar with a lid (1-quart size; a mayonnaise jar is a good choice), tap water.

From Humphrey C: *Home care nursing handbook,* ed 3, Baltimore, 1998, Aspen.

Procedure
1. Fill the jar to the top with tap water.
2. Stand the jar up in the pan, and fill up the pan with enough water to cover the jar. Drop the jar lid into the pan, and be sure it sinks to the bottom.
3. Cover the pan, bring the water to a boil, and boil for 20 minutes.
4. After 20 minutes, remove the pan from heat, cool, and pour off enough water from the pan so that you can handle the jar comfortably or use tongs that also have been boiled. Touching only the outside of the jar, take the jar out of the pan, and set it on a counter.
5. Pour off the remaining water in the pan, remove the jar lid, touching only the outside of the rim, and place it on the jar.

Note: This procedure can be followed to prepare an empty sterile jar and lid. Water can be boiled in another container and poured into the sterile, empty jar, the lid attached and the water stored.

Normal saline. Normal saline is simply water mixed with a certain amount of salt that is compatible with all body fluids. You should make a new batch of normal saline every 24 hours.

Equipment: Table salt (iodized or noniodized), tap water, teaspoon, measuring cup, quart jar with lid, and pan.
Strength: Normal saline: 0.9%
Procedure
1. Wash teaspoon, measuring cup, jar, and lid in hot soapy water, and rinse well in hot water.
2. Boil at least 6 cups of tap water in a pan for 20 minutes and let cool.
3. Pour 4 cups of the boiled water into a clean jar.
4. Add 2 teaspoons of salt, using the clean teaspoon. Replace the jar lid, and shake well to mix the salt with the water.
5. Write the date on which you made the solution on the outside of the jar.

Dakin's solution. Dakin's solution can be made from bleach. Bleach is 5.25% sodium hypochlorite, and full-strength Dakin's solution is 0.5% sodium hypochlorite. The solution is good only for 7 days because it deteriorates.

Equipment: Bleach, sterile water (see procedure above), a pint glass jar with cover, and a teaspoon that has been boiled for 20 minutes.

Strength: half strength (0.25) = 25 mL per pint of sterile water. Full strength (0.50) = 50 mL per pint of sterile water.

Procedure

1. Into the sterile jar, put the amount of bleach desired to achieve the strength ordered.
2. Add enough sterile water to fill to the top. The water does not have to be cooled before adding to the bleach if the solution is to be used immediately. If the solution is to be stored, it is preferable to cool the water before adding to the bleach.
3. Cover with a sterile lid and store in a cool place.

Chloramine-T. Chloramine-T, or chlorozone solution, is similar to Dakin's solution in terms of activity. It is more stable and lasts longer but should not be used in place of Dakin's solution without the permission of the physician. It is used in 1% or 2% solutions applied in the same manner as Dakin's solution. You must have chlorozone tablets (purchased by prescription) to make this solution.

Equipment: Chlorozone tablets, sterile water, and a small container.
Strength: For 1% chlorozone, use one tablet to 1 ounce of water. For 2% chlorozone, use two tablets to 1 ounce of water.
Procedure: Mix chlorozone tablet(s) and water together in a small, clean container.

Acetic acid. Acetic acid can be made with white vinegar because vinegar contains 5% acetic acid. Acetic acid may be used for dressings but should not be used for bladder irrigations; the acid can cause a negative effect on kidney function. Even though the solution can be kept in the refrigerator for 1 week, a fresh solution made daily is preferable.

Equipment: White distilled vinegar, sterile water, 1.5-quart (or larger) glass bowl, jar with lid, tablespoon, measuring cup, and large pan.
Strength: 0.25 acetic acid = 4 tablespoons vinegar in 5 cups of boiled water.

Procedure

1. Wash tablespoon, measuring cup, jar, and lid in hot, soapy water. Rinse well in hot water.
2. Boil at least 6 cups of water in the pan for 20 minutes, and let cool.
3. Add 4 tablespoons of white, distilled vinegar, and mix well.
4. Put the lid on the jar, and write the date on a label on the outside of the jar.

Improvised Equipment

Bed cradle

To alleviate the pressure of the covers over the feet of a bed-bound client, try any of the following:

- Lay a lightweight walker on the bed to support the covers.
- Put a small, open-legged television table under the covers, with the tabletop facing the foot of the bed. This can also serve as a footboard.
- Use an empty cardboard box with the top cut off to allow the client room to move the feet.

Bed table

A bed table can be improvised with the following methods:

- Place the longer end of an adjustable-height ironing board across the bed.
- Cut out the two wide sides of a cardboard or wooden box, and place the box over the client's lap.

Footboards

When footboards are unavailable, high-top canvas basketball sneakers work well in keeping the client's feet aligned to prevent foot drop. They should be worn with cotton socks and rotated with a schedule of 4 hours on and 4 hours off to keep the feet dry and healthy.

Bed rails

- A card table can be used as a bed rail. Simply open two legs and slip them under the mattress. Make a soft cushion against the card table with pillows or blankets. This should not be used with a very active client, but it can be helpful in ensuring the safety of an elderly or sedated client or a young child.
- High-back chairs can be placed against the bed, and heavy items, such as books, can be placed on the chairs to keep them in place.
- To assist clients who need to practice walking with safety, arrange six or eight sturdy chairs, such as dining room chairs, in two rows so that the backs form a walkway. The client can practice walking with the same support as parallel bars would provide.

Modified from Humphrey C: *Home care nursing handbook,* ed 3, Baltimore, 1998, Aspen.

Feeding tubes

- If a client or caregiver has difficulty giving a feeding through the small lumen of the feeding tube because of poor vision and/or tremors, a funnel can be attached to the tube. The feeding mixture is prepared and poured from a see-through glass or plastic measuring cup. This allows for accuracy in the amount of feeding and ensures that the client gets the feeding in a relaxed atmosphere.
- A plastic or wooden golf tee can be used as a plug for a feeding tube that must be clamped between feedings.

Irrigation syringe

- A turkey baster can be used for irrigating wound areas with such solutions as normal saline or Dakin's solution.
- A large syringe can be attached to a rubber catheter to irrigate deep, tunneled wounds.

Elastic stockings

Elastic stockings are easier to put on when x-ray film is placed inside each elastic stocking to keep it open while the client puts it on. Satin-toe socks are helpful in getting the client's feet into stockings and also keep the feet warm.

Soaking of extremities

If the client must soak a hand or foot in a prescribed, nonsterile solution, pour the solution into a plastic bag, and have the client put the extremity in the bag. Fasten the bag with a rubber band and place the bag in a bucket of warm water. The water not only warms the solution but also causes it to rise in the bag to the level of the water in the bucket. The client uses less solution to cover the hand or foot for each soak and saves money.

Making a temporary eye shield*

Many serious eye injuries seen in offices and clinics call for a metal eye shield to protect the eye while the client travels to a hospital or to another physician's office. If one is not available, create a disposable shield by cutting a circle with a 5- to 6-inch diameter out of a client folder. Remove a 1-inch "pie slice" and then pull the sides together with tape to form a slightly conical shape. This makes a sturdy, light-weight eye shield (Figure 15).

---

*Modified from Brewer T: Making a temporary eye shield, *Consultant* 78(12):53, 1988.

Figure 15

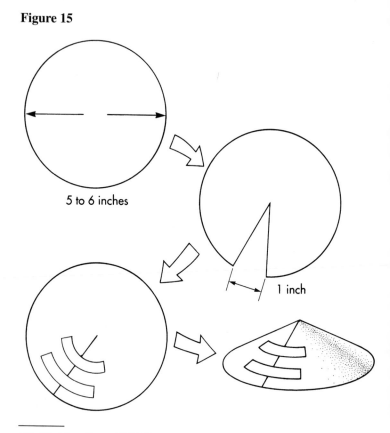

5 to 6 inches

1 inch

*Modified from Brewer T: Making a temporary eye shield, *Consultant* 78(12):53, 1988.

Notes

Specimen Collection Techniques

Specimen source	Amount needed*	Collection device*	Specimen collection and transfer
Wound	As much as possible (after cleaning skin to remove flora)	Cotton-tipped swab or syringe	Have clean test tube or culturette tube on clean paper towel. After swabbing center of wound site, grasp collection tube by holding it with paper towel. Carefully insert swab without touching outside of tube. After washing hands and securing tube's top, transfer tube into bag held by nurse outside room.
Blood	10 ml per culture bottle, from two different venipuncture sites	Syringe and culture media bottles	Perform venipuncture at two different sites to decrease likelihood of both specimens being contaminated by skin flora. Have second nurse at client's door holding culture bottles and swabbing off bottletops with alcohol. Change needles after venipuncture. Inject 10 ml of blood into each bottle. Nurse at doorway secures tops of bottles, labels specimens, and sends to laboratory.
Stool	Small amount, approximate size of a walnut	Clean cup with seal top (not necessary to be sterile) and tongue blade	Place cup on clean paper towel in client's bathroom. Using tongue blade, collect needed amount of feces from client's bedpan. Transfer feces to cup without touching cup's outside surface. Wash hands and place seal on cup. Transfer specimen into clean bag held by nurse outside room.
Urine	1-5 ml	Syringe and sterile cup	Place cup or tube on clean towel in client's bathroom. Use syringe to collect specimen if client has a Foley catheter. Have client follow procedure to obtain a clean voided specimen if not catheterized. Transfer urine into sterile container either by injecting urine from syringe or pouring it from used container. Wash hands and secure top of container. Transfer specimen into clean bag held by nurse outside room.

From Potter PA, Perry AG: *Fundamentals of nursing; concepts, process, and practice*, ed 4, St. Louis, 1997, Mosby.
*Agency policies may differ on type of containers and amount of specimen material required.

Peritoneal Dialysis and Continuous Ambulatory Dialysis

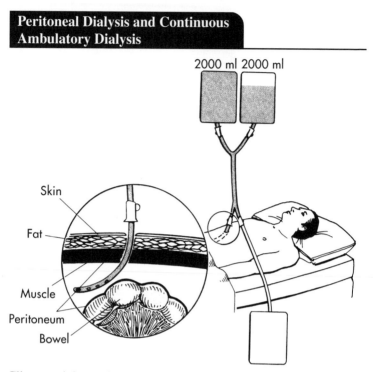

Client receiving peritoneal dialysis. Dialysis fluid is being inserted into peritoneal cavity. *From Phipps WJ et al.:* Medical-surgical nursing: concepts and clinical practice, *ed 5, St. Louis, 1995, Mosby.*

Assessment

1. Obtain client's weight.
2. Obtain vital signs.
3. Assess respiratory rate and auscultate lungs.
4. Measure abdominal girth.
    a. Mark midpoint of client's abdomen. Keep mark as reference for future measurements.
5. Inspect catheter site for erythema, tenderness, and drainage.
6. Measure body temperature.
7. Review dialysis procedure for IPD or CAPD.
8. Review physician's orders:
    a. Verify 12-24 exchanges with specific dialysate volume and composition, as well as specific dwell time and drain time.
    b. Verify dialysis solution and any medications added to solution.

From Perry A, Potter G: *Clinical nursing skills and techniques,* ed 4, St. Louis, 1998, Mosby.

9. Obtain laboratory data as ordered:
   a. PD: every 12 to 24 hours.
   b. CAPD can vary depending on individual needs.
10. Assess client's knowledge of dialysis.

Evaluation

1. Obtain weight.
2. Obtain dialysis fluid balance.
3. Obtain vital signs.
4. Obtain body temperature.
5. Measure abdominal girth.
6. Inspect catheter site for erythema, tenderness, and drainage.
7. Auscultate lungs for crackles.
8. Inspect returned dialysate solution.
9. Observe client performing CAPD.
10. Assess client's comfort level.
11. Monitor lab work.

Expected outcomes

1. Decreased weight.
2. Stable vital signs.
3. Decreased abdominal girth.
4. No erythema, tenderness, drainage at catheter site.
5. No fever.
6. Dialysate return is clear or slightly light yellow.
7. Client is able to discuss principles of asepsis and dialysis.
8. Client or caregiver will perform CAPD.

Unexpected outcomes

1. Increased weight or no weight change
2. Positive fluid balance
3. Decreased blood pressure and tachycardia
4. Increased abdominal girth
5. Erythema, tenderness, drainage at catheter site
6. Fever
7. Dialysate drainage abnormal:
   a. Cloudy
   b. Bright red blood
   c. Brown color or presence of stool
8. Cramps
9. Sudden respiratory distress
10. Poor installation flow
11. Poor drainage

12. Leaking dialysate from peritoneum
13. Leak at catheter site

Recording and reporting

1. Document client's weight, abdominal girth, and dialysis fluid balance before and after PD.
2. Document client's vital signs before, during, after dialysis.
3. Document temperature and status of catheter site.
4. Record color of drainage.
5. Record condition of catheter dressing or if new dressing applied.
6. Note any unexpected outcomes and action taken by nurse and physician.
7. Record presence or absence of pain or discomfort.

Follow-up activities

1. Remove catheter if the following occur:
   a. Signs of local infection
   b. Catheter displacement
2. Stop dialysis and notify physician for:
   a. Change in vital signs
   b. Respiratory distress
   c. Bright red blood
   d. Fecal contents in drainage
   e. Scrotal swelling
   f. Complaints of cramps
   g. Leak of fluid
   h. Inability to drain fluid from catheter

Special considerations

- Fever is early sign of catheter-induced peritonitis.
- Changes in blood pressure and increased respiratory rate may signal intolerance to amount of fluid instilled in peritoneal cavity.
- Large volume of dialysate instilled may give client urge to defecate.
- Client receiving PD should be encouraged to move around in bed. However, movements should avoid stressing catheter or tubing.
- CAPD clients have increased abdominal girth during dwell time of exchange.
- Clients on CAPD may experience fresh weight gain caused by dextrose absorption.
- Follow CDC guidelines for proper disposal of materials.

Teaching considerations
- Teach CAPD clients scrub and exchange procedures according to policy.
- Review teaching plan with client before discharge and during each visit.
- Ask client to correctly demonstrate scrub and exchange procedure.
- Periodically review potential complications and signs and symptoms.
- Instruct client about common symptoms of fluid excess and deficit.
- Review medications and dietary and fluid restrictions.
- Instruct client when and whom to contact in emergency.
- Instruct client to correctly take blood pressure.
- Instruct client to correctly weigh self.
- Instruct client about common symptoms associated with peritonitis.

Home care considerations
CAPD clients must do the following to correctly complete CAPD exchanges:

Achieve goals under planning.

Demonstrate CAPD scrub and aseptic exchange.

State signs of infection.

Adhere to fluid, dietary, and medication therapies.

Perform activities of daily living. CAPD is designed so client can maintain normal daily activities.

Cast Care

So now you or a member of your family is wearing a cast. The cast is only one of several devices used to promote the healing of broken bones. Doctors also use traction and pins, or a combination of the three, to help heal broken bones. The cast has the advantage of being less expensive, requiring little care on your part, and allowing you to move around. The cast also encloses and immobilizes the broken bone and injured soft tissues to prevent movement that could cause further injury and to keep the bone in place for proper healing.

From *Mosby's patient teaching guides,* St. Louis, 1995, Mosby.

Your cast may be made of plaster or of a synthetic material such as fiberglass. Although the plaster cast is heavy, the doctor can mold a plaster cast more easily for a close fit over severe injuries. The synthetic cast is lightweight and easier to move around, making it good for elderly patients. Your cast has a name. If it covers your forearm or lower leg, it is a **short arm** or **short leg** cast. A **long leg** cast covers the whole leg, and a **hanging** cast covers the whole arm and forearm. The **body** cast encircles the chest and abdomen, whereas the **Minerva** cast covers the chest, neck, and head with openings for the ears, face, and arms. The cast that covers the hips and one or both legs is the **hip spica** or **spica** cast.

Things to watch for

Your cast will be warm at first because of the setting process. However, warm areas on the cast later on may indicate infection, and you should notify your doctor at once.

You should watch for increased pain or soreness under the cast, particularly around bony prominences such as the wrist or ankle, that is not relieved by repositioning the body. Check the skin color and temperature periodically. When the tip of a finger or the big toe that protrudes from the cast is squeezed until it is white, the pink color should return within 2 to 4 seconds. If skin color does not return within 4 to 6 seconds or if the skin is red, blue, white, or discolored, notify your doctor. If fingers or toes are cool, cover them. If they do not warm up in 20 minutes, call your doctor. Call your doctor immediately if any of these other symptoms occur:

- An increase in swelling and pain
- A tingling or burning sensation inside the cast
- An inability to move muscles around the cast
- A foul odor detected from the edges of the cast
- Any drainage, which may show through the cast
- Any cracks or breaks in the cast
- Marked loosening of the cast allowing the parts inside the cast to move fairly easily

The first 24 hours

Your cast needs at least 24 hours to dry if it is plaster. Avoid handling it as much as possible. When you do have to move the cast, such as when you change your body position, use only the palms of your hands and support the cast under your joints. You want to avoid putting indentations in the cast that will put pressure on the skin inside. You may use a fan placed 18 to 24 inches from the cast to aid its drying in the first 24 hours. You should be sure to expose the whole cast for drying, and do not cover it for the first 24 hours to aid drying.

Keep the cast and extremity above the level of the heart for at least 48 hours by propping your cast up on firm pillows. Put ice directly over the fractured area for 24 hours, but be sure to enclose the ice in a plastic bag to keep the cast dry. Move the parts of your body above and below the cast regularly to aid circulation and relieve stiffness. Massaging the joints and extremities around the cast will also improve circulation.

How to care for your cast

If you have a plaster cast, do not get the cast wet because it will lose its strength. To keep the cast clean and dry, you should cover it with plastic when bathing, using the toilet (if it is a spica cast), or going out in rain or snow. You may use a damp cloth and scouring powder to clean soiled spots on the cast. Be sure to brush away plaster crumbs or other objects from the edges of the cast, but do not remove any padding.

If you have a synthetic cast and you do not have any open areas under the cast, your doctor may allow you to bathe and swim with it. You should use only a small amount of mild soap around your cast and should rinse under your cast thoroughly. If you swim in a pool or a lake, be sure to rinse both the inside and outside of the cast to flush out any dirt and chemicals. Dry your cast and stockinette thoroughly each time they get wet to avoid excess moisture on your skin. Use a towel to blot moisture off the cast, then dry it with a hair dryer set on low. When your cast does not feel cold and damp, it is dry.

Skin care is very important during the time a cast is worn. Do not insert objects under the cast, because you could scrape the skin or add pressure and cause an infection or sore under the cast. You should use powders and lotions only outside the cast so that the skin stays clean and soft. Powder inside a cast can cake and cause sore areas.

Do not walk on a leg cast for the first 48 hours. If you are allowed to walk on it, be sure to walk on the walking heel. If your arm is in a cast, be sure to use your sling for support and comfort.

Once your cast has been taken off, you should not try to scrub away the flaky skin and old skin cells all at once. Soften and condition your skin with a dampened cloth and Woolite, which contains enzymes that loosen the dead cells so they will wash off easily without injuring the remaining skin cells. Gently wash the skin with water and Woolite, let the Woolite stay on the skin for 5 to 10 minutes, then rinse it off thoroughly. Pat your skin dry—do not rub it, because you could cause a sore to develop. After the skin is dry, apply a moisturizing lotion. Repeat the cleaning and lotion the next day, after which your skin should be nearly normal again.

The part that was in the cast may be sore and weak for several days or longer. You may need to limit use of the part for a period of time (1 to 4 weeks) until the muscles have become stronger. You may also need to take a mild pain medication such as aspirin or acetaminophen for a day or so to relieve the soreness of reuse.

Also, you may have some swelling of the part after the cast is removed. Elevating the part for 1 to 3 days should help relieve the swelling.

Remember, it takes time for the muscles and joints that had been injured and were in the cast to regain their strength, flexibility, and full functions. Try to build up to full use over 1 to 4 weeks, so these tissues have time to adjust to being used again. Easy does it.

Application of Male External Catheter

The external application of a urinary drainage device is a convenient, safe method of draining urine in male clients. The condom catheter is suitable for incontinent or comatose clients who still have complete and spontaneous bladder emptying. The condom is a soft, pliable rubber sheath that slips over the penis. A strip of elastic adhesive is placed around the top of the condom to secure it. The catheter may be attached to a leg drainage bag or a standard urinary drainage bag.

A condom catheter may remain in place for 24 hours, but must be monitored every 4 hours to detect problems. With each catheter change, the nurse cleanses the urethral meatus and penis thoroughly and looks for signs of skin irritation.

Assessment

1. Assess urinary elimination patterns, ability to voluntarily urinate, and continence.
2. Assess mental status of client so appropriate teaching related to condom can be implemented.
3. Assess condition of penis.
4. Assess client's knowledge of the purpose of a condom catheter.

Evaluation

1. Observe urinary drainage.
2. Inspect within 30 minutes after application. Look for swelling and discoloration and ask client about discomfort.

From Perry A, Potter P: *Clinical nursing skills and techniques,* ed 4, St. Louis, 1998, Mosby.

3. Remove condom and inspect skin on penile shaft for signs of breakdown or irritation at least daily during hygiene and when condom is reapplied.

Expected outcomes are based on goals of care:

1. Client is continent with condom catheter intact.
2. Penile shaft is free of skin irritation or breakdown.

Unexpected outcomes that may occur include the following:

1. Skin around penis is reddened and excoriated.
2. Urination is reduced or infrequent.
3. Urine leaks from tubing.
4. Penis swells.

Special considerations

- Condom catheter is suitable for incontinent or comatose male clients with complete and spontaneous bladder emptying.
- Check policy to determine if physician's order is required to apply condom.
- Procedure should be explained, even if client is comatose, because client may be able to hear.
- Some apply thin layer of plasticized skin spray to skin of penile shaft to protect skin from ulceration and irritation caused by rubber condom and adhesive holding it in place.
- Never use adhesive tape because it is too constrictive.
- Have leg assessed every 8 hours for circulatory problems.

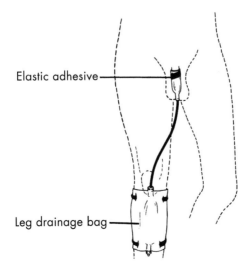

Elastic adhesive

Leg drainage bag

EMERGENCY PROCEDURES

Sequence of CPR in Adults and Children

CPR/Rescue breathing	Maneuver	Summary of ABCD maneuvers		
		Adult (8 years of age and older)	**Child** (1-8 years of age)	**Infant** (less than 1 year of age)
Establish unresponsiveness; activate EMS system or appropriate resuscitation team.				
A. **Open airway** (head tilt–chin lift or jaw thrust)	**Airway**	Head tilt–chin lift (If trauma is present, use jaw thrust.)	Head tilt–chin lift (If trauma is present, use jaw thrust.)	Head tilt–chin lift (If trauma is present, use jaw thrust.)
B. **Check for breathing** (look, listen, and feel)	**Breathing** Initial	2 breaths at 1½-2 sec/breath	2 breaths at 1-1½ sec/breath	2 breaths at 1-1½ sec/breath
If victim is breathing or resumes effective breathing, place in the recovery position.	Subsequent	12 breaths/min (approximate)	20 breaths/min (approximate)	20 breaths/min (approximate)
If victim is not breathing, give 2 slow breaths using pocket mask or bag-valve mask. Allow for exhalation between breaths.	Foreign-body airway obstruction	Heimlich maneuver	Heimlich maneuver	Back blows and chest thrusts
C. **Check pulse** (carotid in child and adult; brachial or femoral in infant)	**Circulation** Pulse check Compression landmarks	Carotid Lower half of sternum	Carotid Lower half of sternum	Brachial or femoral One finger width below intermammary line

Compression method	Heel of one hand, other hand on top	Heel of one hand	Two or three fingers
Compression depth	1½-2 inches	1-1½ inches or approximately one third to one half the depth of chest	½-1 inch or approximately one third to one half the depth of chest
Compression rate	80-100/min	100/min	At least 100/min (newborn: 120/min)
Compression/ventilation ratio	15:2 (single rescuer) 5:1 (two rescuers, pause for ventilation until trachea is intubated)	5:1 (pause for ventilation until trachea is intubated)	5:1 (pause for ventilation until trachea is intubated) 3:1 for intubated newborn (two rescuers)
Defibrillation AED	Per local EMS protocol	Not yet recommended for use in infants and children	

If pulse is present but breathing is absent, provide rescue breathing (1 breath every 5-6 seconds for adult, 1 breath every 3 seconds for infant or child).

If pulse is absent, begin chest compressions interposed with breaths.

If pulse is present but less than 60 beats/min in infant or child with poor perfusion, begin chest compressions. Continue basic life support. Integrate procedures appropriate for newborn resuscitation, pediatric advanced life support, or advanced cardiac life support at earliest opportunity.

D. Defibrillation

Defibrillation using automated external defibrillators (AEDs) is now considered an integral part of basic life support by healthcare providers.

From *Handbook of emergency cardiovascular for healthcare providers*, 1997, Copyright American Heart Association.

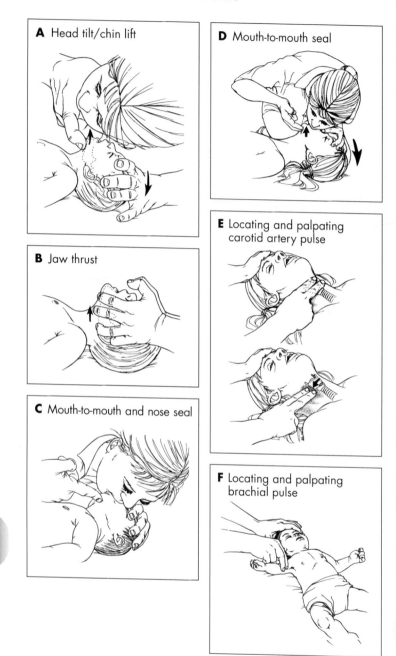

Figure 16 Procedures for CPR, **A** to **H,** and airway obstruction, **I** to **K.**
From Chandra NC, Hazinski MF, editors: Textbook of basic life support for healthcare providers, *Dallas, 1994, American Heart Association.*

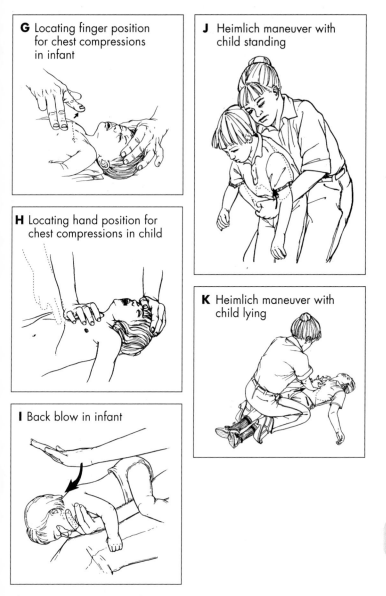

G Locating finger position for chest compressions in infant

H Locating hand position for chest compressions in child

I Back blow in infant

J Heimlich maneuver with child standing

K Heimlich maneuver with child lying

Figure 16, cont'd. Procedures for CPR, **A** to **H,** and airway obstruction, **I** to **K.**

Heimlich Abdominal Thrust Maneuver

1. Stand behind victim.
2. Encircle arms around victim's waist.
3. Place one fist between umbilicus and sternum with thumb against abdomen.
4. Place second hand over fist.
5. Press on abdomen with quick upward thrusts.
6. For infants, the chest thrusts are delivered with two fingers over the breastbone between the nipples. The baby's head should be lower than the chest for thrusts.
7. Start mouth-to-mouth resuscitation if breathing stops.

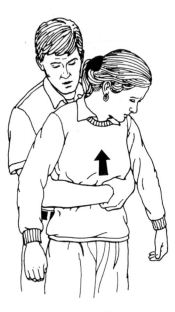

Heimlich abdominal thrust maneuver. Rescuer places fist between umbilicus and xiphoid process with the thumb pressed against the abdomen. Pressure is applied upward.

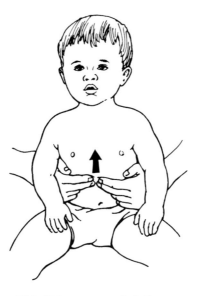

Heimlich maneuver in infants.

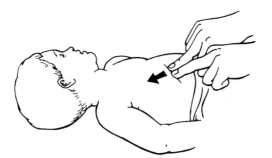

Signs and Symptoms in Early and Late Shock

	Early shock	Late shock
Respiratory system	Hyperventilation; ↑ minute volume; ↓ $Paco_2$; normal Pao_2; bronchodilation	Respirations shallow; breath sounds may suggest congestion; ↑ $Paco_2$, ↓ Pao_2; pulmonary edema; ↓ pulse oximetry
Cardiovascular system	Blood pressure normal to slightly lowered; ↑ diastolic pressure; ↓ pulse pressure; tachycardia; cardiac output normal in hypovolemic shock, slightly decreased in cardiogenic shock, and increased in septic shock; mild vasoconstriction in hypovolemic and cardiogenic shock; vasodilation in septic shock	↓ Blood pressure; ↓ cardiac output; tachycardia continues; vasoconstriction worsens in hypovolemic, cardiogenic, and septic shock
Renal system	Decreased urine output; ↑ urine osmolality; ↓ urine sodium concentration; hypokalemia	Oliguria or complete renal shutdown; hyperkalemia; buildup of waste products
Acid-base balance	Respiratory alkalosis	Metabolic acidosis; respiratory acidosis
Vascular compartment	Fluid shift from interstitial space to intravascular compartment; thirst	Fluid shift from intravascular space to interstitial and intracellular spaces, causing edema
Skin	Minimal to no changes in hypovolemic and cardiogenic shock; warm, flushed skin in septic shock	Cool, clammy skin in hypovolemic, cardiogenic, and septic shock; cool, mottled skin in neurogenic and vasogenic shock
Hematological system	Release of red blood cells (RBCs) from bone marrow to increase vascular volume; platelet aggregation	Disseminated intravascular coagulation (DIC); ↓ hematopoiesis leading to ↓ white blood cells, ↓ hemoglobin, ↓ hematocrit, ↓ platelets
Mental-neurological system	Restless; alert; confused	Lethargy; unconsciousness
GI-hepatic system	No obvious changes	Perfusion decreases; bowel sounds possibly diminished; gastric distension; nausea, vomiting

From Phipps WJ, Sands J, Marek J: *Medical-surgical nursing: concepts and clinical practice*, ed 6, St. Louis, 1999, Mosby.
$Paco_2$, carbon dioxide pressure; Pao_2, oxygen pressure.

Types of Shock

Hypovolemic	Shock from loss of fluid from vascular system (through blood loss or fluid loss)
Cardiogenic	Shock from inability of heart to pump blood to tissues (decreased cardiac output)
Distributive	Shock from massive vasodilation (from interference with sympathetic nervous system or effects of histamine or toxins)

Notes

Clinical Manifestations of Hypovolemic Shock

Parameter (for a 70-kg male)	Class I early	Class II moderate	Class III major or progressive	Class IV severe or profound
Approximate blood volume loss (ml)	Up to 750	750-1500	1500-2000	2000 or more
% of blood volume	Up to 15%	15%-30%	30%-40%	40% or more
Neurological/behavioral status	Slightly anxious	Mildly anxious, restless; muscle fatigue and weakness evident	Agitated, confused; progressive decrease in activity; progressive thirst evident	Stuporous, lethargic, unconscious; dilated pupils may be evident
Heart rate	<100	>100 Mild tachycardia	>120 Tachycardia	140 or higher Irregular pulse, decreased pulse amplitude
Blood pressure	Normal	Normal	Decreased	Severe hypotension
Pulse pressure (mm Hg)	Normal or increased	Decreased	Decreased	Decreased
Respirations	14-20, normal	20-30, normal	30-40, hyperpnea	>35, shallow, irregular
Urine output (ml/hr)	30 or more	20-30	5-15	Negligible
Capillary blanch test	Normal	Slight delay	Defined delay	No refilling observed
Skin	Pale flushed, slightly cool	Slightly cold, pale	Cold and moist	Cold and cyanotic, mottled

From McQuillian KA, Wiles CE: Initial management of traumatic shock. In Cardona DV et al., editors: *Trauma nursing from resuscitation through rehabilitation*, Philadelphia, 1988, WB Saunders.

FIRST AID

First Aid Tips

A physician should be called immediately for all serious injuries or suspected poisoning.

Bruises—Rest injured part. Apply cold compresses for half hour (no ice next to skin). If skin is broken, treat as a cut. For wringer injuries always consult physician without delay.

Scrapes—Use wet gauze or cotton to sponge off gently with clean water and soap.

Bleeding—To control most bleeding, apply a compress directly over a wound. Place the cleanest material available (sterile gauze is best) over the wound and press firmly until the bleeding stops or until a physician reaches the victim. A bandage can also be used to keep the material in place. If blood is spurting out of the wound, it is an indication that an artery has ruptured and, in addition to the direct pressure on the wound, you also should apply firm pressure with your finger at a point located about 2 inches above the wound. Tourniquets are used only when the bleeding cannot be controlled in any other way, such as in cases where a limb has been severed or severely mangled.

Cuts—Minor—Wash with clean water and soap. Hold under running water. Apply sterile gauze dressing. Major—Apply dressing. Press firmly to stop bleeding—use tourniquet only if necessary. Bandage. Secure medical care. *Do not* use iodine or other antiseptics before the physician arrives.

Puncture wounds—Consult physician immediately.

Slivers—Wash with clean water and soap. Remove with tweezers or forceps. Wash again. If large or deep, consult physician.

Nosebleeds—In sitting position blow out from the nose all clot and blood. Insert into the bleeding nostril a wedge of cotton moistened with any of the common nose drops. With the finger against the outside of that nostril apply firm pressure for 5 minutes. If bleeding stops remove packing (no rush, here). Check with a physician if bleeding persists.

From Chemical Specialties Manufacturers Association: *Your child and household safety,* Washington, DC, 1988, The Association.

These are basic first aid principles to be used in case of an emergency until professional help can be obtained or consulted. Any person relying solely upon this information does so at his or her own risk.

Fainting and unconsciousness—Keep in flat position. Loosen clothing around neck. Summon physician. Keep client warm. Keep mouth clear. Give nothing to swallow.

Convulsions—Contact physician. If caused by fever, sponge body with cool water; apply cold cloths to head. Lay on side with hips elevated. Biting of tongue is rare, but be sure that the tongue is not blocking the passage of air to the lung.

Head injuries—*Do not* move unless additional danger would occur to injured person. Consult physician immediately.

Poisoning—See following First Aid Treatment for Poisoning Tool.

Bites or stings—(A) Insect—Remove stinger *at base* if present. Do not squeeze stinger as it is removed. Cold compresses. Consult physician promptly if there is *any* reaction. (B) Animal—Wash with clean water and soap. Hold under running water for 2 or 3 minutes if not bleeding profusely. Apply sterile dressing. Consult physician. If possible, catch or retain the animal and maintain alive for observation regarding rabies. Notify police or health officer. (C) Human—(Can be serious) Wash thoroughly with soap and water. See physician for severe bites. (D) Snake—Nonpoisonous—No treatment necessary. If there is a question, treat as "Poisonous." Poisonous—(Keep calm and work fast.) Complete rest. Apply constricting band above the bite (not too tight). Get victim to physician or hospital immediately.

Burns and scalds—If caused by chemicals: Wash burned area thoroughly with water. Consult physician. Bring chemical container to physician or hospital. Extensive burns—Keep client in flat position. Remove clothing from burned area—*If adherent, leave alone.* Cover with clean cloth. Keep client warm. Take client to hospital or to a physician at once. *Do not* use ointments, greases, powder, etc. Application of cold water or compresses to minor burns relieves pain. Electric burns with shock may require artificial respiration.

Fractures—Any deformity of injured part usually means a fracture. *Do not* move person if fracture of leg or back is suspected. Summon physician at once. If person *must* be moved, immobilize with adequate splints.

Sprains—Elevate injured part. Apply cold compresses for half hour. If swelling is unusual, do not use injured part until seen by physician.

Eyes—To remove foreign bodies, *do not* use a moist cotton swab. Irrigate thoroughly with water. Immediate and copious irrigation with plain water is procedure for most chemicals splashed in eyes. Contact physician or hospital immediately.

Choking—The American Red Cross and the American Heart Association both agree that the recommended first aid for choking victims is the abdominal thrust, also known as the Heimlich maneuver. **Slaps on the back are no longer advised and may even prove detrimental in an attempt to assist a choking victim.**

First Aid Treatment for Poisoning

In all cases except poisonous bites, the principle of first aid is to get the poison **out** or **off,** or to **dilute** it. Always call a **physician, hospital, poison control center,** or **rescue unit promptly.** The following are safe first aid measures for various types of poisoning:

I. Swallowed poison
  A. Dilute chemical or household product poisons by giving water or milk, one or two glassfuls.
  B. Make client vomit if so directed. *But not if:*
    1. Client is unconscious or having seizures.
    2. Swallowed poison was a strong corrosive (lye, strong acid, drain cleaner, etc.).
    3. Swallowed poison contains kerosene, gasoline or other petroleum distillates (unless directed otherwise or containing a dangerous pesticide or chemical which must be removed).
  C. To induce vomiting
    1. Give one tablespoonful (1/2 ounce) of Syrup of Ipecac for a child 1 year of age or older, plus at least 1 cup of water. *Never substitute milk or carbonated fluids.* If no vomiting occurs in 20 minutes, this dose may be repeated once only. Older children and adults can be given 2 tablespoonsful (1 ounce) at one time. After vomiting has ceased, offer a mixture of activated charcoal (2 to 4 tablespoonsful) in a glass of water. Palatable suspensions are available.
    2. If no Ipecac syrup is available, try to induce vomiting by tickling back of throat with a spoon handle or other blunt object, after giving water.
    3. *Do not* give salt or mustard to children.
    4. *Do not* waste time waiting for vomiting, but transport victim promptly to a medical facility. Bring package or container with intact label.

From Chemical Specialties Manufacturers Association: *Your child and household safety,* Washington, DC, 1988, The Association.

II. Fumes or gases—for example, fuel gases, auto exhaust, dense smoke from fires or fumes from poisonous chemical.

A. Get victim into fresh, clean air.

B. Loosen clothing.

C. If victim is not breathing, start artificial respiration promptly. *Do not* stop until victim is breathing well, or help arrives.

D. Have *someone else* call a physician, hospital, poison control center, or rescue unit.

E. Transport victim to a medical facility promptly.

III. Eye

A. Gently wash eye out immediately, using plenty of water (or milk in an emergency), for 5 minutes with eyelids held open.

B. Remove contact lenses if worn; *never* permit the eye to be rubbed.

C. Call physician, hospital, poison control center, or rescue unit and transport victim to a medical facility promptly.

IV. Skin (acids, lye, other caustics, pesticides, etc.)

A. Wash off skin immediately with a large amount of water; use soap if available.

B. Remove any contaminated clothing.

C. Call physician, hospital, poison control center, or rescue unit and transport victim to a medical facility if necessary.

V. Poisonous bites

A. Snakes

    1. Do not let victim walk; keep victim as quiet as possible.

    2. Do not give alcohol.

    3. Call physician, hospital, poison control center, or rescue unit, and transport victim promptly to a medical facility.

    En route, or while awaiting transportation

    4. Apply suction to bite wound with mouth or suction cup.

    5. If victim stops breathing, use artificial respiration.

B. Insects (spiders, scorpions, or unusual reaction to other stinging insects such as bees, wasps, and hornets)

    1. Do not let victim walk or exercise.

    2. Place any available cold substance on bite area to relieve pain.

    3. A paste of Adolph's Meat Tenderizer or baking soda applied to the bite will often reduce the swelling and itching by its enzymatic action.

    4. If victim stops breathing, use artificial respiration.

    5. Call physician, hospital, poison control center, or rescue unit, and transport victim promptly to a medical facility. (Persons with known unusual reactions to insect stings should carry emergency treatment kits and an emergency identity card.)

C. Animal bites

Bat and skunk bites, and other unprovoked animal bites, may be from a rabid animal. Call physician or medical facility; wash wound gently but thoroughly with soap and water.

D. Poisonous marine animals

Apply any cold substance to relieve pain. (For "sting ray," heat is better.) Call physician or medical facility if reaction is severe.

Pediculosis

Identification. Infestation of the head, the hairy parts of the body or clothing (especially along the seams of inner surfaces), with adult lice, larvae, or nits (eggs), which results in severe itching and excoriation of the scalp or body. Secondary infection may occur with ensuing cervical lymphadenitis. Crab lice usually infest the pubic area; they may infest facial hair (including eyelashes), axillae, and body surface.

Incubation period. Under optimal conditions the eggs of lice hatch in 7 to 10 days.

Methods of control

A. Preventive measures:
1. Avoid physical contact with infested individuals and their belongings, especially clothing and bedding.
2. Health education of the public in the value of laundering clothing and bedding in hot water (55° C or 131° F for 20 minutes) or dry cleaning to destroy nits and lice.
3. Regular direct inspection of all primary school children for head lice and, when indicated, of body and clothing, particularly of children in schools, institutions, nursing homes, and summer camps.

B. Control of infested persons, contacts, and the immediate environment:
1. Report to local health authority: Official report not ordinarily justifiable; school authorities should be informed.
2. Isolation: Contact isolation until 24 hours after application of effective insecticide.

Modified from Benenson A: *Control of communicable diseases manual,* ed 16, Washington, DC, 1995, American Public Health Association.

3. Concurrent disinfection: With body lice in members of a family or group, to include clothing, bedding and other appropriate vehicles of transmission (e.g., cosmetic articles), treated by laundering in hot water, by dry cleaning, or by application of an effective chemical insecticide and ovicide. After chemical treatment has been completed, clothes and laundry facilities should be rinsed adequately.

4. Quarantine: None.

5. Immunization of contacts: Does not apply.

6. Investigation of contacts: Examination of household and other close personal contacts, with concurrent treatment as indicated.

7. Specific treatment: For head and pubic lice, 1% permethrin cream rinse (Nix) (not recommended for infants, young children, and pregnant or lactating women), pyrethrins synergized with piperonyl butoxide (A-200 Pyrinate, RID, and XXX), 0.5% malathion (Prioderm) carbaryl, and benzyl benzoate and 1% gamma benzene hexachloride lotions (Lindane, Kwell) are effective. Retreatment after 7 to 10 days is recommended to ensure that no eggs have survived. For body lice: Clothing and bedding should be washed with the hot cycle of an automatic washing machine, or, if not available, dusted with powders containing 1% lindane or, preferably, in view of widespread resistance to lindane, 1% malathion or pyrethrins with piperonyl butoxide or carbaryl, and then laundered before using. Abate (temephos) as a 2% dusting powder is also effective and is recommended by WHO for use in areas where strains of body lice are resistant to malathion.

Removal of a Tick

1. Put on gloves.

2. Use curved forceps or tweezers to remove tick.

3. Grasp tick firmly as close to the skin as possible and pull upward with a steady, even pressure. Do not twist or jerk.

4. Try not to squeeze or crush the body of the tick because its fluids may contain infectious agents.

5. After removal, wash the site with soap and water. Clean with a disinfectant.

6. Contact a physician if signs of a reaction (or symptoms) occur within the next few weeks.

Checklist of Treatment for Animal Bites

1. Cleanse and flush wound immediately (first aid).
2. Thorough wound cleansing under medical supervision.
3. Rabies immune globulin or vaccine as indicated.
4. Tetanus prophylaxis and antibacterial treatment when required.
5. No sutures or wound closure advised unless unavoidable.

From Benenson A: *Control of communicable diseases manual,* ed 16, Washington, DC, 1995, American Public Health Association.

Rabies Postexposure Prophylaxis Guide

The following recommendations are only a guide. In applying them, take into account the animal species involved, the circumstances of the bite or other exposure, vaccination status of the animal, and presence of rabies in the region. Local or state health officials should be consulted if questions arise about the need for rabies prophylaxis.

Species	Condition of animal at time of attack	Treatment
Domestic dog and cat	Healthy and available for 10 days of observation	None, unless animal develops rabies
	Rabid or suspected rabid	HRIG and vaccine
	Unknown (escaped)	Consult public health official. If treatment is indicated, give HRIG and vaccine
Wild carnivores, skunk, fox, bat, coyote, bobcat, raccoon	Regard as rabid unless proven negative by laboratory tests	HRIG and vaccine
Other livestock, rodents, and lagomorphs (hares and rabbits)	Consider individually. Local and state public health officials should be consulted on questions about the need for rabies prophylaxis. Bites of squirrels, hamsters, guinea pigs, gerbils, chipmunks, rats, mice, other rodents, rabbits, and hares almost never call for antirabies prophylaxis.	

From Benenson A: *Control of communicable diseases manual,* ed 16, Washington, DC, 1995, American Public Health Association.

SKIN AND WOUND CARE

Helpful Tips

- Remind clients they can use a hair dryer to dry skin thoroughly. This is especially important in obese clients and for any area that drying well with a towel might be difficult or painful. The heat setting should always be on low and the dryer always kept moving to facilitate air circulation.
- A small, 6-inch hem gauge that is marked in centimeters can be used to measure the size of wounds, or the area of drainage, on a bandage. Carry one in your nursing bag.
- In females who need breast or sternal dressings, instead of using Montgomery straps, a binder, or tape, the client's bra may be used. This holds the dressing in place, is more comfortable, and reduces skin irritation.
- When immobilizers or binders are used, especially those with Velcro bindings or fasteners, a disposable baby diaper liner can be used for padding to prevent skin irritation and breakdown. They are well padded and serve the purpose perfectly.
- Vaseline gauze can be made by using roller gauze and regular petroleum jelly. Accordian pleat (fold back and forth) the gauze in a metal mixing bowl or a shallow glass pan. Put a generous amount of petroleum jelly on top of the gauze, cover with aluminum foil, and bake at 375° F for 25 minutes. If sterile gauze is needed, individual aluminum foil packets can be made. Purchase unsterile dressings, wrap in aluminum foil and bake for 25 minutes at 375° F to sterilize.

Modified from Humphrey C: *Home care nursing,* Norwalk, Conn, 1994, Aspen.

Treatment Options by Ulcer Stage

Ulcer stage	Ulcer status	Dressing*	Comments	Expected change	Adjuvant
I	Intact	None Film, adherent Hydrocolloid	Allows visual assessment. Protects from shear. May not allow visual assessment.	Resolves slowly without epidermal loss over 7 to 14 days.	Turning schedule. Support hydration. Nutritional support. Silicone-based lotion to decrease shear. Pressure-relief mattress or chair cushion.
II	Clean	Composite Hydrocolloid Hydrogel sheet	Viasorb, film plus Telfa. Exudry. Limits shear. Change every 7 days if occlusive seal. Absorbent, requires secondary dressing of gauze or adherent film.	Heals through reepithelialization and epithelial budding.	See previous stage. Manage incontinence.
III	Clean	Hydrocolloid Hydrogel Exudate absorbers Calcium alginate Wound pastes	See stage II. Apply ½-inch thick, cover with gauze or hydrocolloid. Change when strike through is noted on secondary dressing. Cover with gauze or hydrocolloid.	Heals through granulation and reepithelialization. (NOTE: Does not become a stage II ulcer as it heals.)	See previous stages. Electrical stimulation. Evaluate pressure-relief needs.

From Potter PA, Perry AG: *Basic nursing: a critical thinking approach*, ed 4, St. Louis, 1999, Mosby.
NOTE: As with *all* occlusive dressings, wound should *not* be clinically infected.

Continued.

Treatment Options by Ulcer Stage—cont'd

Ulcer Stage	Ulcer Status	Dressing*	Comments	Expected Change	Adjuvant
		Gauze, fluffy Growth factors Adherent film	Use with normal saline. Use with gauze. Will facilitate softening of eschar.		See previous stages. Surgical consult for debridement.
	Eschar	Hydrocolloid Gauze plus ordered solution None	Will facilitate softening of eschar. Absorb drainage. Rarely, if eschar is dry and intact, no dressing is used, allowing eschar to act as physiological cover.	Eschar will lift at the edges as healing progresses. Cross-hatching central area of eschar with a small blade will facilitate release from center.	Surgical consult for closure.
IV	Clean	Hydrogel Hydrocolloid plus hydrocolloid paste/beads Calcium alginate Gauze Growth factors	See stage III Clean. See stage III Clean; critical to treat areas of undermining.	Heals through granulation and reepithelialization. Because of contraction, surface may close more rapidly than base, leaving wound cavity.	See stages I, II, and III Clean.
	Eschar	See stage III Eschar	See stage III Clean. Pack deeply undermined ulcers. Use with gauze.	See stage III Eschar.	See stage III Eschar.

From Potter PA, Perry AG: *Basic nursing: a critical thinking approach*, ed 4, St. Louis, 1999, Mosby.

Performing Wound Irrigation

Steps

1. Assess client's level of pain.
2. Review record for physician's prescription for irrigation of open wound and type of solution to be used.
3. Identify recent recording of signs and symptoms related to client's open wound:
   a. Extent of impairment of skin integrity
   b. Elevation of body temperature
   c. Drainage from wound (amount, color)
   d. Odor
   e. Consistency of drainage
   f. Size of wounds, including depth, length, and width
4. Administer prescribed analgesic 30 to 45 min before starting wound irrigation procedure.
5. Gather equipment at bedside:
   a. Sterile basin
   b. 150- to 500-ml prescribed sterile irrigating solution warmed to body temperature
   c. Sterile irrigation syringe, sterile soft catheter, if needed
   d. Clean basin
   e. Clean gloves (check policy of institution)
   f. Sterile gloves
   g. Waterproof underpad
   h. Sterile dressing tray and supplies for dressing change, including packing, if ordered
   i. Leakproof refuse bag
   j. Gown
6. Explain procedure.
7. Position client comfortably to permit gravitational flow of irrigating solution through wound and into collection basin. Position client so that wound is vertical to collection basin.
8. Warm sterile irrigating solution to approximate body temperature.
9. Form cuff on leakproof refuse bag and place it near bed.
10. Close room door or bed curtains.
11. Place waterproof underpad on bed surface in front of wound.
12. Place clean basin directly under wound.
13. Wash hands.

From Perry A, Potter P: *Clinical nursing skills and techniques,* ed 4, St. Louis, 1998, Mosby.

14. If gown is needed, apply it now.
15. Prepare sterile field using sterile dressing set and supplies.
16. Add sterile basin and pour in estimated volume of warm sterile irrigating solution and set irrigating syringe in basin with solution.
17. Place several strips of adhesive tape within reach and *not* on sterile field.
18. Put on clean gloves and remove soiled dressing and discard in leakproof refuse bag.
19. Remove and discard gloves.
20. Inspect wound and make mental note of healing process, inflammation, drainage, or purulent matter.
21. Apply sterile gloves.
22. Irrigate wound with wide opening:
    a. Fill syringe with irrigating solution.
    b. Hold syringe tip 2.5 cm (1 inch) above upper end of wound.
    c. Using slow, continuous pressure, flush wound.
    d. Repeat Steps 22a through 22c until solution draining into basin is clear.
23. Irrigate deep wound with very small opening:
    a. Attach soft catheter to filled irrigating syringe.
    b. Lubricate tip of catheter with irrigating solution. Gently insert tip of catheter until resistance is felt, and then pull out about 1.2 cm (½ inch) to remove tip from fragile inner wall of wound.
    c. Using slow, continuous pressure, flush wound.
    d. Pinch off catheter just below syringe.
    e. Remove syringe, fill, and reattach to catheter. Repeat until return is clear.
24. Dry wound edges with sterile gauze.
25. Apply sterile dressing.
26. Remove and dispose of gloves.
27. Secure dressing with adhesive tape.
28. Assist client to comfortable position.
29. Dispose of equipment; retain remaining bottle of sterile solution.
30. Wash hands.
31. Inspect dressing periodically.
32. Evaluate skin integrity.
33. Record wound appearance, irrigation, and client response in nurses' notes.

Surgical Wound Classification

Classification	Definition	Examples
Clean wound	Uninfected, primary closure Closed wound drainage system No inflammation present	Total knee arthroplasty Mitral valve replacement Breast biopsy
Clean contaminated wound	Respiratory, alimentary, or genitourinary tract entered without spillage No sign of infection, minor break in sterile technique	Total abdominal hysterectomy Radical prostatectomy Pneumonectomy
Contaminated wound	Major break in aseptic technique Signs of infection Contamination from gastrointestinal tract Open fresh traumatic wound	Appendectomy for ruptured appendix Laparotomy for perforated bowel
Dirty wound	Old trauma with necrotic tissue Preexisting infection Perforated viscera Acute inflammation	Incision and drainage of abscess

From Phipps WJ et al.: *Medical-surgical nursing: concepts and clinical practice,* ed 6, St. Louis, 1999, Mosby.

DIABETES

Testing Blood for Glucose

1. Assist client in determining clean area for storage of equipment and supplies.
2. Wash hands and organize equipment.
3. Explain procedure to client and inquire as to preference of finger and use of lancet injector.
4. Perform, teach, observe calibration of glucose meter, if used:
   Turn machine on.
   Compare number on machine or strip in machine with number on bottle of chemical strips (Figure 17).
   Perform, observe, teach procedures to ready machine for operation; consult user's manual for steps and readiness indicator.
   Machine calibration should be done per manufacturer's instruction/agency policy, with high and low glucose solutions to ensure accuracy. The client should maintain a calibration record.
5. Remove chemical strip from container; client should place face up where it is most accessible.
6. Load lancet in injector, if used, set trigger, prepare alcohol sponge and cottonball for use.

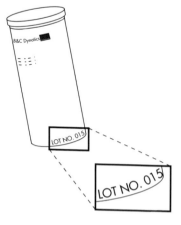

Figure 17

From Johnson JY et al.: *Nurse's guide to home health procedures,* Philadelphia, 1998, Lippincott.

7. If nurse is performing procedure, gloves should be worn. If client is performing procedure, hands should be clean.

8. Hold chosen finger downward and squeeze gently from lower digits to fingertip, or wrap finger in warm wet cloth for 30 seconds or longer.

9. Wipe intended puncture site with alcohol pad.

10. Place injector against side of finger (where there are fewer nerve endings) and release trigger; or stick side of finger with lancet using a darting motion.

11. Hold chemical strip under puncture site and squeeze gently until drop of blood is large enough to drop onto strip and cover indicator square.

12. Push timer button on machine as soon as blood has covered indicator squares, or note position on watch or kitchen timer.

13. Apply pressure to puncture site until bleeding stops, or have client do it, and place lancet in needle disposal unit.

14. When timer or watch indicates 60 seconds or designated time (per machine user's manual) has passed, wipe excess blood from strip.

15. Place into machine, if used, with indicator patch facing reading window (consult user's manual). After an additional 60 seconds have passed, read results from the machine.

16. Or compare colors on strip with those in chart on chemical strip container or insert after the additional 60 seconds (Figure 18).

17. Discard soiled materials and gloves in proper container.

18. Assist client with recording results on glucose flow sheet, and administering insulin, if indicated.

19. Assist client in cleaning equipment and storing in a safe, clean, secure area.

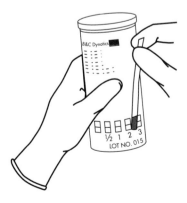

Figure 18

Guidelines for Foot Care for the Client With Diabetes

1. *Never* soak feet.
2. Wash feet daily and dry them well, paying attention to area between toes.
3. Inspect feet daily. Look for the following:
   a. Color changes
   b. Swelling
   c. Cuts
   d. Cracks in the skin
   e. Redness
   f. Blisters
   g. Temperature changes
4. Never walk barefoot. Always wear shoes or slippers.
5. Wear well-fitting shoes and clean socks.
6. After bathing, when toenails are soft, cut nails straight across. Do not cut into the corners. File edges smooth with an emery board. If you have visual problems, have someone else cut toenails for you.
7. If feet are dry, apply lotion or cream; do not put lotion between the toes.
8. Do not perform "bathroom surgery."
9. Do not self-treat corns, calluses, warts, or ingrown toenails. Consult a podiatrist.
10. Bath water should be no warmer than 90° F. Test water temperature on your inner forearm, just as you would a baby's bottle, before immersing hands or feet.
11. Do not use heating pads or hot water bottles.
12. Enhance your circulation by doing the following:
    a. Not smoking
    b. Avoiding crossing legs when sitting
    c. Protecting your hands and feet when exposed to cold
    d. Avoiding tight elastic on socks
    e. Exercising
    f. Using sunscreen
13. **Any foot problem is a medical emergency.** Consult your primary care provider, podiatrist, or diabetes team immediately if any foot problem arises. Delay in seeking care can cost you your feet.

From Phipps WJ et al.: *Medical-surgical nursing: concepts and clinical practice,* ed 6, St. Louis, 1999, Mosby.

Assessment of Feet of the Client With Diabetes

Color: Compare one foot with the other.
Temperature: Compare both feet with upper legs; assess for line of demarcations.
Sensory function: Test for pinprick and vibratory sense (Semmes-Weinstein monofilament).
Reflexes: Test Achilles tendon reflex.
Pulses: Check dorsalis pedis and posterior tibialis.
Lesions: Examine for calluses, cuts, bruises, cracks, or infection.
Self-care: Discuss self-care regimen being used.

From Phipps WJ et al.: *Medical-surgical nursing: concepts and clinical practice,* ed 6, St. Louis, 1999, Mosby.

Risk Categories and Associated Footwear Guidelines

	Clinical findings	Footwear changes
Category 0	Has protective sensation	Education on proper footwear
Category 1	Has lost protective sensation	Add soft insole to shoe of proper contour and fit
Category 2	Has lost protective sensation and has foot deformity	Depth footwear or custom shoe for severe deformity, molded insoles
Category 3	Has lost protective sensation and has history of foot ulcer	Inspect type and condition of footwear and insoles at every visit

From Haire-Joshu D: *Management of diabetes mellitus—perspective of care across the life span,* ed 2, St. Louis, 1996, Mosby.

Insulin Injection Sites

Rotate injection sites as numbered. Make injections 1 inch apart. After sites in one area are used, move to the next area.

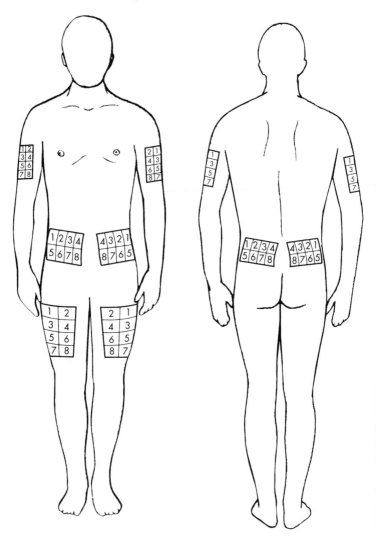

Subcutaneous injection site diagram.

From Potter PA, Perry AG: *Fundamentals of nursing: concepts, process, and practice,* ed 4, St. Louis, 1998, Mosby.

Comparison of Hyperglycemia and Hypoglycemia

Hyperglycemia	Hypoglycemia
Manifestations*	
Blood glucose >500 mg/dl (27.8 mmol/L)	Blood glucose <50 mg/dl (2.8 mmol/L)
Increase in urination	Cold, clammy skin
Increase in appetite followed by lack of appetite	Numbness of fingers, toes, mouth
Weakness, fatigue	Rapid heartbeat
Blurred vision	Emotional changes
Headache	Headache
Glycosuria	Nervousness, tremors
Nausea and vomiting	Faintness, dizziness
Abdominal cramps	Unsteady gait, slurred speech
Progression to DKA or HHNK	Hunger
	Changes in vision
	Seizures, coma
Causes	
Too much food	Alcohol intake with food
Too little or no diabetes medication	Too little food—delayed, omitted, inadequate intake
Inactivity	Too much diabetic medication
Emotional, physical stress	Too much exercise without compensation
Poor absorption of insulin	Diabetes medication or food taken at wrong time
	Loss of weight with change in medication
	Use of β-blockers interfering with recognition of symptoms
Treatment	
Physician's attention	Immediate ingestion of 5-20 g of simple carbohydrates
Continuance of diabetes medication as ordered	Ingestion of another 5-20 g of simple carbohydrates in 15 minutes if no relief obtained
Frequent checking of blood and urine specimens and recording of results	Contacting of physician if no relief obtained
Hourly drinking of fluids	Discussion with physician about medication dosage

From Lewis S et al.: *Medical surgical nursing,* ed 4, St. Louis, 1996, Mosby.

*There is usually a gradual onset of symptoms in hyperglycemia and a rapid onset in hypoglycemia.

Continued.

Comparison of Hyperglycemia and Hypoglycemia—cont'd

Hyperglycemia	Hypoglycemia

Preventive measures

Hyperglycemia	Hypoglycemia
Taking of prescribed dose of medication at proper time	Taking of prescribed dose of medication at proper time
Accurate administration of insulin	Accurate administration of insulin
Maintenance of diet	Ingestion of all ordered diet foods at proper time
Maintenance of good personal hygiene	Provision of compensation for exercise
Adherence to sick-day rules when ill	Ability to recognize and know symptoms and treat them immediately
Checking of blood for glucose as ordered	Carrying of simple carbohydrates
Contacting of physician regarding ketonuria	Education of friends, family, fellow employees about symptoms and treatment
Wearing of diabetic identification	Checking blood glucose as ordered

Notes

Specimen Labeling and Transport

Purpose
- To identify laboratory specimen(s) with appropriate data.
- To safely deliver the specimens to the laboratory for analysis.

Equipment
1. Tape or specimen label; biohazard labels
2. Plastic bags
3. Laboratory requisition
4. Antiseptic wipes
5. Leak- and puncture-proof cooler or container with biohazard sign posted on the outside
6. Disposable nonsterile gloves

Procedure
1. Clarify with the physician the designated laboratory for the delivery of specimens.
2. Clarify with the designated laboratory the color of the test tubes, the specimen collection container, and the client data that are required to process the specimen.
3. Clean blood and body substances from outside of test tube(s) or speci-container(s) with antiseptic wipes as needed.
4. Label the specimen container in the following manner:
   a. Client's name
   b. Test to be performed by the laboratory
   c. Time and date specimen was collected
   d. Initials of the person who collects the specimen
5. Place test tubes or the specimen container in a plastic bag, and **seal** it to prevent possible leakage during transport. Place a biohazard label on the outside of the plastic bag. Double bag the specimen to prevent possible leakage when using ice to refrigerate the specimens or PRN.
6. Place the specimen into a leak- and puncture-proof cooler or container.
7. Place cooler or container on the floorboard of the car during transport.
8. Fill out the laboratory requisition, and transport the specimen.
9. Call the physician with the lab results as soon as they are available.
10. Discard disposable items in a plastic trash bag, and secure.

From Rice R: *Manual of home health nursing procedures,* St. Louis, 1995, Mosby.

Nursing considerations

- Many specimens **must** be delivered to the laboratory within 30 minutes to 1 hour after sampling.
- Consult with the laboratory concerning the type of container or test tube that should be used to collect the specimen and whether the specimen should be refrigerated by placing it on ice; also inquire about a time frame for deliveries. Many laboratories provide courier services to pick up specimens at the client's home.

Documentation guidelines

- Document the following on the visit report: the type of laboratory test ordered by the physician; date and time the specimen was collected; designated laboratory for delivery; and other pertinent findings.
- Document physician notification of laboratory test results on the visit report or appropriate home health agency communique and any subsequent orders.
- Update the client care plan.

ORTHOPEDIC CARE

Range of Motion

- Assess family/primary caregiver's ability, availability, and motivation to assist client with exercises client is unable to perform independently.
- Assist family/primary caregiver to arrange environment to promote exercise program, e.g., space allocation, lighting, temperature.
- Consult physical therapist for additional assistance or exercises and client's response to exercise program.
- Develop schedule for recording the performance of the exercise program.
- Instruct client or caregiver in performing exercise slowly.
- Teach caregiver how to provide adequate support to joint being exercised.
- Instruct to exercise only to point of resistance and to stop if client expresses pain.
- Each exercise should be repeated five times during exercise period.

Modified from Perry AG, Potter PA: *Clinical nursing skills and techniques,* ed 4, St. Louis, 1998, Mosby.

Neck

- *Flexion:* Bring chin to rest on chest (ROM: 45*) (Figure 19).
- *Extension:* Return head to erect position (ROM: 45) (Figure 19).
- *Hyperextension:* Bend head as far back as possible (ROM: 10) (Figure 19).
- *Lateral flexion:* Tilt head as far as possible toward each shoulder (ROM: 40-45) (Figure 20).
- *Rotation:* Rotate head in circular motion (ROM: 360) (Figure 21).

  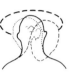

Figure 19 **Figure 20** **Figure 21**

Shoulder

- *Flexion:* Raise arm from side position forward to above head (ROM: 180) (Figure 22).
- *Extension:* Return arm to position at side of body (ROM: 180) (Figure 22).
- *Hyperextension:* Move arm behind body, keeping elbow straight (ROM: 45-60) (Figure 22).
- *Abduction:* Raise arm to side to position above head with palm away from head (ROM: 180) (Figure 23).
- *Adduction:* Lower arm sideways and across body as far as possible (ROM: 320) (Figure 23).

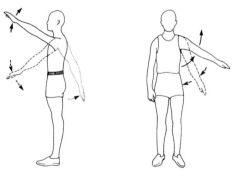

Figure 22 **Figure 23**

---

*Ranges are measured in degrees using a goniometer.

- *Internal rotation:* With elbow flexed, rotate shoulder by moving arm until thumb is turned inward and toward back (ROM: 90) (Figure 24).
- *External rotation:* With elbow flexed, move arm until thumb is upward and lateral to head (ROM: 90) (Figure 24).
- *Circumduction:* Move arm in full circle. Circumduction is a combination of all movements of ball-and-socket joint (ROM: 360) (Figure 25).

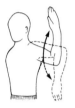
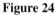

Figure 24   **Figure 25**

Elbow

- *Flexion:* Bend elbow so that lower arm moves toward its shoulder joint and hand is level with shoulder (ROM: 150) (Figure 26).
- *Extension:* Straighten elbow by lowering hand (ROM: 150) (Figure 26).
- *Hyperextension:* Bend lower arm back as far as possible (ROM: 10-20).

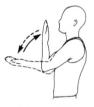

Figure 26

Forearm

- *Supination:* Turn lower arm and hand so palm is up (ROM: 70-90) (Figure 27).
- *Pronation:* Turn lower arm so palm is down (ROM: 70-90) (Figure 27).

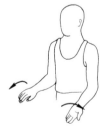

Figure 27

Wrist
- *Flexion:* Move palm toward inner aspect of forearm (ROM: 80-90) (Figure 28).
- *Extension:* Move fingers so fingers, hands, and forearm are in same plane (ROM: 80-90) (Figure 28).
- *Hyperextension:* Bring dorsal surface of hand back as far as possible (ROM: 80-90) (Figure 28).
- *Abduction (radial flexion):* Bend wrist medially toward thumb (ROM: Up to 30) (Figure 29).
- *Adduction (ulnar flexion):* Bend wrist laterally toward fifth finger (ROM: 30-50) (Figure 29).

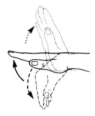

Figure 28

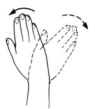

Figure 29

Fingers
- *Flexion:* Make fist (ROM: 90) (Figure 30).
- *Extension:* Straighten fingers (ROM: 90) (Figure 31).
- *Hyperextension:* Bend fingers back as far as possible (ROM: 30-60) (Figure 31).
- *Abduction:* Spread fingers apart (ROM: 30) (Figure 32).
- *Adduction:* Bring fingers together (ROM: 30) (Figure 32).

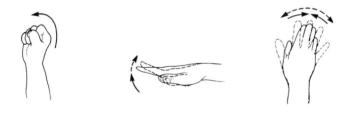

Figure 30 **Figure 31** **Figure 32**

Thumb

- *Flexion:* Move thumb across palmar surface of hand (ROM: 90) (Figure 33).
- *Extension:* Move thumb straight away from hand (ROM: 90).
- *Abduction:* Extend thumb laterally (usually done when placing fingers in abduction and adduction) (ROM: 30).
- *Adduction:* Move thumb back toward hand (ROM: 30).
- *Opposition:* Touch thumb to each finger of same hand (Figure 34).

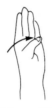

Figure 33

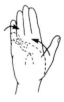

Figure 34

Hip

- *Flexion:* Move leg forward and up (ROM: 90-120) (Figure 35).
- *Extension:* Move leg back beside other leg (ROM: 90-120) (Figure 35).
- *Hyperextension:* Move leg behind body (ROM: 30-50) (Figure 36).
- *Abduction:* Move leg laterally away from body (ROM: 30-50) (Figure 37).
- *Adduction:* Move leg back toward medial position and beyond if possible (ROM: 30-50) (Figure 37).

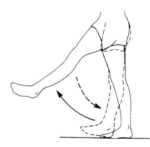

Figure 35

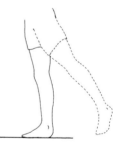

Figure 36

- *Internal rotation:* Turn foot and leg toward other leg (ROM: 90) (Figure 38).
- *External rotation:* Turn foot and leg away from other leg (ROM: 90) (Figure 38).
- *Circumduction:* Move leg in circle (ROM: 360) (Figure 39).

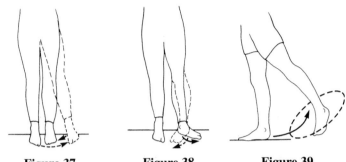

Figure 37   **Figure 38**   **Figure 39**

Knee

- *Flexion:* Bring heel toward back of thigh (ROM: 120-130) (Figure 40).
- *Extension:* Return leg to floor (ROM: 120-130) (Figure 40).

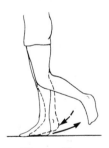

Figure 40

Ankle

- *Dorsal flexion:* Move foot so toes are pointed upward (ROM: 20-30) (Figure 41).
- *Plantar flexion:* Move foot so toes are pointed downward (ROM: 45-50) (Figure 41).

Figure 41

Foot

- *Inversion:* Turn sole of foot medially (ROM: 10 or less) (Figure 42).
- *Eversion:* Turn sole of foot laterally (ROM: 10 or less) (Figure 42).
- *Flexion:* Curl toes downward (ROM: 30-60) (Figure 43).
- *Extension:* Straighten toes (ROM: 30-60) (Figure 43).
- *Abduction:* Spread toes apart (ROM: 15 or less) (Figure 44).
- *Adduction:* Bring toes together (ROM: 15 or less) (Figure 44).

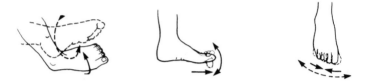

Figure 42   **Figure 43**   **Figure 44**

Special considerations

- It is essential to maintain joint flexibility. Contracted or immobile joints make protective positioning of a client difficult or impossible. It is hard to relieve pressure over bony prominences and to protect the client from pressure sores. Adequate skin care is difficult because it is hard to separate the skin folds adequately. If the client is in a curled or fetal position, chest expansion is restricted, and changes in abdominal pressure make elimination difficult.
- Contractures can begin shortly after onset of immobility. ROM exercises should be started as soon as possible. However, not all clients will require ROM exercises. Assess to determine which joints will get full ROM during client's normal activities and which will not and will require intervention.
- Some clients may need ROM exercises several times a day. Frequency depends on the individual client's medical diagnosis, present health condition, and willingness and ability to perform ROM exercises. Schedule exercises when it is convenient for the client. Bath time is a good time because bath water relaxes muscles, and joints are exposed so they are easy to manipulate and observe.
- When a person is immobile, the hip joint may become affected because full extension of the hip is difficult in all positions except relaxed standing. Partial flexion of the hip may occur. Elevation of the head, use of pillows under the knee, or elevation of the legs all increase flexion of the hip.
- Full extension of the knee while in bed seldom occurs without conscious effort. All positions, except prone, favor flexion. The domi-

nant muscle of the lower leg, the hamstring muscle group, tends to draw the knee up into flexion. Other factors contributing to flexion of the knee include use of pillows under the knee, painful disabilities, and stationary positions.

- The ankle has a high risk for the development of flexion contractures (drop foot) because of gravity and the strength of the plantar flexion group. Plus, the weight of bedclothes contributes to the fatigue of the dorsal flexor muscles. Along with instituting ROM exercises of the ankle, a footboard or pillow may be useful in the prevention of foot-drop. The client is instructed to place the feet against a pillow or footboard and to flex and extend the ankles against a pillow or footboard frequently throughout the day.

Walking With Crutches

Measurement

- Crutch measurement includes three areas: client's height, distance between crutch pad and axilla, and angle of elbow flexion. Use one of two methods: *Standing*—Position crutches with crutch tips at point 4 to 6 inches (14 to 15 cm) to side and 4 to 6 inches in front of client's feet and crutch pads 1½ to 2 inches (4 to 5 cm) below axilla. *Supine*—Crutch pad should be 3 to 4 finger widths under axilla with crutch tips positioned 6 inches (15 cm) lateral to client's heel.
- With either method elbows should be flexed 15 to 30 degrees. Elbow flexion is verified with goniometer.
- In addition to overall *length* of axillary crutch, *height* of handgrip is important. Both dimensions are adjustable on well-made crutch, and this is an important feature for a growing child. Handgrip should be adjusted so that client's elbow is *slightly flexed.* If handgrip is too low, radial nerve can be damaged even if overall crutch length is correct because extra length between handgrip and axillary bar can force bar up into axilla as client stretches down to reach handgrip. If handpiece is too high, client's elbow is sharply flexed and strength and stability of arms are decreased.

Modified from Potter PA, Perry AG: *Fundamentals of nursing,* ed 4, St. Louis, 1997, Mosby.

Teaching the crutch gait

Assist client in crutch walking by choosing appropriate gait.

To use crutches, client supports self with his or her hands and arms; therefore strength in arm and shoulder muscles, ability to balance body in upright position, and stamina are necessary. Type of gait client uses in crutch walking depends on amount of weight client is able to support with one or both legs.

A. The four-point gait is the most stable of crutch gaits because it provides at least three points of support at all times. Requires weight bearing on both legs. Often used when there is paralysis as in spastic children with cerebral palsy. May also be used for arthritic clients.

   Begin in tripod position (Figure 45). Crutches are placed 6 inches (15 cm) in front and 6 inches to side of each foot. This improves client's balance by providing wider base of support. Posture should be erect head and neck, straight vertebrae, and extended hips and knees.

   Crutch and foot position are similar to arm and foot position during normal walking.

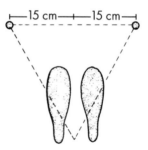

Figure 45

Move right crutch forward 4 to 6 inches (Figure 46).
Move left foot forward to level of left crutch.
Move left crutch forward 4 to 6 inches.
Move right foot forward to level of right crutch.
Repeat above sequence.

B. The three-point gait requires client to bear all weight on one foot. Weight is borne on uninvolved leg, then on both crutches. Affected leg does not touch ground during early phase of three-point gait. May be useful for client with broken leg or sprained ankle.

Begin in tripod position. This improves client's balance by providing wide base of support.
Advance both crutches and affected leg (Figure 47).
Move stronger leg forward.
Repeat sequence.

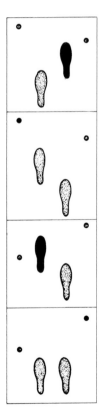

Figure 46

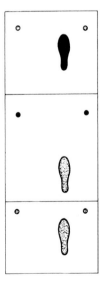

Figure 47

C. The two-point gait requires at least partial weight bearing on each foot, and is faster than the four-point gait. Requires more balance because only two points support the body at one time.

Begin in tripod position. This improves client's balance by providing wider base of support.

Move left crutch and right foot forward (Figure 48). (Crutch movements are similar to arm movement during normal walking.)

Move right crutch and left foot forward.

Repeat sequence.

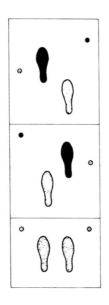

Figure 48

Assist client in swing-to gait and swing-through gait. These are frequently used by clients whose lower extremities are paralyzed or who wear weight-supporting braces on their legs.

The swing-to gait is the easier of the two swinging gaits.

Swing-to gait:

Move both crutches forward.

Lift and swing legs to crutches letting crutches support body weight.

Repeat steps 1 and 2.

Swing-through gait:
Move both crutches forward. Initial placement of crutches is to increase the client's base of support so that when the body swings forward the client is moving the center of gravity toward the additional support provided by the crutches.
Lift and swing legs through and beyond crutches.

Using crutches while walking on stairs

A. Ascending stairs with crutches:

Begin in tripod position.
Transfer body weight to crutches. This prepares client to transfer weight to unaffected leg when ascending first stair.
Advance unaffected leg to stair. The crutch adds support to affected leg. Client then shifts weight from crutches to unaffected leg.
Align both crutches and unaffected leg on stairs to maintain balance and provide wide base of support.
Repeat sequence until client reaches top of stairs.

B. Descending stairs with crutches:

Begin in tripod position.
Transfer body weight to unaffected leg. This prepares client to release support of body weight maintained by crutches.
Move crutches to stair and instruct client to begin to transfer body weight to crutches and move affected leg forward. This maintains client's balance and base of support.
Move unaffected leg to stair and align with crutches. This maintains balance and provides base of support.
Repeat sequence until stairs are descended.

Sitting in a chair when using crutches

As with crutch walking and crutch walking up and down stairs, the procedure for sitting in a chair involves phases and requires the client to transfer weight. First, the client gets positioned at the center front of the chair with the posterior aspect of the legs touching the chair. Second, the client holds both crutches in the hand opposite the affected leg. If both legs are affected, as with a paraplegic who wears weight-supporting braces, the crutches are held on the client's stronger side. With both crutches in one hand the client supports body weight on the unaffected leg and crutches. While still holding the crutches, the client grasps the arm of the chair with the remaining hand and lowers the body. To stand, the procedure is reversed, and the client when fully erect should assume the tripod position before walking.

Walker Use

Walkers are used by clients who are able to bear partial weight. Walkers need to be picked up, so clients need sufficient strength to be able to pick up walker. The four-wheeled model, which does not need to be picked up, is not as stable.

- Stand in center of walker and grasp handgrips on upper bars to balance self before attempting to walk.
- Take step forward into walker. This provides broad base of support between walker and client. Client then moves center of gravity toward the walker.
- Move walker 6 to 8 inches forward and take another step forward with either leg. If there is one-sided weakness, instruct the client after advancing walker to step forward with uninvolved leg, support self with the arms, and follow through with involved leg. If unable to bear weight on one leg, after advancing walker have the client swing on to it, supporting weight on hands.
- Repeat steps.

Modified from Perry AG, Potter PA: *Clinical nursing skills and techniques,* ed 4, St. Louis, 1998, Mosby.

Transferring and Positioning of Immobile Clients

The nurse will frequently encounter a semihelpless, helpless, or immobilized client whose position must be changed or who must be moved up in bed. Proper use of body mechanics can enable the nurse (and a helper) to move, lift, or transfer such a client safely and at the same time avoid musculoskeletal injury.

Prepare the following equipment and supplies:

- **a.** Pillows
- **b.** Footboard
- **c.** Trochanter roll
- **d.** Sandbag
- **e.** Hand rolls
- **f.** Restraints (as appropriate)
- **g.** Side rails

Modified from Perry AG, Potter PA: *Clinical nursing skills and techniques,* ed 4, St. Louis, 1998, Mosby.

Raise level of bed to comfortable working height.
Remove all pillows and devices used in previous position.
Get extra help as needed.
Explain procedure to client.

Moving helpless client up in bed (one person):

a. Place client on back with head of bed flat. Stand on one side of bed.
b. Place pillow at head of bed.
c. Begin at client's feet. Face foot of bed at 45-degree angle. Place feet apart with foot nearest head of bed behind other foot (forward-backward stance). Flex knees and hips as needed to bring arms level with client's legs. Shift weight from front to back leg and slide client's legs diagonally toward head of bed.
d. Move parallel to client's hips. Flex knees and hips as needed to bring arms level with client's hips.
e. Slide client's hips diagonally toward head of bed.
f. Move parallel to client's head and shoulders. Flex knees and hips as needed to bring arms level with client's body.
g. Slide arm closest to head of bed under client's neck, with hand reaching under and supporting client's shoulder.
h. Place other arm under client's chest.
i. Slide client's trunk, shoulders, head, and neck diagonally toward head of bed.
j. Repeat procedure, switching sides until client reaches desired height in bed.
k. Center client in middle of bed, moving body in same three sections.

Assisting client to move up in bed (one person or two):

a. Place client on back.
b. Place pillow at head of bed.
c. Face head of bed.
Each person should have one arm under client's shoulders and one arm under client's thighs.
Alternate position: position one person at client's upper body. Person's arm nearest head of bed should be under client's head and opposite shoulder; other arm should be under client's closest arm and shoulder. Position other person at client's lower torso. This person's arms should be under client's lower back and torso.
d. Place feet apart with foot nearest head of bed behind other foot (forward-backward stance).
e. Ask client to flex knees with feet flat on bed.
f. Instruct client to flex neck, tilting chin toward chest.

g. Instruct client to assist moving by pushing with feet on bed surface.

h. Flex knees and hips, bringing forearms closer to level of bed.

i. Instruct client to push with heels and elevate trunk while breathing out, thus moving toward head of bed on count of 3.

j. On count of 3, rock and shift weight from front to back leg. At the same time, client pushes with heels and elevates trunk.

Positioning client in lateral (side-lying) position:

- Position client to side of bed.
- Turn client onto side:
    To turn helpless client onto side, flex knee that will not be next to mattress. Place one hand on client's hip and one hand on shoulder. Roll client onto side.
- Place pillow under client's head and neck.
- Bring shoulder blade forward.
- Position both arms in slightly flexed position. Upper arm is supported by pillow level with shoulder, other arm by mattress.
- Place tuck-back pillow behind client's back. (Make by folding pillow lengthwise. Smooth area is slightly tucked under client's back.)
- Place pillow under semiflexed upper leg level at hip from groin to foot.
- Place sandbag parallel to plantar surface of dependent foot.

Transferring client from bed to chair:

a. Assist client to sitting position on side of bed. Have chair in position at 45-degree angle to bed.

b. Apply transfer belt and transfer aids, if needed.

c. Ensure that client has stable, nonskid shoes. Weight-bearing, or strong leg forward, weak foot back.

d. Spread feet apart.

e. Flex hips and knees, aligning knees with client's.

f. Grasp transfer belt from underneath, if used, or reach through client's axilla and place hands on client's scapulae.

g. Rock client up to standing position on count of 3 while straightening hips and legs, keeping knees slightly flexed. Client may be instructed to use hands to push up if applicable.

h. Maintain stability of client's weak or paralyzed leg with knee.

i. Pivot on foot farther from chair.

j. Instruct client to use arm rests on chair for support and ease into chair.

k. Flex hips and knees while lowering client into chair.

l. Assess client for proper alignment for sitting position. Provide support for paralyzed extremities. Lap board or sling will support flaccid arm. Stabilize leg with bath blanket or pillow.
m. Praise client progress, effort, performance.

INTRAVENOUS CARE

Intravenous Therapy

Procedure 1: vein selection

1. Wash hands and organize equipment.
2. Explain procedure, including client assistance needed during and after therapy initiation.
3. Encourage client to use bedpan or commode before beginning.
4. Help client into loose-fitting gown or clothing.
5. Ask client which is dominant hand.
6. Tie tourniquet on arm 3 to 5 inches below elbow.
7. Ask client to open and close hand or hang arm at side of bed.
8. Look for vein with fewest curves or junctions and largest diameter (puffiness).
9. Find vein on lower arm, if possible. Check anterior and posterior surfaces.
10. If lower arm veins are unsuitable, look at hand and wrist veins.
11. Look for site with 2 inches of skin surface below it (Figure 49). If a large vein is needed, tie tourniquet just above antecubital area and search upper arm for suitable vein. A doctor's order is usually required before a vein in the lower extremities can be used. For PICC catheter the basilic or cephalic veins are most appropriate.
12. Release tourniquet.
13. Obtain supplies.
14. Select smallest catheter size that meets infusion needs and is appropriate for vein size.
15. Include two appropriately sized catheters and one smaller gauge catheter with other supplies.

From Johnson JY et al.: *Nurses' guide to home health procedures,* Philadelphia, 1998, Lippincott.

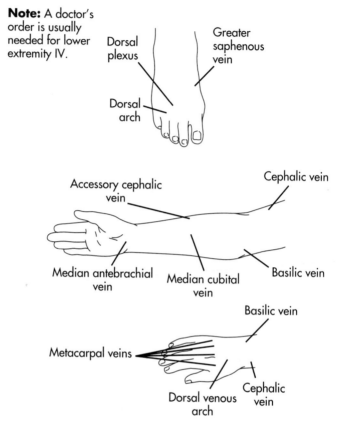

Note: A doctor's order is usually needed for lower extremity IV.

Dorsal plexus

Greater saphenous vein

Dorsal arch

Accessory cephalic vein

Cephalic vein

Median antebrachial vein

Median cubital vein

Basilic vein

Basilic vein

Metacarpal veins

Dorsal venous arch

Cephalic vein

Figure 49

Procedure 2: solution preparation

1. Select vein (see Procedure 1).
2. Open tubing package and check tubing for cracks or flaws. Check ends for covers and verify that regulator clamp is closed (rolled down, clamped off, or screwed closed).
3. Open IV fluid container:

    Bottles: With one hand, hold bottle firmly on counter; with other hand, lift, then pull metal tab down, outward, and around until entire ring is removed (Figure 50); lift metal cap and pull flat rubber pad up and off. MAINTAIN STERILITY OF BOTTLE TOP.

    Bags: Remove outer bag covering; hold bag by neck in one hand; pull down on plastic tab with other hand and remove (Figure 50).

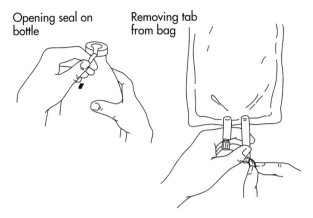

Opening seal on bottle

Removing tab from bag

Figure 50

4. To attach tubing, first remove cap from tubing spikes:
   Bottles: Wipe top with alcohol; push spike into bottle port that is *not* attached to white tube.
   Bags: Push spike into port until flat end of tubing and bag meet.
5. Prime the tubing (remove air):
   Hang bottle or bag on IV pole or wall hook; squeeze and release drip chamber until fluid level reaches ring mark.
   Remove cap from end of tubing.
   Open roller clamp and flush tubing until air is removed.
   Hold rubber medication plugs and in-line filter (if present) upside down and tap while fluid is running.
   Close roller clamp.
6. Replace cap on end of tubing.
7. Apply time strip.
8. Proceed to client with equipment. Drape tubing over pole.

Procedure 3: catheter/IV lock insertion for primary infusion line and IV lock

1. Select vein (see Procedure 1) and prepare solution (see Procedure 2). Place IV tubing beside client.
2. Assist client into a supine or sitting position. Sit alongside of bed or chair.
3. Tear (three 1-inch) tape strips. Cut one piece down center.
4. Prepare needle/catheter for insertion:
   Over-the-needle catheter: Examine the catheter for cracks or flaws. Rotate the catheter on needle.
   Butterfly: Check needle tip for straight edge without bends or chips.

5. Open antimicrobial solution or alcohol pad.
6. Place towel under extremity.
7. Place tourniquet on extremity.
8. Locate largest, most distal vein.
9. Don gloves.
10. With alcohol or antimicrobial solution, clean vein area, beginning at the vein and circling outward in a 2-inch diameter. Repeat with povidone solution. Allow to air dry completely.
11. Encourage client to take slow, deep breaths as you begin.
12. Hold skin taut with one hand while holding catheter with other (Figure 51).

    Over-the-needle catheter: Hold the catheter by holding fingers on opposite sides of needle housing, *not* over catheter hub.

    Butterfly: Pinch "wings" of butterfly together to insert needle.
13. Maintaining sterility, insert catheter into vein with bevel of needle up. Insert needle parallel to straightest section of vein. Puncture skin at a 30-degree angle, 1 cm below site where the vein will be entered (Figure 52).

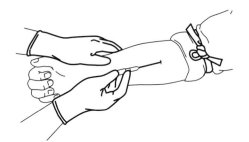

Figure 51

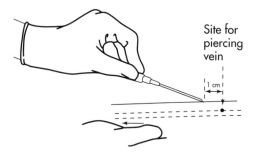

Site for piercing vein

1 cm

Figure 52

14. When needle has entered skin, lower it until it is almost flush with the skin (Figure 53).
15. Following path of vein, insert catheter into side of vein wall. *(If using a needle-stick protective over-the-needle catheter system, insert needle at a 30-degree angle with bevel and push-off tabs in the up position. Place index finger on the push-off tab and thread the catheter to the desired length.)*
16. Watch for first backflow of blood, then push needle gently into vein.

    Over-the-needle catheter: Push needle into vein about ¼ inch after blood is noted. Slide catheter over needle and into vein. Apply digital pressure distal to catheter tip before pulling needle out of vein and skin (Figure 54). IF UNABLE TO INSERT CATHETER FULLY, DO NOT FORCE; WAIT UNTIL FLUID FLOW IS INITIATED.

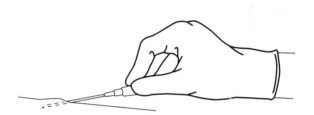

Figure 53

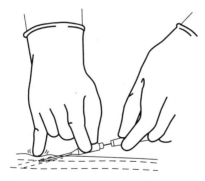

Figure 54

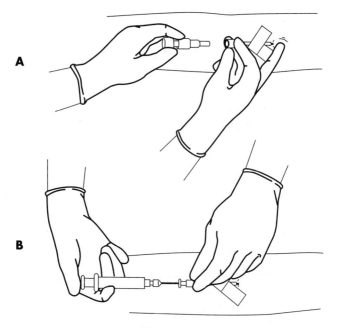

Figure 55

17. Holding catheter securely, remove cap from IV tubing and insert into hub of catheter; with **IV LOCK** twist on infusion plug (Figure 55, *A*).
18. Remove tourniquet.
19. Open roller clamp and allow fluid to flow freely for a few seconds; with **heparin lock,** wipe plug with alcohol and flush with saline (Figure 55, *B*).
20. Monitor for swelling or pain.
21. Tape catheter in position that allows free flow of the fluid. Tape catheter using one of the following methods:
    Over-the-needle catheter: Put small piece of tape under hub of catheter and fold ends straight down towards the insertion site; place a tape strip across the top of the hub to secure hub to skin. DO NOT PLACE TAPE OVER INSERTION SITE.
    Butterfly: Put smallest pieces of tape across "wings" of butterfly; put another tape piece across middle to form an H.
22. Slow IV fluids to a moderate drip.
23. Place ointment over insertion site, if desired, and cover with adhesive bandage, 2 × 2-inch dressing, or transparent dressing (omit ointment with this dressing type).

24. Remove gloves and secure tubing:

    Over-the-needle catheter: Place tape across top of tubing, just below catheter. Loop tubing and tape to dressing. Secure length of tubing to arm with short piece of tape. Tape the tubing/catheter hub junction.

    Butterfly: Coil needle tubing around and on top of IV site. Tape across coil and hub of needle.

    IV lock: Flush with dilute heparin solution (1:10 or 1:100) or saline. Tape across infusion plug.

25. On a piece of tape or label, record needle size, type, date, and time of insertion and your initials. Place label over top of dressing.

26. Apply armboard if needed.

27. Discard gloves and dispose of equipment properly.

28. Regulate IV flow manually or set infusion device at appropriate rate.

29. Review limitations in range of motion with client. Instruct client to notify nurse of problems or discomfort.

30. Remove towel and assist client to a comfortable position.

31. Check infusion accuracy after 5 minutes and again after 15 minutes. Teach client how to check volume every 1 to 2 hours for infusion rate accuracy.

Home Care Teaching for IV Therapy

1. Wash your hands before and after IV care.

2. Check your IV site. If it is red or painful, do not administer IV fluids, and call the home health agency clinical supervisor. Your home health agency's number is _____.

3. Flush your IV catheter with _____ ml of normal saline solution before administering IV fluids or medications, such as antibiotics.

4. When preparing your IV fluids, close the roller clamp on the IV tubing. Then attach the IV tubing to the IV bag without touching the sterile surfaces. *Keep the tubing and connections as germ free as possible.*

5. Squeeze the drip chamber on the IV tubing until it is about ½ full. Always remember to flush air from the IV tubing.

6. If you have an IV pump, follow your nurse's instructions to hook up your IV tubing and to operate the pump.

7. Connect the IV fluids to the catheter. Open the roller clamp. You should see fluid flow through the drip chamber.

From Rice R: *Manual of home health nursing procedures,* St. Louis, 1995, Mosby.

8. Turn on the IV pump or adjust the roller clamp on the IV tubing to adjust the drops per minute as your physician has ordered. Your drops per minute are _____.

9. Watch the rate of flow of your IV fluids every hour, and do not let the bag of IV fluids run dry because this can cause the catheter to clog up.

10. Administer your IV fluids and medications at the correct dose and time.

11. Stop the IV infusion when it has been completed. Irrigate and flush your catheter as your nurse has shown you in order to keep your IV line open. Flush with _____ of normal saline solution and _____ of heparin solution. Check with your nurse because some catheters will not require a heparin flush.

12. If you have a central line, keep your catheter clamped at all times when it is not in use.

13. Change your IV dressing if it becomes loose or soiled.

14. Clean the entry site of your IV with an antiseptic wipe. Start at the center and move outward about 1 to 2 inches in a circular motion. Do this two more times, with fresh antiseptic wipes. Never return to the entry site of your IV with the same wipe because this could spread germs into your IV.

15. Cover your IV with a gauze dressing, and secure it with tape. Tape your IV catheter to prevent tugging or to prevent it from accidentally coming out.

16. If your IV catheter accidently gets torn, clamp it to prevent leakage or air embolism, and notify the home health agency clinical supervisor.

17. If the IV catheter accidentally comes out, cover the site with a gauze dressing to prevent bleeding. Hold pressure to the area for 5 minutes, and then notify the home health agency clinical supervisor.

18. If you should feel short of breath or dizzy, notify the Emergency Medical Services (EMS) for emergency assistance. Your local EMS number is _____.

19. Carefully place used needles in a sharps container. Always avoid touching the needle. Keep your sharps container out of the reach of children. When your sharps container is full, call your home IV supplier for a new sharps container for IV supplies.

20. Record when you hang a bag of IV fluids. Record the date and time.

21. Call the home health agency clinical supervisor if the following circumstances occur:

    Dressing supplies are needed.

    You have questions or problems regarding your IV.

    You are hospitalized.

Collecting Blood Specimens by Venipuncture

The three primary methods of obtaining blood specimens are venipuncture, skin puncture, and arterial stick.

Venipuncture, the most common method, involves inserting a hollow-bore needle into the lumen of a large vein to obtain a specimen. The nurse may use a needle and syringe or a special Vacutainer that allows the drawing of multiple blood samples. Because veins are major sources of blood for laboratory testing and routes for IV fluid or blood replacement, maintaining their integrity is essential. The nurse should be skilled in venipuncture to avoid unnecessary injury to veins.

Skin puncture is the least traumatic method of obtaining a blood specimen. A sterile lancet or needle is used to puncture a vascular area on a finger, toe, or heel. A drop of blood is placed on a test slide or collected within a thin glass capillary tube for laboratory analysis.

The most traumatic form of obtaining blood specimens is arterial stick. A small-gauge needle is inserted directly into the lumen of an artery to collect a specimen. Of all methods for obtaining blood specimens, arterial stick poses the greatest risks.

1. Determine understanding of purpose of procedure and method to be used.
2. Determine if special conditions need to be met before specimen collection (e.g., client to the NPO, specific time for collection after medication or meal).
3. Assess client for possible risk for venipuncture: anticoagulant therapy, low platelet count, bleeding disorders (history of hemophilia or ecchymosis).
4. Determine ability to cooperate with procedure.
5. Assess client for contraindicated sites for venipuncture: presence of IV fluids, hematoma at potential site, history of mastectomy, hemodialysis recipient.
6. Review physician's orders for type of tests.
7. **a.** Obtain appropriate specimen under required conditions (according to agency laboratory policy).
   b. Minimize discomfort at venipuncture site.
   c. Minimize trauma at needle insertion site.
   d. Prevent infection at venipuncture site.
   e. Minimize client's anxiety.

Modified from Perry AG, Potter PA: *Clinical nursing skills and techniques,* ed 4, St. Louis, 1998, Mosby.

8. Prepare equipment and supplies:
   a. Alcohol or antiseptic swab.
   b. Disposable gloves.
   c. Small pillow or folded towel.
   d. Sterile gauze pads (2 × 2).
   e. Rubber tourniquet.
   f. Band-Aid or adhesive tape.
   g. *Syringe method:*
      • Sterile needles (20 to 21 gauge for adults, 23 to 25 gauge for children).
      • Sterile syringe of appropriate size.
   h. *Vacutainer method:*
      • Vacutainer tube with needle holder.
      • Sterile, double-ended needles (20 to 21 gauge for adults, 23 to 25 gauge for children). (Some nurses prefer to use butterfly or scalp vein needles.)
   i. Appropriate blood tubes.
   j. Completed identification labels according to agency policy.
   k. Completed laboratory requisition (date, time, type of test).
9. Explain procedure to client: describe purpose of tests; explain how sensation of tourniquet, alcohol swab, needle stick feel.
10. Wash hands.
11. Bring equipment to bedside.
12. Assist client to supine or semi-Fowler's position with arms extended to form straight line from shoulders to wrists. Place small pillow or towel under upper arm.
13. If client is a child, ask parent to restrain child so venipuncture site is immobilized.
14. Apply disposable gloves.
15. Apply tourniquet 5 to 15 cm (2 to 6 inches) above venipuncture site selected (antecubital fossa site is most often used). Encircle extremity and pull one end of tourniquet tightly over other, looping one end under other. Apply tourniquet so it can be removed by pulling end with single motion.
16. Palpate distal pulse (e.g., radial) below tourniquet. If pulse not palpable, reapply tourniquet more loosely.
17. Keep tourniquet on no longer than 1 to 2 minutes.
18. Ask client to open and close fist several times, finally leaving fist clenched.
19. Quickly inspect extremity for best venipuncture site, looking for straight, prominent vein without swelling or hematoma.
20. Palpate selected vein with index finger. Note if vein is firm and rebounds when palpated or if vein feels rigid and cordlike and rolls when palpated.

21. Select venipuncture site. (If tourniquet is on arm too long, remove, and assess other extremity or wait 60 seconds before reapplying.)
22. Obtain blood sample:
    a. *Syringe method:*
       - Have syringe with appropriate needle securely attached.
       - Cleanse venipuncture site with alcohol swab, moving in circular motion from site for approximately 5 cm (2 inches). Allow to dry.
       - Remove needle cover and inform client "stick" lasting only few seconds will be felt.
       - Place thumb or forefinger of nondominant hand 2.5 cm (1 inch) above or below site and pull skin taut.
       - Hold syringe and needle at 15- to 30-degree angle from client's arm with bevel up.
       - Slowly insert needle into vein.
       - Hold syringe securely and pull back gently on plunger.
       - Look for blood return.
       - Obtain desired amount of blood, keeping needle stabilized.
       - After specimen is obtained, release tourniquet.
       - Apply 2 × 2 gauze pad or antiseptic swab over puncture site without applying pressure and quickly but carefully withdraw needle from vein.
    b. *Vacutainer method:*
       - Attach double-ended needle to Vacutainer tube.
       - Have proper blood specimen tube resting inside Vacutainer but do not puncture rubber stopper.
       - Cleanse venipuncture site with alcohol swab, moving in circular motion out from site for approximately 5 cm (2 inches).
       - Remove needle cover and inform client that "stick" lasting only few seconds will be felt.
       - Place thumb or forefinger of nondominant hand 2.5 cm (1 inch) above or below site and pull skin taut. Stretch skin down until vein is stabilized.
       - Hold Vacutainer at 15- to 30-degree angle from arm with bevel up.
       - Slowly insert needle into vein.
       - Grasp Vacutainer securely and advance specimen tube into needle of holder (do not advance needle in vein).
       - Note flow of blood into tube (should be fairly rapid).
       - After specimen tube is filled, grasp Vacutainer firmly and remove tube. Insert additional specimen tubes as needed.
       - After last tube is filled, release tourniquet.
       - Apply 2 × 2 gauze pad over puncture site without applying pressure and quickly but carefully withdraw needle from vein.

23. Immediately apply pressure over venipuncture site with gauze or antiseptic pad for 2 to 3 minutes or until bleeding stops. *Option:* apply pressure over site and tape gauze dressing securely.

24. For blood obtained by syringe, transfer specimen to tubes. Insert needle through stopper of blood tube and allow vacuum to fill tube. Do not force blood into tube.

    or

    Remove needle from syringe and stopper to each test tube. Gently inject required amount of blood into each tube. Reapply stopper.

25. Take blood tubes containing additives and gently rotate back and forth 8 to 10 times.

26. Inspect puncture site for bleeding and apply adhesive tape with gauze.

27. Check tubes for any sign of external contamination with blood. Decontaminate with 70% alcohol if necessary.

28. Remove disposable gloves after specimen obtained and any spillage cleaned.

29. Assist client to comfortable position.

30. Securely attach properly completed identification label to each tube and affix proper requisition.

31. Dispose of needles, syringe, soiled equipment in proper container. Do not cap needles.

32. Wash hands after procedure.

33. Send or take specimens immediately to laboratory.

34. Reinspect venipuncture site.

35. Determine if client remains anxious or fearful.

36. Check laboratory report for test results.

37. If hematoma develops, obtain order from physician to apply cold compress. After bleeding subsides, order for hot compress can be obtained.

38. Inform clients who are to receive further venipunctures about reasons for tests.

Special considerations

- Check policy regarding designated container for disposal of contaminated needles and syringes.
- If gloves become contaminated with blood, replace with clean pair after proper disposal of contaminated ones. Touch nothing and do not handle supplies with contaminated gloves.
- Infants and young children need to be restrained, as do restless, confused, or combative clients. Check policy on need for physician's order if restraint is necessary. Parent may hold child to facilitate cooperation and decrease anxiety.

- Samples taken from vein near IV infusion may be diluted or contain concentrations of IV fluids. Postmastectomy client may have reduced lymphatic drainage in arm on operative side, increasing risk of infection from needle sticks. Arteriovenous shunt should never be used to obtain specimens because of risks of clotting and bleeding. Hematoma indicates existing injury to vessel's wall.
- If drawing sample for blood alcohol level, use only antiseptic swab to ensure accurate test results.
- Clients receiving anticoagulants require pressure over site for at least 5 minutes.
- If child needs to be restrained during procedure, let parents choose if they want to assist. Person restraining client should speak in calm, reassuring tone. By leaning across child, nurse maintains body and eye contact, which can help reduce fear.
- If client has large distended veins, tourniquet may not be needed.
- Clients undergoing frequent venipunctures may have preferred or undesirable site. Most commonly used vein is median cubital in antecubital fossa. In children, use veins on dorsal aspect of foot or scalp veins. Avoid vessels that pulsate; this indicates artery.
- If vein cannot be palpated or viewed easily, remove tourniquet and apply warm, wet compress over extremity for 10 to 20 minutes. Heat causes local vasodilation.
- With experience nurse will feel "pop" as needle enters vein. If plunger is pulled back too quickly, pressure may cause vein to collapse.
- Instruct client to briefly apply pressure to venipuncture site. Clients with bleeding disorders or on anticoagulant therapy should apply pressure for at least 5 minutes.
- Instruct client to notify nurse, agency, or physician if persistent or recurrent bleeding or expanding hematoma occurs at venipuncture site.

Vascular Access Devices

Clients with chronic diseases often need long-term IV therapy, which requires safe, repeated access to the venous system for administration of drugs, fluids, nutrition, and blood products. Frequent venipuncture and multiple IV lines pose problems and risks, including infection, pain, and bruising. Clients with chronic diseases are generally more susceptible to infection and bleeding. Clients receiving multiple doses of chemotherapeutic drugs experience vein sclerosis or hardening. Eventually, no suitable peripheral veins remain for drug administration.

The need for safe and convenient long-term IV therapy has led to the development of VADs, which are catheters, cannulas, or infusion ports designed for long-term, repeated access to the venous or arterial systems. The nurse must be able to maintain the integrity of central venous catheters and implanted infusion ports and educate clients about the care of catheters for home use.

Home health nurses frequently administer parenteral nutrition and chemotherapy in the home using VADs. The trend in the care of oncology clients is expanded home health services. VADs allow clients to go home earlier and to receive continued care rather than remain in acute-care settings for several weeks.

Nurses play a role in identifying clients who may benefit from VADs. For example, a client with severe nutritional deficiencies may need long-term parenteral nutrition. The nurse may be the first to recognize the client's intolerance to oral or enteral feedings.

The types of VADs and their therapeutic uses vary according to the diagnosis. Nurses must have the necessary knowledge, skill, and judgment to maintain and troubleshoot VADs. Client education is also important. Clients and families learn to change dressings around catheters and to recognize signs of complications such as infection, bleeding, or leakage at insertion sites.

To manage long-term IV therapy effectively the nurse must know the types of VADs, including central venous catheters, external catheters, and implanted infusion ports.

Central venous catheters are inserted by the physician into a large vein, typically the superior vena cava that leads to the right atrium of the heart (Figure 56). The large vessel lumen minimizes the risks of vessel irritation, inflammation, or sclerosis that commonly occur when smaller peripheral veins are used.

Atrial catheters are surgically inserted with the client in the operating room under general or local anesthesia. First a tunnel is made through subcutaneous tissue, usually between the clavicle and nipple.

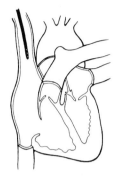

Figure 56

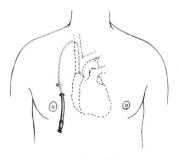

Figure 57

The tunnel allows the catheter to remain in place longer because it creates space between the end of the catheter and the actual vein. The risk of infection is less. Then the catheter tip is inserted through the cephalic, internal, or external jugular vein, or a similar large vein, and is threaded into the right atrium (Figure 57). These catheters have single or double lumens; i.e., one or two hollow tubes extend within the inside of the catheter and allow for administration of more than one type of infusion simultaneously.

A second type of external catheter is the small-gauge central venous catheter, which is inserted directly through the skin and into the subclavian vein of the neck or the basilic vein in the antecubital fossa of the arm. The catheter is threaded into the right atrium but can be used for only a short time. Intermittent or continuous intravenous infusions can be given.

The third type of VAD is the implanted infusion port, which consists of a self-sealing injection port housed in a plastic or metal case

(Figure 58) and connected to a silicone venous catheter. The port is also now available with a double-lumen catheter. The physician implants the infusion port under sterile conditions in an operating room with the client under local anesthesia. The infusion port usually rests in a subcutaneous pocket in the infraclavicular fossa, and the catheter is inserted into a large vein and threaded into the right atrium (Figure 59). The port can be easily palpated to determine placement. Specially designed Huber needles (straight or with 90-degree angles) are inserted through the skin to enter the port (Figure 60). Implanted infusion ports are used for administration of injections and for continuous infusions of all types: medications, chemotherapy, parenteral nutrition, and blood products. The nurse or client heparinizes the port every 4 weeks when not in use to maintain its patency.

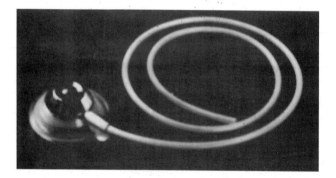

Figure 58

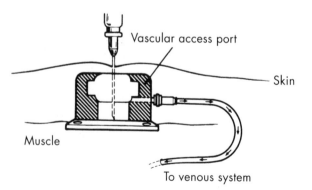

Figure 59

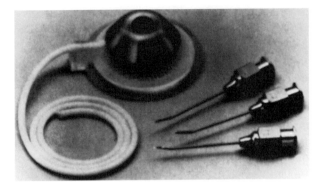

Figure 60

Care of VADs is simple as long as nurses and clients are aware of the purpose and function of the devices and the two most common complications, infection and clotting. In the home, most clients learn to use clean technique for dressing changes and catheter care. Within 2 to 3 weeks an adhesive bandage is sufficient to cover catheter insertion sites. Clients can learn to initiate infusions, heparinize devices, and discontinue infusions.

Criteria for Admission of Client to Home Infusion Therapy

1. Physician orders will be obtained before initiating treatment.
2. The client/caregiver will be informed about the treatment, risks, and responsibilities pertaining to the prescribed therapies and must sign the appropriate consent form before the institution of therapy.
3. The client/caregiver must assume full responsibility for purchasing all infusion supplies, medications, and solutions.
4. The client and caregiver are expected to participate in the management of the infusion treatment as agreed to in the consent form.
5. The IV program manager determines whether or not the agency has sufficient resources and/or expertise for safe administration.

Modified from VNA Health Care: *Infusion therapy admission policy,* Plainville, Conn, 1998, The Author.

Central Venous Catheter Management

Central venous catheters (CVC) are required for clients with a variety of medical conditions that include cancer and bowel disease. These catheters are used for long-term venous access and spare the patient repeated venipunctures. Central venous catheters are commonly used in the home to administer all types of IV therapy, including antimicrobial agents, hyperalimentation, chemotherapy, narcotics, and blood components. Central venous catheters are also used for blood sampling.

Common CVC catheters used in home care are subclavian catheters (e.g., Hohn catheter, or Deseret triple lumen catheters); tunneled catheters (e.g., Hickman-Broviac catheters or Groshong catheters); implantable vascular access devices (IVAD) (e.g., Port-a-Cath); and peripheral venous access systems (e.g., PAS port or PICC line). Use 1-inch needles whenever injections are made through the Luer-Lok injection cap because this reduces the possibility of damaging the catheter. Consult the manufacturer's recommendations if you are using a *needleless* system to access the central venous catheter and to initiate IV therapy.

Blood sampling

Equipment
1. Blood specimen tubes
2. Occlusion hemostat or Kelly-Bulldog clamp if needed (most central venous catheters have preattached clamps)
3. 20 cc and 10 cc syringes with 1-inch, 20-gauge needles for blood sampling
4. Laboratory requisition, labels
5. Antiseptic (povidone-iodine) and alcohol wipes
6. Disposable nonsterile gloves, sharps container

Procedure
1. Explain the procedure to the client/caregiver.
2. Assemble the equipment at a convenient work area.
3. Assist the client to a comfortable position to access the catheter.
4. Review the orders for laboratory specimens, and obtain the correct blood tubes.
5. Clean the injection cap(s) with an antiseptic, then use an alcohol wipe and air dry.

From Rice R: *Manual of home health nursing procedures,* St. Louis, 1995, Mosby.

6. Release the clamp. (Most Hickman and Broviac catheters come with preattached clamps and reinforced clamping sleeves. The Groshong catheter does not have a clamp.)

7. Gently aspirate 7 ml of blood from the catheter. Place needle-syringe with blood in a sharps container.

8. Insert a 20 cc syringe into the injection cap. Gently withdraw the appropriate amount of blood needed for blood sampling.

9. Follow the procedure for *Irrigation* in order to clear the line and to prevent occlusion.

10. Clamp the catheter over the reinforced clamping sleeve or the tape tab.

11. Label and prepare the blood tube(s) for transport.

12. Provide client comfort measures.

13. Clean and replace the equipment. Discard disposable items in a plastic trash bag, and secure.

Cap change

Equipment

1. Injection cap(s), tape

2. Occlusion hemostat or Kelly-Bulldog clamp (many central venous catheters are preattached clamps)

3. Sterile normal saline solution

4. 3 cc syringe with 1-inch, 23-gauge needle

5. Antiseptic wipes, alcohol wipes

6. Disposable nonsterile gloves (See *Infection Control*)

Procedure

1. Follow steps 1 through 3 of the procedure for *Blood Sampling*.

2. Make sure the catheter is clamped with an occlusion hemostat if the catheter does not have a preattached clamp. (The Groshong catheter does not have a clamp.)

3. Untape the connection between the injection cap and the catheter (taping the connection helps prevent the cap from becoming dislodged). *Do not* cut the tape with scissors as you may damage the catheter.

4. Grasp the end of the catheter between the index finger and the thumb. Clean the connection with antiseptic and then an alcohol wipe, and air dry (Figure 61).

5. Open the package containing the replacement cap. Using the aseptic technique, prime the injection cap with 1 ml of normal saline solution; then replace the cap in the package, until you are ready to use it.

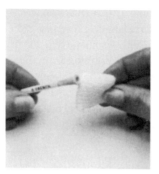

Figure 61 Cleaning the catheter connection. *Courtesy Bard Access Systems, Salt Lake City, Utah.*

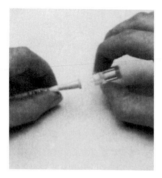

Figure 62 Attaching the new injection cap to the catheter. *Courtesy Bard Access Systems, Salt Lake City, Utah.*

6. Unscrew the old injection cap, and discard it. Pick up the new cap, touching only the outside rubber port. Then remove the protective covering from the end of the new injection cap, and discard it.
7. Screw the new injection cap onto the catheter. Be careful not to touch the tip of the catheter or the injection cap (Figure 62).
8. Release the clamp for a minute to make sure that the cap is on correctly and that the connection is not leaking. Then reclamp the catheter over the reinforced clamping sleeve or over the tape tab if the catheter is not being used.
9. Tape the connection, making tabs on the ends of the tape by folding back ½ inch. (The tabs on the end of the tape will enable you to remove it very easily.) Write the date and time of the cap change on the tape.
10. Follow steps 12 and 13 of the procedure for *Blood Sampling*.

Dressing change

Equipment

1. Disposable CVC dressing tray (includes alcohol swab sticks (3), antiseptic swabsticks (3), benzoin swabstick (1), antibiotic ointment, tape, and face mask)
2. Two transparent adhesive dressings
3. Disposable nonsterile and sterile gloves, sharps container (see *Infection Control*)

Procedure

1. Follow steps 1 through 3 of the procedure for *Blood Sampling.*
2. Place the dressing tray on a clean, dry surface. Unwrap the tray, including the sterile gloves, without touching the inner sterile contents.
3. Don nonsterile gloves and the face mask. Remove the old dressing, being careful not to dislodge the catheter. Discard the dressing.
4. Examine the catheter exit site for signs of infection (redness or drainage). Report to the physician as appropriate.
5. Discard the nonsterile gloves. Don the sterile gloves. Use the aseptic technique to clean the catheter exit site in the following manner:
   a. Remove the antiseptic swabstick from its package; clean the area with the antiseptic swabstick, starting at the catheter exit site and moving outward in a spiral motion to cover an area 4 to 6 cm in diameter (Figure 63); discard the swab, and select a new one (never go back to the catheter exit site with a swabstick or a wipe that has touched skin away from the site)

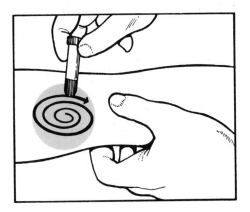

Figure 63 Cleaning the venipuncture site. *From LaRocca J:* Handbook of home care IV therapy, *St. Louis, 1994, Mosby.*

    b. Repeat step 5*a* two additional times with antiseptic swab-sticks; then air dry

    c. Clean the area thoroughly with alcohol swabsticks as de-scribed in step 5*a;* then air dry

6. Apply the benzoin swab to the perimeters of the dressing as a skin preparation.

7. Apply transparent adhesive dressing. If desired, picture frame the perimeters of dressing with tape (Figure 64).

8. Loop the catheter, with the cap pointing upward, on the dress-ing. Secure with tape to prevent tugging or accidental dislodge-ment.

9. Date and time the dressing change on the tape.

10. Perform injection *Cap Change* and catheter *Irrigation* as needed (see procedures for CVC injection *Cap Change* and *Irrigation*).

11. Instruct the client to contact the home health agency if the dress-ing becomes loosened or soiled.

12. Follow steps 12 through 13 of the procedure for *Blood Sampling.*

Irrigation and heparinization

Equipment

1. 100 u/ml heparin solution

2. Sterile normal saline solution

3. 3 cc syringes with 1-inch 23-gauge needle

4. Antiseptic (povidone-iodine) and alcohol wipes

5. Disposable nonsterile gloves, sharps container (see *Infection Control*)

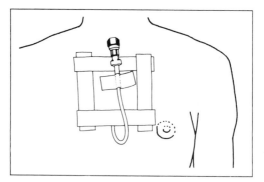

Figure 64 Securing the transparent adhesive dressing. *Courtesy Bard Access Systems, Salt Lake City, Utah.*

Procedure
1. Follow steps 1 through 3 of the procedure for *Blood Sampling*.
2. Clean the injection cap(s) with an antiseptic then with alcohol wipe. Air dry.
3. Release the clamp from the catheter. (Most Hickman and Broviac catheters come with preattached clamps and reinforced clamping sleeves. The Groshong catheter does not have a clamp.)
4. Irrigate the lumen with 2.5 ml of normal saline solution; then flush with 2.5 ml of heparin solution. Inject the heparin into the catheter no faster than ½ ml per second.
5. Maintain positive pressure on the syringe plunger as you withdraw the needle to prevent a backflow of blood into the catheter tip and to ensure a heparin lock.
6. Clamp the catheter.
7. Loop the catheter with the cap pointing upward on the dressing. Secure with tape to prevent tugging or accidental dislodgement.
8. Follow steps 12 and 13 of the procedure for *Blood Sampling*.

Nursing considerations
If the catheter cannot be irrigated, do not force the solution into the catheter.
Instruct the client to change his or her body position, to cough, to deep breathe, or to raise his or her arm above the head. If you are still unable to irrigate and flush the catheter, notify the home health agency clinical supervisor and physician for further orders.
Refer to specific catheter procedures for further irrigation guidelines. Groshong catheters do not require heparinization.

Documentation guidelines
Document the following on the visit report:

- The procedure and client toleration
- The condition of the catheter exit site including any signs of redness, swelling, or drainage
- Irrigation and patency of the catheter lumen(s)
- Blood sampling and designated laboratory for delivery
- Any client/caregiver instructions, including the ability to safely manage the Groshong catheter at home
- Other pertinent findings
  Document IV medications/solutions infused on the medication or IV record.
  Update the client care plan.

Declotting a Port-A-Cath

Purpose
- To declot and clear the Port-A-Cath with thrombolytic agents

General information
Adhere to the manufacturer's recommendations for administration of thrombolytic agents. According to the Intravenous Nursing Society in the *Intravenous Nursing Standards of Practice,* the volume of the thrombolytic agent instilled should approximate the volume of the catheter, assuring that the agent is retained in the catheter and is not instilled into the bloodstream.

Equipment
1. Thrombolytic agent (e.g., Urokinase) as prescribed by the physician
2. Sterile normal saline solution
3. 3 cc syringes with 1-inch needles, straight noncoring needle with integrated extension tubing and clamp for IVAD
4. Antiseptic (povidone-iodine) and alcohol wipes
5. Disposable nonsterile gloves, sharps container (See *Infection Control*)

Procedure
1. Explain the procedure to the client/caregiver.
2. Assemble the equipment at a convenient work area.
3. Assist the client to a comfortable position to access the catheter.
4. Clean the injection cap(s) or the area of skin over the Port-A-Cath septum with antiseptic followed by alcohol wipe; then air dry.
5. Follow specific catheter protocols to access the catheter.
6. Draw up 1 ml of Urokinase and 1 ml normal saline solution into a 3 cc syringe.
7. Connect the syringe to the integrated extension tubing on a noncoring needle. Unclamp the tubing.
8. Slowly inject the Urokinase into the occluded lumen and port of the Port-A-Cath. Wait 10 minutes.
9. Attempt aspiration of the residual clot.
10. Repeat the procedure with a 20-minute dwell time if patency is not achieved.

From Rice R: *Manual of home health nursing procedures,* St. Louis, 1995, Mosby.

11. Notify the physician if you are unable to aspirate the catheter. Otherwise follow the procedure for *Irrigation and Heparinization.*
12. Provide client comfort measures.
13. Clean and replace the equipment. Discard disposable items in a plastic trash bag, and secure. Place the used needles and syringes in a sharps container.

Documentation guidelines
Document the following on the visit report:

- The procedure and patient toleration
- Patency of the Port-A-Cath
- Condition of the catheter exit site
- Other pertinent findings

Document the thrombolytic agent on the medication record.
Update the client care plan.

Groshong Catheter Management

Purpose
- To administer intravenous (IV) fluids
- To sample blood for laboratory analysis
- To maintain patency of the catheter
- To prevent infection

General information
The Groshong Catheter is a long-term, central venous access device. It can be used to administer total parenteral nutrition, chemotherapy, IV fluids, blood and blood products, and antibiotic therapy; it may also be used for blood sampling.

From Rice R: *Manual of home health nursing procedures,* St. Louis, 1995, Mosby.

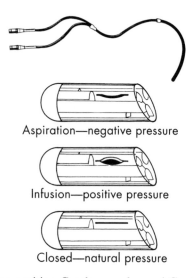

Aspiration—negative pressure

Infusion—positive pressure

Closed—natural pressure

Figure 65 Three-position Groshong valve and Groshong central venous catheter. *Courtesy Bard Access Systems, Salt Lake City, Utah.*

A small diameter, silicone rubber catheter, the Groshong has a patented, three-position valve that eliminates the need for heparinization and clamping (Figure 65). The tip of the catheter is placed in the superior vena cava via one of the large central veins (e.g., right subclavian) and tunneled subcutaneously to the exit site (upper abdominal area).

The Groshong catheter has a small dacron cuff that fibroses to the surrounding tissue. This secures the catheter in place and acts as a physical barrier for bacterial migration. The three-position valve near the closed tip opens outward during infusion and inward during blood withdrawal. The valve automatically closes when it is not in use. As a result of hydrostatic pressure, venous blood pressure is not sufficient to spontaneously open the valve inward; this prevents blood from backing up into the lumen and occluding the catheter with a clot.

Equipment
1. Sterile normal saline solution
2. 10, 20, or 30 cc syringes with 1-inch needles
3. Blood specimen tubes
4. Laboratory requisition, labels
5. Antiseptic (povidone-iodine) and alcohol wipes
6. Disposable nonsterile gloves, sharps container (See *Infection Control*)

Blood sampling

Procedure

1. Explain the procedure to the client/caregiver.
2. Assemble the equipment at a convenient work area.
3. Assist the client to a comfortable position to access the catheter.
4. Ask the client/caregiver if there are any problems with the catheter. Evaluate the dressing and injection cap change.
5. Review the order for the laboratory specimens, and obtain correct blood tubes.
6. Remove the injection cap from the end of the catheter and clean it with antiseptic followed by alcohol wipes. Then air dry.
7. Connect 10 cc syringe, and then aspirate 5 to 10 ml of blood (slowly withdraw the blood). Discard syringe into a sharps container.
8. Attach a 20 cc syringe directly to the catheter tubing, and withdraw the amount of blood needed for lab analysis.
9. Flush the Groshong catheter with 20 ml of normal saline solution, giving 1 ml at a time for the first 10 ml. Then briskly push the remaining 10 ml to remove residual blood.
10. Maintain positive pressure on the syringe plunger as the syringe is removed.
11. Using the aseptic technique, attach a new sterile injection cap. (See procedure for *Central Venous Catheter Management.*)
12. Label and prepare the blood tube(s) for transport.
13. Provide client comfort measures.
14. Clean and replace the equipment. Discard disposable items in a plastic trash bag, and secure.

Irrigation

Procedure

1. Follow steps 1 through 4 of the procedure for *Blood Sampling.*
2. Clean the injection cap with antiseptic, followed by alcohol wipe. Then air dry.
3. Draw up the required amount of normal saline solution in syringe.
4. Gently insert the syringe needle into the injection cap; then irrigate the catheter in the following manner:
   a. Briskly irrigate Groshong catheter with 10 ml of normal saline solution
      (1) Before and after antibiotic therapy
      (2) Weekly, when the catheter is not in use

    b. Briskly irrigate the Groshong catheter with 20 ml of normal saline solution

      (1) After blood sample withdrawal

      (2) After blood transfusions

      (3) After administration of blood products

      (4) If blood is observed in the catheter

    c. Irrigate the Groshong catheter with 30 ml of normal saline solution

      (1) After total parenteral nutrition infusion

5. Maintain positive pressure on the syringe plunger as the needle is removed from the injection cap.

6. Follow steps 11 through 14 of the procedure for *Blood Sampling.*

Nursing considerations

Routine clamping of the Groshong catheter is not needed. Heparin is not required to keep the catheter open.

Documentation guidelines

Document the following on the visit report:

- The procedure and client toleration
- Blood sampling and designated laboratory for delivery
- Amount of normal saline solution used for irrigation
- Condition of catheter exit site
- Dressing and cap change (if done)
- Any client/caregiver instructions, including the ability to safely manage the Groshong catheter at home
- Other pertinent findings

    Document IV medications/solutions infused on the medication or IV record.

    Update the client care plan.

Implantable Vascular Access Device Management

Purpose
- To administer intravenous (IV) fluids
- To sample blood for laboratory analysis
- To maintain the patency of the Implantable Vascular Access Device (IVAD)
- To prevent infection

General information
The IVAD is implanted under the skin with the attached catheter surgically tunneled into the cephalic or external jugular vein. The catheter tip sits in the superior vena cava near the right atrium, much like other central venous catheters. Flush the port of the IVAD with 10 ml of normal saline solution after intravenous infusion or blood sampling. Then heparinize with 5 ml heparin solution. Heparinize the IVAD every 30 days when it is not in use.

Equipment
1. (1) right-angle noncoring needle with integrated 6-inch extension tubing with clamp
2. 100 u/ml heparin solution
3. Sterile normal saline solution
4. 5 cc syringes, 10 cc syringes, and (1) 20 cc syringe for blood sampling
5. Blood specimen tubes
6. Laboratory requisition, labels
7. Antiseptic (povidone-iodine) and alcohol wipes
8. Disposable sterile gloves, sharps container (See *Infection Control*)

Blood sampling
Procedure
1. Explain the procedure to the client/caregiver.
2. Review the orders for laboratory specimen, and obtain the correct blood tubes.
3. Assemble the equipment at a convenient work area.
4. Assist the client to a comfortable position to access the IVAD.

From Rice R: *Manual of home health nursing procedures,* St. Louis, 1995, Mosby.

5. Cleanse the skin over the IVAD septum (injection site) with antiseptic wipes. Start at the site of the needle entrance, and work in a circular motion 4 to 6 cm outward. Discard the wipe.
6. Repeat step 5 two additional times, with antiseptic wipes.
7. Clean the area with an alcohol wipe; then air dry.
8. Attach the syringe with 10 ml of normal saline solution to the extension tubing; prime the extension tubing and noncoring needle. (Only special noncoring needles can be used when entering the port.)
9. Palpate the location of the IVAD septum to access the portal septum.
10. Firmly push the needle through the skin and portal septum at a 90-degree angle, until it hits the bottom of the portal chamber (Figure 66). You may hear a click as the needle touches the bottom of the portal chamber.
11. Flush the system with 10 ml normal saline solution to confirm that fluid flows through the system.
12. Aspirate 5 ml of blood for discard.
13. Clamp the extension tubing, remove the syringe, and discard it in a sharps container.

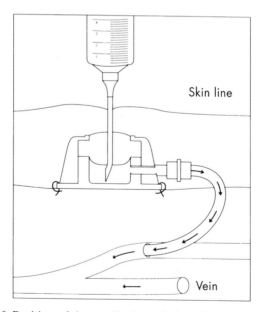

Figure 66 Position of the needle through the skin. *Courtesy Sims Deltec, St. Paul, Minn.*

14. Attach a 20 cc syringe. Unclamp the extension tubing, withdraw the appropriate amount of blood for a sample.
15. Repeat steps 13 and 14 until the appropriate amount of blood sample is obtained.
16. When the blood sampling is completed, clamp the tubing, and remove the syringe. Discard the syringe in a sharps container.
17. Attach the syringe containing 10 ml of normal saline solution. Unclamp the extension tubing, and irrigate the IVAD.
18. Clamp the extension tubing, and remove the syringe. Discard the syringe.
19. Attach the syringe containing the 5 ml of heparin solution. Unclamp the extension tubing, and flush the system.
20. Maintain positive pressure on the syringe plunger as you remove the syringe to prevent backflow of blood into the portal septum and to ensure a heparin lock (Figure 67). Hold the port in place, while removing the needle. Discard the needle, tubing, and syringe.
21. Cleanse the injection site with an antiseptic wipe, followed by an alcohol wipe; then air dry.
22. Label and prepare the blood tube(s) for transport.
23. Provide client comfort measures.
24. Clean and replace the equipment. Discard disposable items in a plastic trash bag, and secure. Place the used needles and syringes in a sharps container.

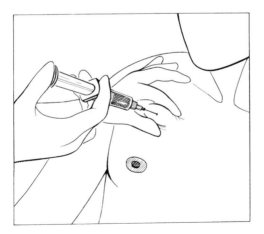

Figure 67 Maintaining positive pressure as needle is withdrawn. *Courtesy Sims Deltec, St. Paul, Minn.*

Bolus injection

Procedure

1. Access the IVAD as described in the procedure for *Blood Sampling.*
2. Flush the system with 10 ml of normal saline solution to ensure patency. Secure the noncoring needle with tape.
3. Clamp the extension tubing, and remove the syringe. Discard the syringe.
4. Attach the syringe with the drug to be injected into the extension tubing.
5. Inject the medication.
6. When the injection is complete, clamp the extension tubing. Remove the syringe, and discard it.
7. Irrigate the IVAD with 10 ml of normal saline solution followed by 5 ml heparin flush. (Be careful to clamp the tubing when exchanging syringes.)
8. Maintain positive pressure on the syringe plunger as you withdraw the noncoring needle to prevent backflow of blood into the portal septum and to ensure a heparin lock.
9. Follow steps 23 and 24 of the procedure for *Blood Sampling.*

Continuous infusion

Procedure

1. Access the IVAD as described in the procedure for *Blood Sampling.* Use a right-angle, noncoring needle with an extension tubing.
2. Clamp the extension tubing.
3. Attach the syringe with 10 ml of normal saline solution to the extension tubing. Unclamp the extension tubing, and flush the portal septum.
4. Clamp the extension tubing, and remove syringe.
5. Connect the IV set or infusion to the extension tubing.
6. Unclamp the extension tubing and begin infusion.
7. Secure the needle placement with sterile Steri-Strips or with ½ inch of tape. Roll a 2 × 2 gauze under the needle to stabilize it if needed. Apply transparent adhesive dressing, and tape all connections.
8. Loop the extension tubing on the dressing, and secure it with tape.
9. Follow steps 23 and 24 of the procedure for *Blood Sampling.*

Nursing considerations
Use a sterile needle and tubing for each bolus access.
Change the sterile needle and tubing for continuous infusion every 5 to 7 days.
Follow the manufacturer's recommendations for blood sampling for PAS PORT and PICC lines.
A dressing is not required when the port is not being accessed.

Documentation guidelines
Document the following on the visit report:

- The procedure and client toleration
- Blood sampling and designated laboratory for delivery
- Patency of the IVAD
- Condition of the skin over the IVAD
- Any client/caregiver instructions, and ability to safely manage the IVAD at home
- Other pertinent findings
    Document IV medications/solutions infused on the medication or IV record.
    Update the client care plan.

Multiple Lumen Nontunneled Catheter Management

Purpose
To administer intravenous (IV) fluids
To sample blood for laboratory analysis

General information
The multiple or triple lumen catheter typically has three ports. The white and blue lumens are of equal diameter (Figure 68). The red-rust colored lumen is slightly larger and should be used for infusion of blood and for obtaining blood specimens. This central venous catheter is for short-term use only.

Irrigate all accessed ports of the multiple lumen catheter with normal saline solution followed by heparin flush before or after use and daily to maintain patency of the lumens. Follow the manufacturer's recommendations for a *needleless* system.

From Rice R: *Manual of home health nursing procedures,* St. Louis, 1995, Mosby.

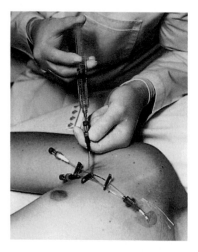

Figure 68 Triple-lumen catheter. *From Perry AG, Potter PA:* Clinical nursing skills and techniques, *ed 3, St. Louis, 1994, Mosby.*

Blood sampling

Equipment
1. Sterile normal saline solution
2. 100 u/ml heparin solution
3. Syringes with 1-inch, 20-gauge needle
4. Blood tubes
5. Laboratory requisitions and labels
6. Antiseptic (povidone-iodine) and alcohol wipes
7. Disposable nonsterile gloves, sharps container (See *Infection Control*)

Procedure
1. Explain the procedure to the client/caregiver.
2. Assemble the equipment at a convenient work area.
3. Assist the client to a comfortable position to access the IV.
4. Review the physician's order for lab specimens, and obtain the correct blood tubes.
5. Stop infusions through all ports being used for IV infusion.
6. Clean the injection cap of the red-rust–colored lumen with antiseptic followed by alcohol wipes; then air dry.
7. Unclamp the lumen.
8. Draw the blood specimen in the following manner:
   a. Attach 12 cc syringe, withdraw at least 6 ml of blood, and discard the syringe and needle into a sharps container

   b. Attach the syringe—the size required for obtaining speci-mens; withdraw enough blood for the specimens needed (use this method for drawing antibiotic levels)

9. Push the needle of the syringe with the blood sample into a rub-ber stopper of a test tube for collection. Discard used needle and syringe in a sharps container.

10. Irrigate the lumen with 10 ml of normal saline solution, and then flush with 2.5 ml of heparin solution.

11. Maintain positive pressure on the syringe plunger as you with-draw the needle to prevent a backflow of blood into the catheter tip and to ensure a heparin lock. Then clamp the lumen with the slide guard.

12. Resume infusion(s) to the other lumens if they are stopped.

13. Label and prepare the test tube(s) for transport.

14. Provide client comfort measures.

15. Clean and replace the equipment. Discard disposable items in a plastic trash bag, and secure. Place the used needles and sy-ringes in a sharps container.

Intermittent infusion

Equipment

1. Sterile normal saline solution
2. 100 u/ml heparin solution
3. (3) 5 cc syringes with 1-inch needle
4. Antiseptic (povidone-iodine) and alcohol wipes
5. Disposable nonsterile gloves, sharps container (See *Infection Control*)

Procedure

1. Follow steps 1 through 3 of the procedure for *Blood Sampling*.
2. Clean the injection cap with an antiseptic wipe, followed by alcohol wipes; then air dry.
3. Unclamp the selected lumen for infusion.
4. Flush the lumen with 5 ml of normal saline solution.
5. Begin infusion, using a small-bore needle to puncture the injec-tion cap.
6. Secure the needle to the injection cap with tape.
7. Tape the connection, making tabs on the ends of the tape by folding back ½ inch. (The tabs on the end of the tape will enable you to remove it easily.)
8. Irrigate catheter lumen with 5 ml of normal saline solution; then flush with 2.5 ml heparin solution when infusion is complete.

9. Maintain a positive pressure on the syringe plunger as you re-move the needle to prevent a backflow of blood into the catheter tip cap and to ensure a heparin lock.
10. Clamp the lumen with the slide guard.
11. Follow steps 14 and 15 of the procedure for *Blood Sampling.*

Nursing considerations

Irrigate all accessed ports of the multiple lumen catheter with nor-mal saline solution, followed by the heparin flush before and af-ter use and daily to maintain patency of lumens.

It may not be possible to aspirate blood if it is drawn too quickly or if the syringe used is smaller than 20 cc.

It may be necessary to clamp the lumen with the slide guard and to remove the Luer-Lok injection cap to obtain blood.

Do not draw clotting studies (PT, PTT) from the catheter.

Draw clotting studies peripherally before the catheter is heparinized because circulating heparin affects the PTT results up to 4 hours after the catheter has been heparinized.

Documentation guidelines

Document the following on the visit report:
- The procedure and client toleration
- Catheter exit site and the condition of the catheter, including the patency of all lumens
- Blood sampling and designated laboratory for delivery
- Any client/caregiver instructions, and ability to safely manage the multiple lumen catheter at home
- Other pertinent findings
  Document IV medications/solutions infused on the medication or IV record.
  Update the client care plan.

Peripheral Insertion of a Central Venous Catheter

Purpose
- To provide guidelines and a standardization of procedure for the peripheral insertion of a central venous catheter (PICC) line

General information
Insertion of PICC lines should be done by a PICC-certified nurse. Before the PICC line is placed, the client's chart should be reviewed for the (1) physician's order; (2) site restrictions; (3) coagulation status; and (4) medical allergies. A postinsertion chest x-ray is recommended to verify the catheter tip position. A client permit is required before placement.

PICC lines can be used for administration of blood products, chemotherapy, antibiotics, fluids, and controlled narcotic infusions (Figure 69). Superior vena cava placement is required for the infusion of total parenteral nutrition (TPN) or of any irritating or sclerosing agents.

PICC lines should never be used for high-pressure injection (i.e., diagnostic procedure or bolus emergency drugs). Do not use a syringe smaller than 3 cc with PICC lines. The alarm feature of infusion pumps should not exceed 40 psi for 3 French catheters or larger.

From Barnes Home IV Therapy Department, Barnes Hospital at Washington University Medical Center.

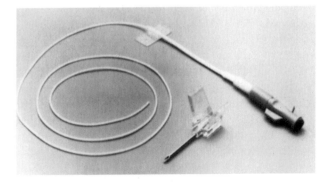

Figure 69 PICC line. *Courtesy Vygon Corporation, East Rutherford, NJ.*

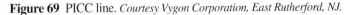

Equipment

1. PICC tray (single lumen 3 French or double lumen 4 French each)
2. Two sterile 5 cc syringes with needles
3. Sterile Luer-Lok injection cap or reflux valve
4. Sterile 3-inch Luer-Lok extension set
5. Vial 10 ml, 100 u/ml heparin solution
6. Vial 10 ml bacteriostatic 0.9% sodium chloride
7. 10 × 12 transparent occlusive dressing
8. Tourniquet
9. Two 2 × 2 gauze dressings
10. Four 4 × 4 gauze dressings
11. Antiseptic (povidone-iodine) and alcohol wipes
12. Two pair of disposable sterile gloves, a mask with an eye shield, a gown, sharps container (See *Infection Control*)

Procedure

1. Explain the procedure to the client/caregiver. Obtain a written consent for the procedure.
2. Assemble the equipment at a convenient work area.
3. Assist the client to a comfortable position to insert the IV.
4. Evaluate the antecubital veins for venipuncture.
5. Using a tape measure, measure the client for the desired final catheter tip location. Position the client's arm at a 45-90–degree angle from the body.

   a. *Subclavian vein:* Measure and record the distance from the insertion site to the sternal notch.

   b. *Superior vena cava* (SVC): If 1 inch of the catheter is to be left out at exit site, measure from 1 inch below the insertion site to the second intercostal space; if the intercostal spaces are not palpable, one third of the distance from the sternal notch to the xiphoid process may be used as an estimate; a catheter entering from the left arm will be slightly longer because it crosses over the chest and into the SVC, which is along the right border of the sternum; (a post insertion x-ray examination is required to verify superior vena cava placement; therefore, SVC placement should be done while the patient is in the hospital)

   c. *Midaxillary:* Measure from the insertion site to the desired tip location, allowing for the amount of the catheter that is to be left out from the exit site as appropriate

   Measure the bilateral arm circumference midway between the elbow and the shoulder.

6. Clean the work area, scrub the hands, and put on a mask and eye protection. Open a sterile PICC tray, and add sterile items to the PICC tray.

7. Prepare the client for the following procedure:
   a. Head of the bed is as flat as possible
   b. Linen protector is under the arm to be cannulated
   c. Provide adequate work space and lighting
   d. Tourniquet is in place but is not tied

8. Don sterile gloves and gown.

9. Place a large sterile drape under the client's arm.

10. Prep the insertion site for 3 minutes with alcohol wipes, and follow in 3 minutes with Betadine wipes. Vigorously cleanse the antecubital area from the center outward in a circular motion.

11. Draw up 5 ml of normal saline solution and 5 ml of heparin flush. Prime the extension tubing.

12. Place a fenestrated drape over the prepared puncture site, and add sterile 4 × 4s around the site as needed to absorb the blood flow.

13. Tighten the tourniquet, and don a second set of sterile gloves.

14. Perform venipuncture in the following manner:
    a. Venipuncture is verified by a flashback of blood into the hub or the syringe (if used)
    b. Advance the introducer sheath into the vein approximately ¼ inch
    c. Remove the needle; to control the blood flow, apply pressure above the introducer with the fifth finger or with 2 × 2s, and occlude the end of the introducer
    d. Release the tourniquet with a 4 × 4

15. The catheter is advanced in the following manner:
    a. Thread the catheter through the introducer with forceps in short, controlled steps
    b. After 5 to 7 inches of the catheter is placed, remove the introducer, and peel it away; allow 3 inches of catheter to remain outside the vein to facilitate removal of the introducer
    c. Advance the remainder of the catheter

16. If the catheter is placed centrally, instruct the client to touch his or her chin to the shoulder of the arm being cannulated to promote insertion while threading in the catheter.

17. The catheter guidewire is removed in the following manner:
    a. Stabilize the catheter with one hand, and gently pull out the guidewire; **do not pull vigorously or suddenly**
    b. After the guidewire is removed, immediately place the thumb over the hub to prevent an ingress of air

    c. Place the extension set with the syringe attached on the hub, and secure the connection

    d. Flush 3 ml of saline solution into the catheter; withdraw blood into the extension set to confirm that the catheter tip is within the vascular system; flush the remaining saline solution into the catheter

    e. Heparinize the catheter with 3 to 5 ml of 100 u/ml heparin solution

18. Apply a sterile occlusive dressing in the following manner:

    a. Cleanse the site with antiseptic wipes

    b. Pull the catheter out 1-inch and L-shape to prevent kinking and occlusion at the bend of the arm; secure with Steri-Strips

    c. Place 2 × 2 gauze pads folded under the length of the hub and extension tubing

    d. Cover with two 10 cm × 14 cm transparent dressings so that the site is covered from 1½ inches above the exit site

19. Provide client comfort measures.

20. Clean and replace the equipment. Discard disposable items in a plastic trash bag, and secure. Place the used needles and syringes in a sharps container.

Documentation guidelines

Document the following on the visit report:

- The client verification and/or chart review of allergy
- The procedure and client toleration
- Catheter type, gauge, lot number, total length, and length inserted
- Insertion site used
- Catheter tip position
- Application of occlusive dressing
- Complications or problems encountered
- Other pertinent findings

Update the client care plan.

Peripheral Intravenous Management

Purpose
- To administer intravenous (IV) fluids
- To hydrate the client
- To sample blood for laboratory analysis
- To heparin lock an IV for intermittent infusion of fluids and/or medications

General information
When choosing a site to start an IV, select the largest convenient vein most distal to an extremity. Choose a site below the client's elbow to increase comfort. Avoid cannulation over joints or previous IV sites because this predisposes to infiltration. The wing-tip or scalp needle is useful for accessing small or fragile veins for blood sampling. Heparin lock the IV for intermittent infusion of IV fluids and/or medications.

Equipment
1. IV administration set
2. IV fluids as prescribed by the physician
3. Tourniquet
4. Arm board (optional)
5. Number 20 to 22 needle, catheter or wing-tip needle with integrated extension tubing
6. Transparent adhesive dressing or 2 × 2 gauze dressing
7. Hypoallergenic tape
8. IV pole
9. Blood specimen tubes, 5 to 10 cc syringes with a 1-inch, 20-gauge needle, laboratory requisition, labels for blood sampling
10. Antiseptic (povidone-iodine) and alcohol wipes
11. Disposable nonsterile gloves, sharps container (See *Infection Control*)

Insertion of a peripheral IV and initiation of hydration fluids
Procedure
1. Explain the procedure to the client/caregiver.
2. Assemble the equipment at a convenient work area.
3. Assist the client to a comfortable position to initiate or to access the IV.

From Rice R: *Manual of home health nursing procedures,* St. Louis, 1995, Mosby.

4. Use an aseptic technique to set up IV fluids in the following manner:
   a. Clamp the tubing with the flow regulator
   b. Spike the container with tubing: hang the container on the IV pole
   c. Squeeze the drip chamber until it is half full
   d. Open the flow regulator, and prime the tubing; reclamp the tubing to prevent fluid flow
   e. Time tape IV bag if the pump is not used
5. Apply a tourniquet, and select the vein.
6. Cleanse the selected site with antiseptic wipes. Start at the point of needle insertion, and clean outward in a circular motion, approximately 3 to 4 cm. Repeat with alcohol wipes; then air dry.
7. Stretch the skin tight. Insert the needle with the bevel up at a 30-degree angle and parallel to the skin. Decrease the angle, and move the needle forward until the needle enters the vein.
8. Observe for blood flow to indicate correct needle placement.
9. Pull the needle back slightly; advance the catheter, and release the tourniquet.
10. Attach the IV tubing to the catheter hub. Open the flow regulator.
11. Slowly start the IV infusion. Assess the site for infiltration. If infiltration occurs, discontinue the IV, and restart the IV at an alternative site. Adjust the prescribed flow rate once the correct placement of the catheter has been established.
12. Tape the catheter to prevent accidental dislodgement. Avoid taping directly over the catheter because this may impede blood flow.
13. Apply transparent adhesive or 2 × 2 gauze dressing. Picture frame dressing with tape to secure the site so that early signs of phlebitis or infiltration can be detected.
14. Secure the IV tubing to the client's arm with tape to prevent tugging.
15. Instruct the client/caregiver in the management of home IV therapy.
16. Provide client comfort measures.
17. Clean and replace the equipment. Discard disposable items in a plastic trash bag, and discard. Place the used needles and syringes in a sharps container.

Nursing considerations

If the venipuncture is unsuccessful, reattempt it with a new catheter. If unsuccessful after 3 attempts, notify the physician.

Label the catheter insertion site with the catheter gauge, the date and time of insertion, and the initials of the nurse.

Inserting a wing-tip needle for blood sampling

Procedure

1. Follow steps 1 through 5 of the procedure for *Insertion of a Peripheral IV and Initiation of Hydration Fluids.* Keep the cap on the needle. Attach the 10 cc syringe to the hub of the integrated extension tubing on the wing-tip needle.
2. Remove the cap from the wing-tip needle. Point the needle in the direction of the blood flow, and hold it at a 45-degree angle above the skin, with the bevel facing up.
3. Pinch the wings tightly together. Pierce the client's skin at a point slightly to one side of the vein, approximately ½ inch below the spot where you plan to puncture the vein wall.
4. Decrease the needle angle, until the needle is almost level with the skin surface, and direct it toward the selected vein.
5. Puncture the vein. Observe for blood backflow.
6. Lift the bevel of the needle off the vein floor, and advance it, until the needle is inserted into the vein.
7. Remove the tourniquet.
8. Withdraw the blood sample into the syringe.
9. Discontinue the IV once the blood sample has been obtained.
10. Apply 2 × 2 gauze dressing or adhesive bandage to the venipuncture site.
11. Attach needle onto syringe with blood sample. Then push needle through the rubber stopper to fill the blood specimen tube(s). Label blood tubes and transport.
12. Follow steps 16 through 17 of the procedure for *Insertion of a Peripheral IV and Initiation of Hydration Fluids.*

Nursing considerations

If the wing-tip needle has an integrated extension set with a two-way needle hub, attach the vacutainer to the two-way needle hub.
Slide the blood specimen tube(s) into the vacutainer and onto the two-way needle once the vein is accessed to obtain blood samples.

Managing a heparin lock: initiating the lock

Equipment

1. (1) Luer-Lok injection cap
2. Sterile normal saline solution
3. 100 u/ml heparin solution
4. Number 20 to 22 catheter and venipuncture supplies
5. Sterile 3 cc syringes with 23- to 25-gauge needles
6. Kelly clamp

7. Antiseptic (povidone-iodine) and alcohol wipes
8. Disposable nonsterile gloves, sharps container (See *Infection Control*)

Procedure

1. Follow steps 1 through 3 of the procedure for *Insertion of a Peripheral IV and Initiation of Hydration Fluids.*
2. Draw up 1 ml of heparin solution and 2 ml of normal saline solution into separate syringes.
3. Cleanse the rubber stopper on the Luer-Lok injection cap with antiseptic, followed by alcohol wipes; then air dry.
4. Prime the Luer-Lok injection cap with normal saline solution.
5. Perform venipuncture. See the procedure for *Insertion of a Peripheral IV.*
6. Attach the saline-filled Luer-Lok injection cap into the cannula. Then flush with 2 ml of normal saline solution.
7. Observe the catheter exit site for signs of infiltration or leakage. If the catheter is patent, flush the Luer-Lok injection cap with 1 ml of heparin solution.
8. Maintain the positive pressure on the syringe plunger as you withdraw the needle to prevent the backflow of blood into the catheter tip and to ensure a heparin lock.
9. Tape to secure the catheter and to prevent accidental dislodgement.
10. Apply a 2 × 2 gauze or transparent adhesive dressing. Picture frame with tape as needed to secure the dressing. Date and time the dressing.
11. Follow steps 16 and 17 of the procedure for *Insertion of a Peripheral IV, and Initiation of Hydration Fluids.*

Managing a heparin lock: converting a continuous infusion to a heparin lock

Equipment

1. Sterile Luer-Lok injection cap
2. Sterile normal saline solution
3. 100 u/ml heparin solution
4. Kelly clamp
5. Sterile 3 cc syringes with 23- and 24-gauge needles
6. Antiseptic (povidone-iodine) and alcohol wipes
7. Disposable nonsterile gloves, sharps container (See *Infection Control*)

Procedure
1. Follow steps 1 through 3 of the procedure for *Insertion of a Peripheral IV, and Initiation of Hydration Fluids.*
2. Clamp off the intravenous tubing with a flow regulator.
3. Disconnect the tubing, using a Kelly clamp to stabilize the catheter hub.
4. Remove the protective covering from the Luer-Lok injection cap and aseptically insert it into the hub of the catheter.
5. Slowly flush with 2 ml of normal saline solution, and assess for infiltration to ascertain the catheter position. Flush with 1 ml of heparin solution if no swelling or leakage is noted.
6. Maintain positive pressure on the syringe plunger as you withdraw the needle to prevent backflow into the catheter tip and to ensure a heparin lock.
7. Follow steps 16 and 17 of the procedure for *Insertion of a Peripheral IV, and Initiation of Hydration Fluids.*

Managing a heparin lock: discontinuing a continuous infusion

Equipment
1. Same as the procedure for *Converting a Continuous Infusion to a Heparin Lock*

Procedure
1. Follow steps 1 through 3 of the procedure for *Insertion of a Peripheral IV, and Initiation of Hydration Fluids.*
2. Draw up 2 ml of normal saline solution and 1 ml of heparin solution in separate syringes.
3. Clamp off the IV tubing with the flow regulator.
4. Remove the needle and tubing from the heparin lock by one of the following methods:
   a. Remove the needle from the Luer-Lok injection cap; carefully remove the needle from the end of the tubing, and place it in the sharps container; discard the tubing and IV bag
   b. Cut the IV tubing 3 inches above the needle; place the needle and the connecting tubing in a sharps container; discard the remainder of the tubing and IV bag
5. Irrigate the Luer-Lok injection cap and the IV catheter with 2 ml normal saline solution. Then flush with 1 ml of heparin solution.
6. Maintain positive pressure on the syringe plunger as you withdraw the needle to prevent backflow of blood into the catheter tip and to ensure a heparin lock.

7. Evaluate for dressing change.
8. Follow steps 16 and 17 of the procedure for *Insertion of a Peripheral IV, and Initiation of Hydration Fluids.*

Documentation guidelines

Document the following on the visit report:

- The procedure and client toleration
- Type and number of the catheter that has been inserted
- Condition of the catheter exit site
- Blood specimen drawn and designated laboratory for delivery
- Any client/caregiver instructions, and the ability to safely manage home IV therapy
- Other pertinent findings

Document IV medications/solutions infused on the medication or IV record.

Update the client care plan.

Troubleshooting IV Therapy

1. If the infusion slows or stops, look for swelling, pain, or hardness around the needle or catheter site. If you notice any of these symptoms, stop the infusion and immediately notify your home health nurse or physician. If these signs and symptoms are not present, do the following:
   a. Check for twisted tubing or for pressure on tubing
   b. See if you have moved or bent your arm with the IV in it; if so, return your arm to its original position
   c. If the flow rate remains slow or has stopped, turn the regulator off, and contact your home health nurse
2. If you experience symptoms such as coughing, shortness of breath, increased rate of breathing, headache, facial flushing, rapid pulse rate, or dizziness, this could mean you are experiencing a condition called circulatory overload and have received too much fluid. Stop the infusion, and immediately call your home health nurse or physician. If the situation is an emergency, call an ambulance directly.
3. If you experience symptoms such as extreme shortness of breath, anxiety, lips and nailbeds turning blue, pulse increasing rapidly, or

From Rice R: *Manual of home health nursing procedures,* St. Louis, 1995, Mosby.

faintness, this could mean that air has entered the blood stream. **This is a medical emergency.** You should be placed on your left side, with head down. Have someone *immediately* call you an ambulance and then stay with you until the ambulance arrives.

4. Symptoms such as an abrupt rise in temperature, chills, complaints of backache or headache, nausea and vomiting, a flushed face, or dizziness may be caused by exposure to contaminated equipment or solutions. Discontinue IV therapy and call your home health nurse or physician. (If symptoms are severe, go to a hospital emergency department.) Save the equipment and IV solution so that it can be analyzed in a laboratory.

5. If the catheter breaks, clamp the line and notify your home health nurse or physician.

AIDS

Aerosolized Pentamidine Administration

Purpose
- To treat mild to moderate pneumocystis carinii pneumonia
- For prophylaxis treatment in acquired immunodeficiency syndrome (AIDS) clients

General information
Aerosolized pentamidine isethionate is administered to prevent AIDS-related pneumocystis carinii pneumonia. The therapeutic goal of the administration of pentamidine is to produce adequate drug levels in alveoli throughout all areas of the lungs while minimizing systemic and pulmonary side effects.

The first dose is administered under the direct supervision of a physician while the client is in a monitored setting. The nurse must stay with the client during subsequent treatments at home.

Evaluate the client for tuberculosis before administering the treatment. Health care workers and clients may be at risk for exposure to tuberculosis in situations where cough-inducing procedures are performed. If tuberculosis is diagnosed, the client should be started on antituberculosis medication before receiving pentamidine aerosol treatments.

From Rice R: *Manual of home health nursing procedures,* St. Louis, 1995, Mosby.

Equipment

1. Jet nebulizer with finger control device (includes a reservoir, hydrophobic filter and a series of one-way valves for effective particle dispersion throughout the lungs)
2. Oxygen with air flow meter or compressed air
3. Pentamidine isothionate, 300 mg or as ordered by the physician
4. 12 cc syringe with 18-gauge needle
5. Sterile water
6. 50 psi gas flow source (pressurized gas cylinder)
7. Glass of hot or cold liquid sipped by client during the procedure to moisten upper airway
8. Bronchodilator in case of emergency
9. Personal protective equipment, which includes a personal respiration mask that would trap most particles and provide some protection against tuberculosis, eyewear that provides a seal around the eyes (goggles), disposable gowns, and nonsterile disposable gloves (See *Infection Control*)

Procedure

1. Explain the procedure to the client.
2. Verify the medication with the client's medication record.
3. Assemble the equipment at a convenient work area. Perform the treatment near a window with the window open to the outside air. Keep family members out of the room during the treatment.
4. Assess breath sounds and heart and respiratory rate before and after the treatment. Also take the client's blood pressure before and after treatment.
5. Draw up 6 ml of sterile water in a syringe, and inject it into the 300 mg vial of pentamidine.
6. Shake the pentamidine until all the solute dissolves in the solution. (Pentamidine does not dissolve well in saline.)
7. Withdraw the solution from the pentamidine vial, and place it in the jet nebulizer.
8. Follow the manufacturer's instructions to set up the gas flow to nebulize the medication. Pressurized air or oxygen may be used as a gas source at 50 psi. Use pressurized air with CO_2 retainers. Instruct the client in the use of the finger control device.
9. Position the client in a high Fowler's position. (Consult with the physician regarding client positioning for treatment; some sources suggest that aerosol distribution is more uniform when the drug is administered with the client in a supine position.)
10. Assist the client to perform mouth care before and after the treatment.

11. Instruct the client to put the mouthpiece in the mouth, and adjust gas flow for a good mist (approximately 7 L/min).
12. Instruct the client to breathe through the mouth and to alternate breathing patterns: from normal to high and low breathing levels of lung capacity.
13. Nebulize the entire treatment for maximal therapeutic effect (approximately 40 to 45 minutes).
14. **Always** turn off the power source before the client removes the mouthpiece to minimize environmental contamination with the pentamidine.
15. The treatment may be stopped when the following occurs:
    a. The client becomes fatigued; allow a short rest period
    b. The client complains of a burning sensation in the back of the throat; offer a drink and then resume aerosolization
    c. The client experiences shortness of breath or wheezing; give the client 2 to 4 puffs of bronchodilator before resuming neb-ulization; consult with the physician, and consider the bron-chodilator treatment to precede the next pentamidine treatment
16. Provide client comfort measures.
17. Clean and replace the equipment. Discard disposable items in a plastic trash bag, and secure. Discard any solution that remains after the treatment. (Nebulizer systems may be used for 48 hours before discarding.)

Nursing considerations

If the client's cardiopulmonary status is unstable, if the client com-plains of chest pain, if the client has a fever or rash, if the client is not responsive to bronchodilator therapy, or if nausea and vomiting occur, immediately discontinue the treatment, stabilize the client, and notify the physician and home health agency clinical supervisor. Coughing can be minimized by having the client sip liquids during the treatment.

Documentation guidelines

Document the following on the visit report:

- The procedure and client toleration
- Cardiopulmonary status before and after the treatment
- Any adverse side effects
- Any client/caregiver instructions and compliance with the procedure
- Other pertinent findings
    Document medications on the medication record.
    Update the client care plan.

Guidelines—Infection Control for Home Health Care of Persons With AIDS and Other Infectious Diseases

The infection control guidelines for persons with acquired immune deficiency syndrome (AIDS) and their caregivers below are based on Centers for Disease Control (CDC) recommendations and epidemiological data. The guidelines have provided the basis for the infection control policy and procedures at the AIDS Home Care and Hospice Program in San Francisco.

Hand washing

Hand washing is the single most important way to prevent the spread of an infectious organism. Soap and water should be used at all times. Hand washing should be done before and after all aspects of client care, including preparation and serving of meals to clients in their homes. If running water is not available, gloves should be worn. Hand washing is advised afer removing and disposing of gloves.

Gloves

Gloves serve to block the transmission of any infectious agent to a potential host. The caregiver should wear gloves in the following situations:

- When caring for open skin lesions or wounds
- When handling secretions or excretions, such as emesis, urine, stool, blood, or wound secretions
- When handling soiled diapers, incontinence pads, linens, or clothing
- When providing oral care, if contact with oral lesions or blood is likely
- When providing perineal care to the person who is incontinent, or to a woman who is menstruating or who has postpartum bleeding

Gloves *are not required* when bathing AIDS clients without skin lesions, when assisting AIDS clients with transfers or ambulation, when feeding AIDS clients, or when talking with or counseling an AIDS client.

Protective smocks

Protective smocks are not required for routine caregiving, but aprons or gowns may be used if soiling of the caregiver or his or her clothing is likely.

From Hughes A, Martin J, Franks P: *AIDS home care and hospice manual,* VNA of San Francisco, 1987, AIDS Home Care and Hospice Program.

Handling of needles and other sharp instruments

Needles, scalpels, and other sharp instruments must be handled with particular caution because the virus is capable of being transmitted through blood contact. *Needles should not be recapped* or resheathed afer use but disposed of intact in a puncture-resistant container. These containers may be available through supply companies. Household metal tins or heavy plastic bottles may be substituted. To prevent injury, the container should be discarded and replaced when it is three-fourths filled.

Disposal of supplies

Soiled disposable supplies used in the care of the person with AIDS (gloves, diapers, incontinence pads, toilet paper, dressing supplies, respiratory therapy tubing, or nebulizers) may be placed in a heavy-duty plastic bag that can be securely fastened at the top. If a heavy-duty plastic bag is not available, double bagging should be done. Removal of these plastic bags, as well as the sharps containers, should be in conformity with local solid waste disposal regulations used by the community. Usually this is the regular trash disposal system. The local public health department should be aware of these regulations and be able to assist in their interpretation and implementation.

Environmental safety

Environmental safety is maintained by usual household cleaning methods. Standard household detergents are appropriate to maintain a safe environment for the person with AIDS and other members of his or her household.

For floor or counter surfaces soiled by secretions or excretions, removal of surface debris and cleansing with hot soapy water, followed by disinfecting with 10% bleach solution (1 part bleach: 9 parts water) is adequate. The bleach solution also can be used to disinfect the toilet, tub, and shower after routine cleaning.

Bedpans and commodes should be cleaned regularly with household detergents and hot water. Soiled linens or clothing may be laundered in the household or laundromat washing machine. One cup of bleach along with the regular detergent should be added to water prior to placing clothes in the washer. (This procedure will help prevent discoloring of clothes.)

Items that are shared with other clients, such as toilets, showers, or bedpans, do not require different handling or cleansing. The cleaning procedures described earlier are sufficient: removing surface debris; cleaning with hot soapy water; and disinfecting with a 10% bleach solution. This procedure should be done between clients if a client is incontinent, has diarrhea, or has open genital lesions.

The dishes of the person with AIDS can be cleaned with those of other household members using hot soapy water. Utensils do not need to be isolated.

Weekly cleaning of the interior surface of the refrigerator, as well as the bathroom fixtures (toilet, shower, and bathtub), will help to control the growth of molds or fungi. Routine household cleaning agents can be used.

Pets

Pets may pose a particular threat to the person with AIDS. Organisms sometimes present in the excrement of cats, birds, and fish may cause serious illness because the immune system of the person is compromised. As a result, for clients who wish to keep pets, someone other than the person with AIDS should be responsible for cleaning the bird cage, cat litter box, or fish tank.

Pregnant caregivers and AIDS

Women who are pregnant or who may be pregnant should be excused from providing direct care to a person with AIDS. The rationale for this policy is that persons with AIDS are prone to two viruses—cytomegalovirus and herpesvirus—that have been known to cause serious birth defects and spontaneous abortions (miscarriages). Although the infection control guidelines discussed earlier would prevent caregivers from acquiring these infections if followed, the serious, harmful effects to the fetus of these viruses require particular caution. Further support for this position is found in the restriction of pregnant women from other potential occupational exposures, such as radiation therapy, that pose a threat to the fetus.

Durable medical equipment and AIDS

The management and cleaning of durable medical equipment (DME) is an issue of particular concern for home health care providers caring for persons with AIDS. The CDC has issued no specific guidelines for the provision or cleaning of DME used in the home of a person with AIDS. However, the CDC has recommended the use of a 10% bleach solution wipe down of *soiled* DME that cannot be sterilized by ethyl oxide or autoclaved. Most DME used at home for clients with AIDS (hospital beds, commodes, walkers, wheelchairs) cannot be autoclaved or sterilized.

San Francisco vendors who were surveyed reported that before DME is returned to the supplier, the DME is expected first to be cleaned by usual cleaning methods (using household detergents with hot water following the removal of any surface debris). The DME is then labeled "AIDS." The supplier disinfects it with a 10% bleach solution. After disinfection, the DME is returned to the inventory for general circulation—*its use is not restricted to AIDS clients.*

Dealing With Loss of Appetite, Nausea, and Vomiting in AIDS

Loss of appetite and nausea and vomiting are common symptoms of HIV infection, opportunistic infections, and treatment. There are a variety of ways to relieve nausea and vomiting and help increase appetite.

Loss of appetite

Loss of appetite can be a serious problem; it can lead to malnutrition and severe weight loss. When your body is trying to fight infection, it needs nutrition. It needs enough protein and calories to function at its best, to give you energy, and to help reduce the effects of the disease and its treatment.

Eating enough of the right kinds of foods can be difficult when you do not feel like eating at all. Here are some tips to help you increase your appetite:

- Take a walk before mealtime. Mild exercise can stimulate your appetite.
- Avoid drinking liquids before a meal, because they can fill you up. If you want to drink, drink juices or milk—something nutritious.
- Eat with family or friends if possible. If eating is a social event, it will seem less of a chore.
- Eat a variety of foods. Spice up your food with herbs, spices, and sauces. Use butter, bacon bits, croutons, wine sauces, and marinades to provide taste-pleasing meals.
- Do not fill up on salads or "diet" foods. Eat vegetables and fruits along with meats, poultry, and fish to make sure you get enough calories and nutrition.
- Eat smaller meals more often, especially if you fill up before you have eaten all your meal.

If you still are not getting enough calories or protein, your health care provider may recommend dietary supplements that can be added to milk, soup, or pudding.

From *Mosby's patient teaching guides,* St. Louis, 1995, Mosby.

Nausea and vomiting

Nausea and vomiting are common side effects of many treatments and infections. Doctors frequently prescribe an *antiemetic* to combat this. The antiemetic usually is given a few hours before the treatment and then every 3 or 4 hours after the treatment for a day or two. It may take some experimenting with dosage and timing to come up with the best schedule for you.

The following are other remedies and preventive measures you can try to help prevent or alleviate nausea and vomiting:

- Eat soda crackers and suck on sour candy balls throughout the day to relive queasiness.
- Choose cold or room-temperature foods instead of hot ones; hot and warm foods seem to cause nausea.
- Avoid salty, fatty, and sweet foods or any food with strong odors— opt instead for bland, creamy foods, such as cottage cheese, toast, and mashed potatoes.
- Stay away from nauseating odors, sights, and sounds. Get as much fresh air as possible. A leisurely walk can help alleviate nausea.
- Don't eat right before your treatment. Eat lightly for a few hours after your treatment.
- Try relaxation therapy, self-hypnosis, or imagery to alleviate nausea-inducing tension.
- Distract yourself with a book, TV, or activity.
- Sleep during episodes of nausea if possible.

If vomiting does occur, eat or drink nothing until your stomach has settled, usually a few hours after the last vomiting episode. Then begin sipping clear liquids or sucking on ice cubes. If you tolerate the liquids, you may begin eating bland foods a few hours after your started the liquids.

Safety Tips for the Caregivers of Persons With Confusion or Impaired Judgment Associated with AIDS

The mental status of a person with HIV infection may change suddenly, leading the person to exhibit symptoms ranging from confusion and forgetfulness to severe dementia and psychosis.

The person who has confusion or impaired judgment may be unable to remember where dangers lie or to judge what is dangerous (steps,

From *Mosby's patient teaching guides,* St. Louis, 1995, Mosby.

stoves, medications). Fatigue and inability to make the body do what one wants also can lead to injury. Therefore it is important that this person live in an environment that has been made as safe as possible. The following are some safety guidelines to use in your home:

- Keep clutter out of the hallway and off stairs or anywhere the person is likely to walk. Remove small rugs that could cause tripping.
- Remove breakables and dangerous objects (matches, knives, guns).
- Keep medications in a locked cabinet or drawer.
- Limit access to potentially dangerous areas (bathrooms, basement) by locking doors if the person tends to wander. Have the person wear an identification bracelet in case he or she wanders outside.
- Dress the person appropriately for the season.
- Put name labels in clothing. Make sure clothing is not too baggy and that shoes fit well and have nonskid soles.
- Keep the person's bed low. If he or she falls out, you may want to place the mattress on the floor or install side rails.
- Make sure rooms are well lit, especially in the evening. Nightlights can help prevent falls.
- Have someone stay with the person who is severely confused or agitated or place the person in a day-care center.
- Encourage rest periods if the person tires easily.
- Keep exit doors locked. Consider some type of exit alarm, such as a bell attached to the door.
- Consider a mat alarm under a bedside rug to alert others of the person getting up during the night.

It is also helpful to do the following:

- Have the person rest frequently. Do not let the person get fatigued.
- Avoid crowded places, such as shopping malls and stadiums.
- Have someone with the person when he or she goes outdoors.
- Keep meal times quiet and calm.
- Limit the number of visitors.
- Have the person do one activity at a time.
- Keep activities siimple—this will minimize fatigue.
- Plan activities ahead of time.
- Ensure that medications are taken as prescribed.
- Keep a calendar of activities visible on the wall. Cross off days as they pass.
- Maintain a photo album with labeled pictures of family members, friends, home, and so on.
- Include the person in family activities and conversations.

- Remember to treat the person with respect and maintain his or her privacy.
- Discuss all medication use with the health care provider.

Some things to avoid during periods of confusion include the following:

- Alcohol
- Contact sports
- Horseback riding
- Swimming
- Hunting
- Power tools or sharp implements
- Driving
- Riding recreational vehicles, such as bicycles, skateboards, motorcycles, or snowmobiles
- Cooking without supervision

Use of Antiretroviral Drugs

No drug cures infection with the human immunodeficiency virus (HIV). However, a number of drugs have been shown to reduce the rate at which HIV multiplies within the body. Each of these drugs seems to be reasonably effective for certain time periods. However, after some time passes, the drug seems to lose some or all of its ability to prevent multiplication of the virus. When this occurs, you may be switched to another antiretroviral drug or you may be given a second drug to take with the first drug. The length of time it takes for a drug to lose its potency varies with each person. For some this takes only a few months, whereas others obtain benefit from the same antiretroviral drug for years.

Because it is not clear why some people do well for only a short time and others do well for a long time, your response to the drugs will be watched closely. Your doctor will schedule you to return for examination and blood testing on a regular basis. It is important that you keep your medical appointments so that your doctor can determine if your drug therapy is working. If it is not, your physician will want to change drugs or add another drug to the one you are taking.

Antiretroviral drugs are powerful and may cause physical reactions, called side effects, even while they are doing their job of preventing HIV from multiplying. Some of the side effects are temporary and go away after a few weeks. Other side effects will continue as long as you

---

From *Mosby's patient teaching guides,* St. Louis, 1995, Mosby.

take the drugs. Most of these side effects can be described as being un-comfortable or inconvenient but not harmful. Other side effects, how-ever, may be permanently damaging or even life-threatening. There-fore, it is important that you learn what to expect when you take these drugs. You are the best judge of how you feel and what is happening to your body. The physicians and nurses caring for you need your assis-tance in watching for potentially harmful side effects. Therefore, the following guide has been prepared to help you understand and report your symptoms.

If you are taking AZT (zidovudine)—possible side effects: what you should do

Nausea or vomiting: usually disappears within 4 to 6 weeks of starting the drug. Report these symptoms to your health care provider if they last longer than this, cause you to lose weight, or return after being absent.

Headache: usually disappears within 4 to 6 weeks of starting the drug. Report this symptom to your health care provider if it persists past 6 weeks, does not respond to usual pain-relieving remedies, or re-turns after being absent.

Fatigue: usually disappears within 4 to 6 weeks. You can cope with it by reducing the amount you expect to accomplish and by getting plenty of rest. Report this symptom to your health care provider if fa-tigue persists past 6 weeks, returns after being absent, or interferes with your ability to live your life.

Muscle pain, severe upper abdominal pain, shortness of breath, un-usual bleeding or bruising, sore throat, fever, injury that will not heal: these indicate more serious reactions; report any of these symptoms to your health care provider.

If you are taking ddI (didanosine)—possible side effects: what you should do

Diarrhea: a fairly common side effect; discuss remedies with your health care provider at the next visit. Report this symptom sooner if the diarrhea is severe, lasts for several days, or causes you to lose weight.

Upper abdominal pain, persistent nausea and vomiting; pain, tin-gling, or numbness in your hands or feet; convulsions; shortness of breath; mental confusion; unusual bleeding or bruising: report these symptoms to your health care provider as soon as possible.

If you are taking ddC (zalcitabine)—possible side effects: what you should do

Canker sores in mouth; rashes and itching skin: see your dentist; avoid using soaps or powders that may further dry or irritate the skin; use lotions to moisturize the skin. Report these symptoms to your health care provider if they persist.

Upper abdominal pain; persistent nausea and vomiting; pain, tingling, or numbness in your hands or feet; convulsions; shortness of breath; mental confusion; unusual bleeding or bruising: report these symptoms to your health care provider as soon as possible.

Other reactions while taking antiretrovirals

All three of these drugs may cause side effects that are not listed here in some people, because individuals respond differently to different drugs. In addition, unusual symptoms may be related to other infections and not to the drugs that you are taking. Symptoms that are disabling or that interfere with your ability to live a reasonably normal life should be reported to your health care provider as soon as possible. Also, symptoms that involve pain, weakness, unusual weight loss, or bleeding should be reported soon. Problems that are merely annoying can usually wait until the next scheduled visit.

Diagnosis of Infection in HIV-Exposed Infants

Age	Test	If test is positive	If test is negative
1 month	HIV culture or PCR[1]	Repeat test to confirm diagnosis of infection	Repeat test at age 3 to 6 months
3 to 6 months	HIV culture or PCR[1]	Repeat test to confirm diagnosis of infection	Test with ELISA at age 15 months
15 months	ELISA	Repeat test at age 18 months	Repeat test at age 18 months
18 months or older	ELISA	Child is infected[2]	Child is not infected[3]

[1] If HIV culture and PCR are unavailable, p24 antigen testing may be used after 1 month of age.

[2] Serological diagnosis of HIV infection requires two sets of confirmed HIV serologic assays (ELISA/Western blot) performed at least 1 month apart after 15 months of age.

[3] Confirmation of seronegativity requires two sets of negative ELISAs after 15 months of age in a child with normal clinical and immunoglobulin evaluation.

NOTE: This chart presents recommendations only for the items reviewed by the HIV panel.

From Dunn S: *Primary care consultant,* St. Louis, 1998, Mosby.

HIV and AIDS Infection in Children and Teens

What is the difference between HIV infection and AIDS in children?

Acquired immunodeficiency syndrome (AIDS) is an illness that is caused by a virus known as the human immunodeficiency virus (HIV). HIV causes the body's immune system to break down so that it cannot fight off infections. This eventually results in AIDS.

How can you tell if a child has the HIV infection?

Most children with HIV infection do not look or act any different from children who do not have HIV infection or AIDS. However, there are some symptoms that children with HIV infection may have. These symptoms include the following:

- Problems gaining weight
- Swollen glands in several places in the body
- Infections of the blood that do not get better
- Diarrhea that will not go away
- A large liver and spleen
- Developmental problems, such as a delay in saying words or talking
- "Thrush" infection in the mouth that will not go away.

If you think a child has any of these symptoms or you are worried that the child may have HIV infection, have the child checked by his or her doctor.

Facts about HIV and AIDS in children and teens

- The most common way HIV infection is spread to children is from an HIV-infected mother during pregnancy or at birth.
- Not every child born to a mother who has HIV infection will become HIV infected. For women with HIV who do not take zidovudine (AZT) during pregnancy, about 25% of children (1 our of 4) will become HIV infected. However, for women with HIV who **do** take AZT during pregnancy, only about 8% of children born to them will become HIV infected. This means that **most** children born to a mother who has HIV infection will **not** become infected with HIV.
- HIV is spread by coming in contact with blood, semen, or vaginal secretions from a person with HIV infection.

From Ball J: *Mosby's pediatric patient teaching guides,* St. Louis, 1998, Mosby.

- Children who have HIV infection are living longer and are surviving into school age and teenage years. This is mostly the result of new medications and earlier treatment for HIV infection.
- Teenagers can become HIV infected by injecting drugs and having unsafe sex.
- About 50% of people who die with AIDS became infected during adolescence.
- Since 1985, the blood supply is considered safe. This means that it is very rare for children to get HIV by receiving blood or blood products.

How can children be protected from getting HIV infection?

Children need to learn to protect themselves from HIV infection. As difficult as it may be to talk to your children about sex and drugs, the fact is that HIV is most commonly spread by having unsafe sex and by injecting drugs. It is important to teach your children the following:

- **Do not have unprotected sex.** If you are having sex with another person, always use condoms plus contraceptive foam or jelly that contains nonoxynol-9. Condoms should also be used when having sex means entering other parts of the body besides the vagina (mouth or anus).
- **Do not inject drugs.** If you do inject drugs, use your own needles. Do not share "works" (needles and syringes) with anyone.

What are some of the safety measures needed for children who have HIV or AIDS?

- **Avoid people with infections.** Avoid having the child with HIV infection around children who have chickenpox, measles, colds, or the flu. If the child with HIV is around any child with a contagious disease such as chickenpox or measles, the child's doctor should be called.
- **Get immunized.** Children with HIV should get all of their baby shots or immunizations on time. This includes getting a flu shot every year. These immunizations will help them fight off many common illnesses.

Are children who do not have HIV able to get infected when playing with a child who has HIV?

Children cannot get HIV or AIDS from playing next to or touching a child who has HIV infection. HIV is spread by coming in contact with blood, semen, or vaginal fluids from a person with HIV infection. All children, whether they have HIV or not, should be taught some common rules:

- Avoid contact with the blood and body fluids of other people.
- Tell an adult if another child is bleeding, and let the adult take care of the bleeding.

HIV-Associated Conditions in Pediatric HIV Infection

Failure to thrive
Generalized lymphadenopathy
Hepatomegaly
Splenomegaly
Persistent oral candidiasis
Parotitis
Recurrent or chronic diarrhea
Encephalopathy
Lymphoid interstitial pneumonitis (LIP)
Hepatitis
Cardiomyopathy
Nephropathy
Recurrent bacterial infections
Opportunistic infections (recurrent viral infections [herpes simplex, herpes zoster], fungal, parasitic)
Malignancies (lymphoma)

From *Managing early HIV infection: quick reference guide,* USDHHS, AHCPR, Pub. #94-0573, 1994, Rockville, Md.

Testing and Preventive Therapy for Tuberculosis Infection in HIV-Infected Individuals

The reemergence of tuberculosis (TB) as a major public health concern is especially important for HIV-infected individuals because the immunosuppression caused by the virus permits *Mycobacterium tuberculosis* infection to progress at an accelerated pace, and they are more likely to develop active TB. TB merits special consideration in the treatment of HIV-infected clients because it is readily communicable to others, management is different for HIV-infected clients than for non–HIV-infected clients, and, unlike many other opportunistic infections, it is preventable and may be curable if treated promptly.

From *Managing early HIV infection: quick reference guide,* USDHHS, AHCPR, Pub. #94-0573, 1994, Rockville, Md.

Screening

- The medical history for all HIV-infected individuals should include the following steps: (a) assessment of previous TB infection or disease, past treatment or preventive therapy, and history of exposure to *M. tuberculosis;* (b) assessment of the risk for *M. tuberculosis* infection, including predisposing social conditions (e.g., household contacts, country of origin, homelessness, history of incarceration, residence in a congregate living situation); and (c) suggestive symptoms (e.g., cough, hemoptysis, fever, night sweats, weight loss). During the physical examination, the provider should seek indications of active disease (e.g., abnormal pulmonary signs, documented weight loss).
- The medical history for all HIV-infected individuals should also include an assessment of health and social conditions that may affect an individual's ability to complete a course of therapy, specifically, repeated failure to keep medical appointments, alcoholism, mental illness, and substance use.
- All HIV-infected individuals, including those who have received BCG vaccination, should be screened, using purified protein derivative (PPD) for infection with *M. tuberculosis* during their initial evaluation.
- All HIV-infected individuals should be screened for anergy using two control antigens in addition to PPD during their initial evaluation.
- All HIV-infected individuals who are PPD-positive or anergic should receive a chest x-ray and clinical evaluation, and those who have symptoms suggestive of TB should receive a chest x-ray, regardless of their PPD or anergy status.
- PPD and anergy testing should be repeated annually in persons who are neither PPD-positive nor anergic on initial evaluation. Persons who reside in areas where TB prevalence is high should be tested every 6 months.
- All PPD-negative or anergic HIV-infected individuals who have recently been exposed to persons with suspected or confirmed TB should be immediately tested with PPD and anergy antigens. Repeat testing should be performed in 3 months.
- PPD testing should be performed by the Mantoux method, using an intradermal injection of 0.1 ml 5 TU PPD (intermediate strength).
- Reactions should be assessed by a trained observer between 48 and 72 hours after injection. Reactions of 5 mm or greater induration should be considered positive in persons with HIV infection, regardless of prior BCG vaccination.
- Two of the following three antigens can be used for anergy testing: candida, mumps, or tetanus toxoid. Any degree of induration observed in response to intradermal injection of these antigens constitutes a positive reaction and indicates that the individual is not anergic.

- Chest x-rays should be obtained to exclude the presence of active pulmonary TB in all HIV-infected individuals who are PPD-positive, anergic, or have symptoms suggestive of TB.
- If the chest x-ray reveals any abnormality, multiple sputum smears and cultures should be performed.
- If a sputum smear is positive, the client should be started on anti-TB therapy immediately, pending culture results. Acid-fast bacillus (AFB) isolation should be initiated promptly if the client is coughing. If the sputum smears are negative and if there is no other etiology for the abnormal chest x-ray, bronchoscopy should be performed and empiric anti-TB therapy should be initiated, pending the results of the mycobacterial culture. AFB isolation should be maintained until the diagnosis is confirmed by a smear or culture.
- In many of these clinical situations, diagnostic evaluation and management will need to be individualized. Consultation with an infectious disease or pulmonary specialist may be necessary.

Preventive therapy

An important consideration during drug selection is the relative likelihood of drug-resistant organisms and drug toxicity. Following are other key elements important to the planning and implementation of the affective therapy:

Drug-susceptibility tests should be performed on the first-isolated *Mycobacterium* sp. (to prevent the development of MDR-TB).

Before the results of the susceptibility tests are known, the client should be started on a four-drug regimen, consisting of INH, rifampin, pyrazinamide, and ethambutol or streptomycin, which together are 95% effective in combating the infection. The use of multiple medications reduces the possibility of the organism becoming drug resistant.

Once drug susceptibility results are available, the regimen should be adjusted accordingly.

Client compliance and the adverse effects of the prescribed regimen should be monitored closely because the incidence of both is high.

Despite all the agents available to combat TB and the efforts mounted to detect and treat victims of the disease, treatment has been made difficult by two problems previously mentioned: client noncompliance with therapy and the growing incidence of drug-resistant organisms.

Preventive Therapy content from Lilley L, Aucker R: *Pharmacology and the nursing process,* ed 2, St. Louis, 1999, Mosby.

SPECIAL TRAINING

Bowel and Bladder Training

Bowel and bladder training refers to a program to assist in controlling urinary and bowel elimination. Urinary or bowel incontinence may be a result of decreased cerebral function, such as lack of awareness, medications, lack of control over sphincter muscle, trauma, surgical procedures, and medical disorders. The training program focuses on stool evacuation and bladder emptying at set times that are as close to the usual elimination patterns as possible.

Interventions

Bowel elimination

1. Assess bowel patterns for usual habits, stool characteristics, and frequency of incontinence.
2. Establish time for daily defecation, preferably 30 minutes to 1 hour after meal.
3. Inform client of need for 2 to 3 L of fluids per day if permitted.
4. Encourage bowel movement at regular times by offering warm fluids, abdominal massage, and digital stimulation of anal area; allow 1 hour for defecation.
5. Administer enema at regular times to empty bowel until next scheduled defecation; suppositories may also be used.
6. Tell client to avoid foods that produce gas and foods that might produce diarrhea and stool incontinence.
7. Encourage a routine time each day for bowel elimination; provide bathroom facilities, bedpan, or commode at that time.
8. Revise training program if it is not successful; report failure to achieve goals.

Bladder elimination

1. Assess urinary patterns for usual habits, characteristics, and frequency of incontinence.
2. Establish schedule for micturition; allow specific amounts of fluid during and between meals.
3. Restrict fluid intake after 9 PM or after retiring.
4. Schedule voiding every 2 hours during the day and every 4 hours during the night; extend periods of time between voidings when continence is established.

From Jaffe M, Skidmore-Roth L: *Home health nursing care plans,* ed 2, St. Louis, 1995, Mosby.

5. Tell client to avoid drinks containing caffeine and diuretics.
6. Monitor intake and output ratio.
7. Palpate for bladder distention that may cause incontinence.
8. Advise client to strengthen perineal muscles with Kegel exercises, tensing muscles by pressing buttocks together and holding for 3 to 5 minutes and repeat 10 times per hour; answer a call to void immediately.
9. Catheterize if program is unsuccessful; revise training program.

Fecal Impaction

When an impaction is present, the fecal mass may be too large or hard to be passed voluntarily. Suppositories and enemas may be ordered to promote evacuation of stool. However, if the enema fails to promote defecation, the nurse must use the fingers to break up and remove the fecal mass. This procedure can be uncomfortable and embarrassing for the client. Excessive rectal manipulation may cause irritation to the mucosa, bleeding, and stimulation of the vagus nerve, which can cause a reflex slowing of the heart rate.

1. Assemble supplies needed before beginning procedure:
   a. Disposable gloves
   b. Water-soluble lubricant
   c. Waterproof absorbent pad
   d. Bedpan
   e. Bedpan cover
   f. Bath blanket or cotton blanket
   g. Face cloth, towel, basin
2. Explain procedure to client. Indicate that manipulation of rectum can cause discomfort.
3. Wash hands.
4. Obtain assistance to help change client's position, if necessary. Assist client to left side-lying position with knees flexed.
5. Provide for privacy: close door to room, drape bath blanket over client so client is minimally exposed.
6. Drape client's trunk and lower extremities with bath blanket.
7. Place waterproof pad under buttocks.
8. Place bedpan next to client.
9. Don disposable gloves.

Modified from Perry AG, Potter PA: *Clinical nursing skills and techniques,* ed 4, St. Louis, 1998, Mosby.

10. Lubricate glove's index finger with lubricating jelly.
11. Insert index finger into rectum and advance finger slowly along rectal wall toward umbilicus.
12. Gently loosen fecal mass by massaging around it. Work finger into hardened mass.
13. Work stool downward toward end of rectum. Remove small sections of feces.
14. Periodically assess heart rate and look for signs of fatigue. Stop procedure if heart rate drops or rhythm changes.
15. Continue to clear rectum of feces and allow client to rest at intervals.
16. After disimpaction, provide washcloth and towel to wash buttocks and anal area.
17. Remove bedpan and dispose of feces. Remove gloves by turning inside out and discarding in proper receptacle.
18. Assist client to toilet or clean bedpan.
19. Wash hands. (Procedure may be followed by enema or cathartic.)
20. Perform rectal examination for stool.
21. Reassess vital signs and compare to baseline values.
22. Assess bowel sounds.
23. Abdomen is soft and nontender.

Expected outcomes
1. Impacted stool is successfully removed.
2. Client is able to subsequently evacuate stool voluntarily.
3. Vital signs remain normal.

Special considerations
- Some allow only physician to perform this procedure. Check policy manuals.
- Physician may order oil-retention enema several hours before this procedure to soften stool for easier extraction.
- Physician may order analgesic to be administered before procedure.
- Physician may order procedure to be followed by administration of cleansing enema or cathartics.
- If constipation and subsequent impaction is diet related, teach client about high-fiber nutritional products to increase bulk.
- If necessary, teach ancillary caregivers about the effects of immobility, hydration, nutrition on normal bowel elimination.

Ostomy Care

Purpose
- To maintain cleanliness and good skin care
- To permit examination of the skin around the stoma
- To provide education for client self-care
- To assist in controlling odors
- To prevent leakage
- To promote as independent a lifestyle as possible

Equipment
1. Ostomy appliance
2. Protective cover
3. Plastic bag or Chux
4. Soap and warm water, basin, washcloth, and towels
5. Disposable nonsterile gloves

Procedure
1. Explain the procedure to the client/caregiver.
2. Assemble the equipment at a convenient work area.
3. Place the client in a comfortable position with the abdominal area exposed.
4. Place a plastic bag or Chux under the client if he or she is bed-bound.
5. Remove the appliance and discard it.
6. Cleanse peristomal area with soap and water. Use a spiral pattern at the stoma site, and work outward. Rinse, pat dry.
7. Examine the stoma for integrity versus any signs of necrosis or infection. Report any abnormal findings to the physician.
8. Position the appliance to fit well around the stoma. (The appliance will depend on the type of stoma.)
9. Provide client comfort measures.
10. Clean and replace the equipment. Discard disposable items in a plastic trash bag, and secure.

Nursing considerations
Consider referral to the enterstomal therapist to establish stoma and persistomal care regimen.

Reassure the client, and be supportive.

From Rice R: *Manual of home health nursing procedures,* St. Louis, 1995, Mosby.

Encourage the client to talk about his or her feelings of the altered body image, sexuality, or self-esteem.

Help the client to adjust to life with a stoma, and encourage her or him to return to normal patterns of socialization.

Documentation guidelines
Document the following on the visit report:

- The procedure and client toleration
- Color, shape, and size of stoma
- Type of stoma
- Condition of the surrounding skin
- Function, character, and amount of drainage
- Any client/caregiver instructions and compliance with the procedure, including the client's reaction to and ability to perform ostomy care
- Other pertinent findings

Update the client care plan.

Contraindications to Colostomy Irrigation

- Ascending colostomies
- Temporary colostomies
- Disease in remaining colon (diverticulosis, inflammatory disease)
- Infant or child
- Physical limitations (arthritis, paralysis)
- Mental limitations (confusion, dementia, retardation)
- Inadequate sanitary facilities
- Stomal abnormalities (prolapse, hernia)

From Potter A, Perry A: *Fundamentals of nursing: concepts, process, and practice,* ed 4, St. Louis, 1997, Mosby.

Pouching a Colostomy or Ileostomy

1. Assess condition of existing pouch/skin barrier for leakage and note appearance of underlying stoma and surgical incision. Question client about discomfort at or around stoma. (Gloves may be necessary.)
2. Note amount of drainage from stoma.
3. Assess skin around stoma, noting scars, folds, or protuberance of skin.
4. Determine client's knowledge and understanding of ostomy.
5. Collect appropriate equipment:
   a. Skin barriers (wafers such as Stomahesive, Hollihesive, or paste or powder)
   b. Ostomy pouch (Figure 70)
   c. Clamp or closing device
   d. Hypoallergenic tape and/or belt
   e. Washcloth, towel, wash basin with warm water
   f. Skin cleanser (Sween or Bard) or mild soap
   g. Disposable gloves

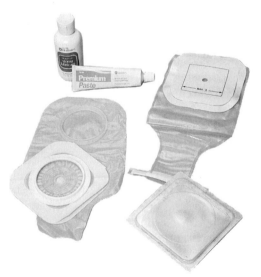

Figure 70

From Potter P, Perry A: *Fundamentals of nursing: concepts, process and practice,* ed 4, St. Louis, 1997, Mosby.

6. Select optimum time to change pouch/skin barrier (e.g., when client is comfortable, between meals, or before administration of medications that may affect bowel function).

7. Explain procedure (if client is unfamiliar with technique); otherwise allow client to organize steps for pouch change. Be sure client observes procedure.

8. Position client supine or sitting for pouch application; if able to stand, help client assume standing position.

9. Wash hands and apply gloves.

10. Close room curtains or door.

11. If pouch is full, remove clamp and empty contents through bottom into bedpan.

12. Remove old appliance as one piece.

13. Wash skin gently with skin cleanser or with regular soap and water. Remove secretions from skin.

14. Rinse soap off thoroughly. Blot dry.

15. If blood appears after washing, reassure client that small amount is normal. Clarify what is abnormal.

16. Observe condition of skin and stoma. Encourage client to make these observations daily. Remeasure the stoma size.

17. If abdominal crease is present or if contour is irregular, fill in with paste-type barrier.

18. Allow paste to dry for 1-2 min.

19. If abdominal contour is flat or after paste has dried, prepare skin barrier using skin sealant or karaya paste. Cut hole in skin barrier slightly larger than stoma, up to $\frac{1}{8}$ in. Cut radial slits from center of hole. Cut rounded corners on edges of skin barrier.

20. Prepare ostomy pouch; for non-precut pouches, cut hole in center of faceplate $\frac{1}{8}$ inch larger than hole in barrier (Figure 71).

21. Remove paper backing from pouch faceplate (Figure 72) and apply to shiny, noncovered side of barrier.

22. Remove backing from barrier and apply it and pouch (Figure 73) as unit to skin. Smooth out from center. Hold in place for 1-3 min. Apply in position that facilitates emptying.

23. Apply hypoallergenic tape and/or belt as needed to edges of faceplate over skin barrier.

24. Fold bottom edges of pouch over to fit clamp or closing device. Secure clamp.

25. Dispose of old appliance in plastic bag and dispose in trash chute. (Be sure this is not a reusable appliance because it should be washed and reused several times.)

26. Remove soiled gloves and dispose in proper receptacle.

27. Wash hands.
28. Assist client to comfortable position if necessary.
29. Record pertinent information: type of pouch and skin barrier, amount and appearance of feces, condition of stoma and surrounding skin, client's ability to do ostomy self-care.

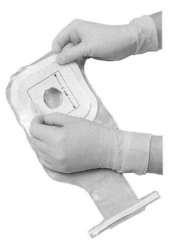

Figure 71

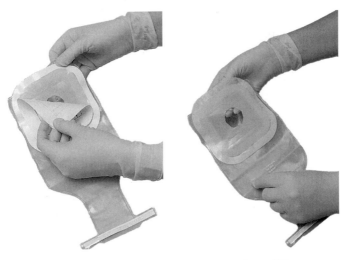

Figure 72   **Figure 73**

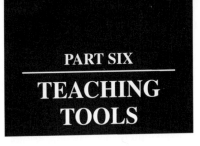

PART SIX

TEACHING TOOLS

ANTICIPATORY GUIDANCE

Preventing Respiratory Infections

Respiratory infections can be a serious complication for anyone with a chronic lung disease. Unfortunately, people with chronic lung diseases are more susceptible to respiratory infections; even an ordinary cold that causes only sniffles in someone else can turn into pneumonia. Because of this, clients must make every effort to prevent infection. The client must also learn the early danger signs and the importance of seeing a doctor at once when any symptoms appear. Some specific guidelines for clients follow.

Preventing infection

Follow your doctor's orders. Take your medications exactly as ordered. Perform chest physiotherapy as directed. If oxygen therapy is prescribed, take it as ordered.

Take care of yourself every day. Drink at least six glasses of water daily (unless your doctor tells you differently). Eat a nutritious, well-balanced diet. Sleep 7 or 8 hours every night. Take several short rests during the day. Learn to conserve your energy and avoid getting too tired.

Stay away from people who have colds and flu, if at all possible. If this cannot be avoided, wear a disposable mask (available at medical supply companies and many grocery stores) when around people with colds or flu.

Avoid air pollution, including tobacco smoke, wood or oil smoke, car exhaust, and industrial pollution.

Take special precautions with your personal hygiene. Wash your hands before taking your medication or handling your oxygen equipment.

From *Mosby's patient teaching guides,* St. Louis, 1995, Mosby.

Wash your hands after handling soiled tissues and before and after using the bathroom. Always rinse your oral inhaler after each use. Ask your doctor about flu vaccines.

Detecting infections

Symptoms of respiratory infections can appear suddenly and worsen quickly. When an infection develops, it is important to start treatment right away. Your doctor may decide to prescribe antibiotics or other drugs to get the infection under control before it becomes serious. (**Do not try to treat yourself.** Over-the-counter cold remedies may worsen the problem, so do not use them unless your doctor tells you it is okay.) Call your doctor immediately if any of these signs occur:

Fever

Increased coughing, wheezing, or trouble breathing

Mucus changes in any of these ways: the mucus is thicker; the amount is either more or less than usual; it has a foul odor; or the color is green, yellow, brown, pink, or red

Stuffy nose, sneezing, or sore throat

Increased fatigue or weakness

Weight gain or loss of more than 5 pounds within a week

Swollen ankles or feet

Confusion, memory loss, or persistent drowsiness

Infection Control

Infection occurs as a result of transmission of an infectious agent to a susceptible host. Home health nurses must keep in mind that an infected individual will not necessarily show signs or symptoms of the infection but may nonetheless be capable of infecting others. Below are common signs and symptoms of infection.

Signs and symptoms of infection
Inflammatory response
- Redness
- Heat
- Swelling
- Pain

From *Mosby's home health nursing pocket consultant*, St. Louis, 1995, Mosby.

Other possible signs and symptoms
- Sore throat, cough
- Sputum production, change in color or amount of sputum
- Elevated temperature
- Tachycardia, tachypnea
- Rash, dermatitis of the skin
- Loose stool, diarrhea
- Nausea, vomiting
- Weight loss (inappropriate)
- Green or yellow exudates or drainage from the wound bed
- Burning or painful urination

Understanding mechanisms of transmission provides insight into the management of communicable diseases. The following procedures will reduce the transmission of communicable disease:

- The infectious agent is eradicated by a method of disinfection/ sterilization.
- The infectious agent is prevented from entering the host (actual or potential).
- Prevalence of the infectious agent is reduced by enhancing host response by means of antibiotic administration or immunizations.
- The infectious agent's reservoir is neutralized.

These procedures, along with a philosophy that all clients should be treated as though they have an infectious disease, form the basis for infection control guidelines recommended by the Centers for Disease Control (CDC).

Universal precautions

Universal precautions are those actions taken to prevent transmission of microorganisms from one person to another. They include care of hands, care of inanimate objects or articles used, and use of barriers and techniques to protect against transmission to client or caregiver.

Since a health history and physical assessment cannot reliably identify all clients who have a communicable disease, the CDC and Occupational Safety and Health Administration (OSHA) recommend that universal blood and body fluid precautions be followed with all clients. All health care workers should wear gloves when touching mucous membrane or nonintact skin of all clients (e.g., wound care, suctioning care). Masks, goggles, and gowns should be worn if aerosolization or splashes are likely to occur.

Provision of care

- Routine precautions should be taken when there is any possibility of exposure to blood or body fluids of any client (wound care, suctioning, any care involving body orifices or injections). Aprons or gowns are required for procedures involving extensive contact with blood or body fluids. Gloves are required when handling items soiled with blood or body fluids (soiled linens, dressings, catheter/enema equipment).
- Immediately after contact with blood or body fluids all contaminated skin surfaces should be washed completely. Hands should be washed with soap and water immediately after gloves are removed. Wearing gloves does not eliminate the necessity for hand washing after each client contact. Do not reuse disposable gloves. Gloves should be changed between contact with clients to prevent cross-contamination. General utility gloves should not be worn if they are peeling, cracked, or discolored, as this is evidence of deterioration.
- All health care workers who perform or assist in invasive procedures must use extraordinary care to prevent injuries caused by needles, glucose monitoring lancets, and other sharp instruments or devices. After use, disposable syringes, needles, and other sharp items should be placed in a puncture-resistant container for disposal. To prevent needlestick injuries, needles should not be recapped, purposely bent or broken, removed from disposable syringes, or otherwise bent by hand.
- Although saliva has not been implicated in HIV transmission, mouthpieces or other ventilation devices should be available for employees to minimize the risk involved in emergency mouth-to-mouth resuscitation.
- Health care workers who have exudative lesions, weeping dermatitis, or breaks in the skin should wear gloves when doing any procedural treatment for the client or family.

Disinfection (at the home health agency)

- Wash all equipment thoroughly with soap and water, rinse, and dry.
- Always read the label of the disinfectant and follow directions. After washing equipment with soap and water, disinfect, rinse, and dry. According to OSHA, after initial cleanup one of the following disinfectants should be used for cleaning equipment exposed to blood or body substances:

    Chemical germicides that are approved for use as hospital disinfectants and are tuberculocidal when used at recommended dilutions

Products registered by the Environmental Protection Agency (EPA) as being effective against HIV with an accepted "HIV (AIDS Virus)" label

A solution of 5.25% sodium hypochlorite (household bleach) diluted between 1:10 and 1:100 with water; mix a fresh supply of bleach every day for effective disinfection

- *Remember:* Disinfectants are designed for inanimate objects and are damaging to the skin. Wear gloves to protect the hands and goggles if there is a possibility of splashes to the eye. Disinfectants should be used in a well-ventilated room. If possible, totally submerge contaminated articles in the disinfecting solution for the required period of time.
- Since most durable medical equipment (DME) used in the home cannot be autoclaved, disinfection is recommended. Submerge or wipe down DME with soap and water and disinfect. Remember, bleach is caustic to metal.

Disposal techniques for waste: environmental considerations

- Sharps: Injection needles with syringes, glucometer lancets, vacutainer needles, etc., should be contained in a puncture-resistant container marked with the biohazard symbol and sealed to prevent leakage.
- Blood, body fluids, and secretions generated by clients in their own homes may be disposed of via the sanitary sewer.
- All antineoplastic chemotherapeutic wastes are considered a hazardous waste by most health departments and must be neutralized by dilution. Review regulations with local health departments and the EPA.

Special precautions in home care

These guidelines are based on practical adaptations of universal/body substance isolation (BSI) precautions for home health nurses and may be individualized to meet specific client needs.

Provision of care for clients with communicable diseases

- Explain all procedures and their rationale to clients. Respect clients' rights to privacy and confidentiality.
- Wash hands with soap and water before and after client care and during care if soiled.
- Wear gloves on both hands whenever there is any possibility of contact with blood or body substances (oral or body secretions, feces, urine, vomitus, tissues, wound or other drainage). Change gloves between procedures as appropriate.

- Wear a mask if clients are coughing productively or when suctioning. Masks may be worn if the client has active TB, influenza, mumps, measles, chickenpox, or pertussis.
- Routinely wipe down the bell/diaphragm of the stethoscope with an alcohol prep-pad between clients.
- Do not recap used syringes/needles; place them in a puncture-resistant container for storage.
- Wipe down blood specimen tubes with a 10% bleach solution, if possible; otherwise, use an alcohol prep-pad. Label tube "blood precautions" and store in a sealed plastic bag for laboratory delivery.
- Do not replace any contaminated equipment in the nursing bag until it has been disinfected.

Guidelines for Preventing and Controlling Nosocomial Infections

Control of external environment (Exogenous sources of infection)

Health care providers
1. In good health—do not care for clients when ill
2. Keep immunizations current
3. Practice effective hand washing between each client
   If skin dry, rough, or broken, seek appropriate attention
   If active herpes simplex infection of hand (herpetic whitlow), do not give direct client care until lesion healed
4. Wear gloves when contact with any body substance is anticipated

Housekeeping and sanitation
1. Bed linens not shaken in air or thrown on floor
2. Proper disposal of wastes—solid and liquid
3. Proper cleaning and sterilization of contaminated articles
4. Proper ventilation for adequate air exchanges
   Modern hospitals—clients' room air is under negative pressure
   Negative pressure keeps air from clients' rooms from moving into hallways
5. Proper mopping and damp dusting to remove dust and other environmental reservoirs of infection

From Phipps WJ et al.: *Medical-surgical nursing: concepts and clinical practice,* ed 6, St. Louis, 1999, Mosby.

Control of internal environment
(endogenous sources of infection)

1. Preventive measures aimed at increasing client's defense mechanisms and thus reducing risk of infection

   Teach client about good nutrition

   Teach client about personal hygiene, especially hand washing

2. Be aware that normal flora of client can be disrupted when client is receiving antibiotics or chemotherapy and colonization may occur

   Give antibiotics on time as scheduled

   Teach client about appropriate use of antibiotics and dangers of taking them when not prescribed by physician

Notes

Insulin Adjustment During Jet Travel Across Multiple Time Zones

Daily insulin regimen	Day of departure	First morning at destination	10 hours after morning dose	Second day at destination
Eastbound				
Single-dose schedule	Usual dose	⅔ usual dose	Remaining ⅓ AM dose if blood sugar over 240	Usual dose
Two-dose schedule	Usual morning and evening doses	⅔ usual morning dose	Usual evening dose plus remaining ⅓ of AM dose if blood sugar over 240	Usual two doses

Daily insulin regimen	Day of departure	18 hours after departure	First day at destination
Westbound			
Single-dose schedule	Usual dose	⅓ usual dose followed by snack if blood sugar over 240	Usual dose
Two-dose schedule	Usual morning and evening doses	⅓ usual AM dose followed by snack if blood sugar over 240	Usual two doses

Reprinted with permission from Edward A. Benson, MD, Virginia Mason Clinic, Seattle, Wash.

Safe Use of Medicines by Older People

Most people, and especially the elderly, use medicines at some point during their lifetime. When used correctly, medicines can be of great value. They can help heal wounds, stop the spread of infections, bring on sleep, and ease pain, both physical and mental. But when used incorrectly, drugs have the ability to injure the client or change the effects of other medicines being taken at the same time.

Drugs can be divided into two major groups; over-the-counter drugs (also called patent medicines), which can be bought without a doctor's prescription; and prescription drugs, which can be ordered only by a doctor and sold only by a pharmacist (druggist). Prescription drugs are usually more powerful and have more side effects than over-the-counter medicines.

People over 65 make up 11% of the American population, yet they take 25% of all prescription drugs sold in this country. One reason for this more frequent use of drugs by older people is that, as a group, they tend to have more long-term illnesses than younger people. Also, advancing age sometimes brings with it changes in physical abilities, eating habits, and social contacts. The result of these changes—whether it is aching muscles, constipation from lack of certain foods, or depression after the loss of a relative or friend—may often lead an older person to seek medical help. Drug treatment may be suggested to help overcome many of these physical and emotional problems.

Safe drug use requires both a well-informed doctor and a well-informed client. New information about drugs and about how they affect the older user is coming to light daily. For this reason, those taking drugs should occasionally review with a doctor their need for each medicine.

In general, drugs given to older people act differently than they do when given to young or middle-aged people. This is probably the result of the normal changes in body makeup that occur with age. For example, as the body grows older, the percent of water and lean tissue (mainly muscle) decreases, while the percent of fat tissue increases. These changes can affect the length of time a drug stays in the body, how a drug will act in the body, and the amount of drug absorbed by body tissues.

The kidneys and the liver are two important organs responsible for breaking down and removing most drugs from the body. With age, the

From U.S. Department of Health and Human Services, Public Health Service, National Institutes of Health, Rockville, Md. Fact sheet, *Safe use of medicines by older people,* 1990.

kidneys and the liver often begin to function less efficiently, and thus drugs leave the body more slowly. This may account for the fact that older people tend to have more undesirable reactions to drugs than do younger people.

Because older people can often have a number of physical problems at the same time, it is very common for them to be taking many different drugs. Two or more medicines taken at the same time can sometimes react with each other and produce harmful effects. For this reason, it is important to tell each doctor you go to about other drugs you are taking. This will allow the doctor to prescribe the safest medicines for your situation.

By taking an active part in learning about the drugs you take and their possible side effects, you can help bring about safer and faster treatment results. Some basic rules for safe drug use are as follows:

1. Take exactly the amount of drug prescribed by your doctor and follow the dosage schedule as closely as possible.

2. Medicines do not produce the same effects in all people. For this reason, you should never take drugs prescribed for a friend or relative, even though your symptoms may be the same.

3. Always tell your doctor about past problems you had with drugs, and be sure to mention other drugs (including over-the-counter medicines) you are taking.

4. It may help to keep a daily record of the drugs you are taking, especially if your treatment schedule is complicated or you are taking more than one drug at a time.

5. If child-proof containers are hard for you to handle, ask your pharmacist for easy-to-open containers. Always be sure, however, that such containers are out of the reach of children.

6. Make sure that you understand the directions printed on the drug container and that the name of the medicine is clearly printed. This will help you to avoid taking the wrong medicine or following the wrong schedule. Ask your pharmacist to use large type on the label if you find the regular labels hard to read.

7. Throw out old medicines, since many drugs lose their effectiveness over time.

8. Ask your doctor about side effects that may occur, about special rules for storage, and about which foods or beverages, if any, to avoid.

9. Always call your doctor promptly if you notice unusual reactions.

Hazards of Polypharmacy

What is polypharmacy?

Polypharmacy is a term used to describe the use of many medications at the same time. Polypharmacy is not always dangerous. There are times that medications taken at the same time work well together to treat a problem. However, there are other times when polypharmacy can put a person at risk, especially an older person.

Why are older persons at risk for polypharmacy?

Medication errors. Older persons may be taking medications to treat several unrelated conditions. The more medications a person must take, the greater the chance that the wrong medication or the wrong dose of medication is taken or that the medication is taken at the wrong time of the day.

Drug side effects. The more medications a person takes, the greater the risk of suffering from side effects of the drugs. There are many side effects that can have significant effects on the older adult. For instance, the side effect of a medication may be dizziness or weakness. Such a side effect in an older adult or frail individual could result in a fall and further injury.

Drug interactions. Some medications do not always mix well with other medications. Sometimes a combination of two drugs causes an increased risk of unexpected and unwanted effects. Sometimes, when more than one health care provider is prescribing medications, it is possible that they are unaware of other medications a patient may be taking.

Age. Older adults can react in unexpected ways to a medication. A medication taken by an older adult may cause effects different from those experienced by a younger adult taking the same medication. Sometimes the medication has stronger effects, or it may not leave the body as quickly. When there are many medications being taken, the overall effects may be very different.

From Mosby: *Mosby's patient teaching guides,* St. Louis, 1995, Mosby.

Who is at greatest risk for polypharmacy?

People (over the age of 65) who are taking four or more medications, whether they are over-the-counter medications or prescriptions, are at risk for polypharmacy. The older the individual and the greater number of medications taken, the greater the risk for polypharmacy.

How can I prevent polypharmacy problems?

There are several important things you can do to prevent problems from polypharmacy.

- Be sure that you have one health care provider who is aware of all the medications that have been prescribed to you. If you see more than one health care provider, be sure your primary provider is aware of the other medications you will be taking.
- Carry a list of all the medications you take. Be sure other health care providers see this list before a new prescription is written for you.
- When you have your prescription filled, talk with the pharmacist about the medications you are taking and how they interact.
- Follow the medication instructions. Do not increase or decrease a dose or change the time you take your medication without talking with your primary health care provider.
- Use medication containers that are color coded for different medications. Make a list so that you can refer to this every day.
- Be sure to bring in all medications you are taking (both prescription and over-the-counter) when you are admitted to the hospital.

It is up to you to help coordinate the number and the type of medications you are taking. If you are taking several medications, be aware of the risk of polypharmacy and how this may actually harm you and make you sick or at risk for injury. It is your responsibility to let your primary health care provider know about *all* of the medications you are taking, both prescription and over-the-counter medications. Ask your health care provider to review all of your medications and make sure that they will not be harmful when used in combination.

From Novak JC, Broom BL: *Ingalls & Salerno's maternal and child health nursing,* ed 9, St. Louis, 1999, Mosby.

Exercise Tips for Pregnant Women

Exercise is considered safe for healthy women with uncomplicated pregnancies. It may also contribute to enhanced feelings of well-being and a quicker return to fitness after delivery. Curtailing the exercise of a previously active woman may negatively affect her physical, emotional, and mental health. Regular exercise at least 3 times per week is preferable to intermittent activity. Walking, golfing, bowling, dancing, and swimming, when not done to the point of fatigue, are safe activities. Horseback riding, skiing, endurance exercises, and contact sports are not recommended for pregnant women.

The following suggestions for exercise habits are general guidelines based on recommendations of the American College of Obstetricians and Gynecologists and the American College of Sports Medicine:

- Avoid heat stress, especially during early pregnancy. Do not exercise during high heat or humidity or when an elevated body temperature exists. Wear appropriate clothing and drink adequate fluids before and after each exercise session.
- Limit exercise periods to 30 to 45 minutes.
- After the fourth month, do not exercise in the supine position because of the risk of supine hypotensive syndrome.
- Sit or lie down after exercising. Standing may cause increased venous pooling in the lower extremities.
- Do not exceed 70% of safe maximum attainable heart rate (SHR). SHR is usually defined as 220 minus the woman's age. For example, a 30-year-old, pregnant woman should aim for a pulse rate not higher than $(220 - 30) \times .7$, or 133 beats/minute. Maternal heart rate should not exceed 140 beats/minute unless the woman is well-conditioned before pregnancy.

From Novak JC, Broom BL: *Ingalls & Salerno's maternal and child health nursing,* ed 9, St. Louis, 1999, Mosby.

Kegel Exercises and Pregnancy

Frequent exercises involving the pelvic floor may facilitate childbirth, promote healing, aid in the restoration of perineal muscle tone, and help prevent stress incontinence.

- The mother can be taught these exercises during the prenatal period and can benefit from their daily performance for the rest of her life.
- The pubococcygeal muscle can be identified as the one she uses to stop a stream of urine when voiding.
- Ask the woman to think of perineal muscles as an elevator on the "first floor," which she should slowly raise by contraction to the "fourth floor" and lower by slowly relaxing the muscles.
- A series of 10 Kegel exercises should be repeated 6 to 8 times each day.

From Novak JC, Broom BL: *Ingalls & Salerno's Maternal and Child Health Nursing,* ed 9, St. Louis, 1999, Mosby.

THERAPEUTIC INTERVENTIONS

Breathing Exercises to Relieve Dyspnea

The feeling of not being able to get enough air into your lungs is frightening. Shortness of breath or difficulty breathing—called dyspnea—is a problem for people with chronic lung diseases. However, there are several things clients can do to help themselves breathe more easily. Some suggested client guidelines follow.

Avoiding trouble

Breathing pollutants can aggravate dyspnea. Avoid heavy traffic and smog as much as possible. Do not use aerosol sprays. Stay away from products that produce fumes, such as paint, kerosene, and cleaning agents.

Cold weather can trigger dyspnea. If you must go outside when it is cold, cover your mouth with a scarf or mask.

Very dry air increases dyspnea and thickens the mucus in your lungs. A portable room humidifier is helpful, especially in the winter.

From *Mosby's patient teaching guides,* St. Louis, 1995, Mosby.

Physical exertion brings on dyspnea. Learn to conserve your energy by resting frequently, alternating light and heavy tasks, and minimizing movement. Instead of standing, sit. Instead of pushing or lifting objects, pull. Be creative in managing tasks—for example, a cart or child's wagon can be used to haul groceries, and wheels can be installed on furniture that is frequently moved.

Breathing exercises

There are two simple exercises that can help you breathe more easily. You can do pursed lip breathing anywhere. With abdominal breathing, you will need to lie down. Practice them daily so when you are having problems with dyspnea, you will immediately know what to do.

Pursed lip breathing

Pursed lip breathing will help get rid of the stale air trapped inside the lungs. It will slow down your breathing so it is more efficient. (Breathing fast only makes the dyspnea worse.)

1. Breathe in slowly through your nose. Hold your breath for three seconds (count to yourself by saying one 100, two 100, three 100). Be sure to breathe through your nose to avoid gulping air.
2. Purse your lips as if you were going to whistle or give someone a kiss.
3. Breathe out slowly through your pursed lips for 6 seconds (count one 100, two 100, three 100, four 100, five 100, six 100.) The sound you make breathing out will be like a soft whistle.

Abdominal breathing

Abdominal breathing will also slow down your breathing to make it more effective. It also helps relax your entire body and is a wonderful technique to use before you go to sleep.

1. Lie on your back in a comfortable position with a pillow under your head. Place another pillow under your knees to help relax your abdomen.
2. Rest one hand on your abdomen just below your rib cage. Rest the other hand on your chest.
3. Slowly breathe in and out through your nose using your abdominal muscles. The hand resting on your abdomen will rise when you breathe in, and it will fall when you breathe out. The hand on the chest should be almost still.

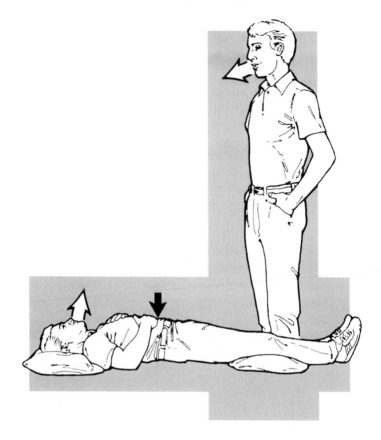

Note: Some medications (e.g., ipratropium bromide) are better administered by using closed mouth technique or a spacer. Some of the atropine-containing MDIs (metered dose inhalers) may cause pupillary dilation if sprayed in the eyes, which can be disabling.

If possible, watch clients do this entire procedure. If they are not properly performing the procedure, they may not be receiving their proper medication dosage.

If clients are using a fast-acting bronchodilator (e.g., metaproterenol, albuterol) instruct them to wait 2 to 5 minutes between puffs to allow the medication time to open the bronchi so the next puff can go deeper into the lungs.

There are also inexpensive arthritic aids available for people who have difficulty compressing the MDI.

Aerosol Therapy (Nebulizer)

Client teaching information

Take your treatment for _____ minutes or until medication is gone.

Do not overuse. If you feel you need the treatment more often than ordered, be sure to call your doctor.

Instruct clients to follow these simple steps:
1. Sit up straight in a chair that will give back support.
2. Make sure the equipment is clean, dry, and located at table height.
3. Put the medication in as directed.
4. Turn the machine on and check for a mist at the mouthpiece.
5. Put your lips around the mouthpiece to form a seal.
   Inhale through your mouth only. If this is hard for you to do, you may need a nose clip.
   Hold your breath for two seconds.
   Exhale slowly and completely through your mouth.
6. Never hold in a cough during the treatment. Stop and cough. Turn the machine off or tip the nebulizer cup sideways until you are ready to start again. Then continue your treatment.
7. Drink water or rinse your mouth during the treatment if your mouth becomes dry.
8. Notify your doctor if you have any discomfort during or after the treatment.
9. Do not allow anyone else to use the machine.
10. Do not use your machine if you have any doubts that it is not working properly. If you are in the hospital when this happens, notify your nurse or therapist. If you are at home, call your supplier.
11. Rinse out your medication containers and mouthpiece after each use.
12. Keep the machine covered with a clean towel when not in use.
13. Rinse your mouth before and after each treatment for cleanliness and comfort.

Cleaning your equipment

All equipment that you use to breathe in medication must be cleaned every day. If germs (bacteria) are not cleaned from your

---

Modified from *Living with lung disease*, American Lung Association of Connecticut, 1989.

equipment, they may cause an infection. An infection would make extra work for your heart and lungs and make it harder for you to breathe.

Your supplier is responsible for providing you with written instructions concerning the appropriate method for cleaning your equipment.

Step Approach for Therapeutic Management of Asthma

Step 4, severe	For long-term prophylaxis control, a high dose corticosteroid inhaler *plus* a long-acting beta$_2$ agonist tablet, or inhaler or a long-acting theophylline *plus* corticosteroid oral (2 mg/kg/day, not exceeding 60 mg/day) daily should be utilized. A short-acting beta$_2$ agonist inhaler is available for symptom control.
Step 3, moderate	Intermediate dose corticosteroid inhaler *plus* a long-acting beta$_2$ agonist inhaler, tablets or long-acting theophylline daily. A short-acting beta$_2$ agonist inhaler is available for symptom control.
Step 2, mild (persistent)	Low dose corticosteroid inhaler or nedocromil daily. Children may start with cromolyn or nedocromil. Zafirlukast, zileuton, or a long-acting theophylline product are alternatives for clients 12 years old or older. A short-acting beta$_2$ agonist inhaler is available for symptom control.
Step 1, mild (intermittent)	Short-acting beta$_2$ agonist inhaler is available for symptom control. If inhaler is used more than twice weekly, consider Step 2 therapy.

From Expert Panel Report II: Guidelines for the Diagnosis and Management of Asthma, National Asthma Education and Prevention Program, February 1997.

Metered Dose Inhaler

Client information

A metered dose inhaler (MDI) is a handheld pressurized device that delivers a premeasured amount of medication to your lungs.

1. Assemble the MDI for use according to package directions.
2. Shake the MDI.
3. Open mouth wide.
4. Place MDI about 1 inch in front of your lips. Do not close lips around mouthpiece.
5. Exhale fully.
6. Press your MDI once as you begin to inhale slowly and deeply.
7. Hold your breath for 5 to 10 seconds if possible at the peak of your deep breath.
8. Exhale slowly through pursed lips.
9. Repeat steps 5 through 7 for each puff as ordered by your doctor. Wait 2 to 5 minutes between puffs if using a fast-acting bronchodilator.
10. If you use both a bronchodilator and other medication MDIs, always use the bronchodilator first. It is most effective to allow 15 minutes between two medications.
11. Rinse your mouth out with water after using steroid sprays.
12. To check the amount of medicine left in your MDI, place the canister in water.

Do not overuse your MDI. Use only as ordered by your doctor.

Instructor information

The medication brochure may not reflect current information regarding appropriate instructions for use. It is important to review these concepts carefully with the client for most effective results.

Some clients have difficulty coordinating their breathing with pressing the MDI. Various types of spacers allow the aerosolized particles to collect in a chamber. The client then inhales from the chamber. Assemble and use as instructed on package insert. If clients will be using a spacer, alter the instructions for use (especially step 4) to correspond with the package insert.

Note: Some medications (e.g., ipratropium bromide) are better administered by using closed mouth technique or a spacer. Some of the

Modified from *Living with lung disease,* American Lung Association of Connecticut, 1989.

atropine-containing MDIs may cause pupillary dilation if sprayed in the eyes, which can be disabling.

If possible, watch clients do this entire procedure. If they are not properly performing the procedure, they may not be receiving their proper medication dosage.

If clients are using a fast-acting bronchodilator (e.g., metaproterenol, albuterol) instruct them to wait 2 to 5 minutes between puffs to allow the medication time to open the bronchi so the next puff can go deeper into the lungs.

There are also inexpensive arthritic aids available for people who have difficulty compressing the MDI.

Using an Inhaler

It is important that the client be instructed in the correct use of a metered dose nebulizer before it is needed to relieve an asthma attack. The prescriber will indicate whether the Closed-Mouth or the Open-Mouth Technique is to be used. If it is optional, encourage the client to use the Open-Mouth Technique for better inhalation of the drug. If used incorrectly, the dose may be dispersed into the air or even swallowed. Since only 10% of an inhaled dose reaches the lungs under the best of conditions, the ability to use the metered dose nebulizer appropriately is essential for the client.

A placebo nebulizer should be used for demonstration. This will enable the client to repeat the demonstration a number of times until the nebulizer can be easily and correctly used.

The closed-mouth technique

1. Shake the container for 2 to 5 seconds.
2. Hold the nebulizer with the drug container upside down (Figure 74).
3. Place the mouthpiece in the mouth, closing lips tightly around it.
4. Exhale steadily and completely through nose.
5. Inhale slowly and deeply, and at the same time press the container down on the mouthpiece (Figure 75).
6. Hold breath for as long as possible before exhaling and remove mouthpiece from your mouth (Figures 77 and 78).

From McKenry LM, Salerno E: *Mosby's pharmacology in nursing,* ed 20, St. Louis, 1998, Mosby.

7. Wait 15 seconds.
8. Repeat steps 1 through 6 above.
9. If no relief is achieved after 5 minutes and condition worsens, contact prescriber.

The open-mouth technique

1. Shake the container for 2 to 5 seconds.
2. Hold the nebulizer with the drug container upside down (See Figure 74).
3. Hold the mouthpiece two fingerwidths (about 1½ inches) in front of widely opened mouth. Hold container upright (Figure 76).
4. Exhale deeply, then inhale slowly through mouth and at the same time press down firmly on the container. Continue to breathe deeply.

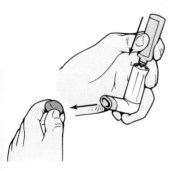

Figure 74

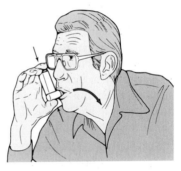

Figure 75

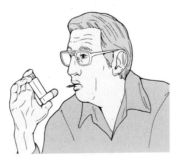

Figure 76

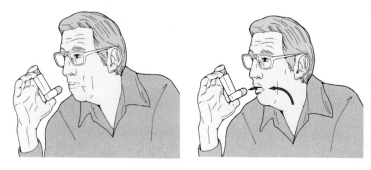

Figure 77   **Figure 78**

5. Hold breath for a few seconds (Figure 77), then exhale slowly (Figure 78). Wait approximately 15 seconds, and then repeat steps 3 to 5 for second inhalation. (Keep eyes closed—temporary blurring of vision may occur if the aerosol is sprayed into the eyes.)

Many practitioners are now advising the use of a spacer, a small tube that fits into the inhaler mouthpiece and goes into the client's mouth, to enhance the delivery of nebulized agent to the bronchioles.

Advise client that rinsing the mouth after using the nebulizer prevents systemic absorption and minimizes dryness of the mouth. The mouthpiece should be rinsed at least once daily to avoid clogging. Stress the importance of keeping the equipment clean to prevent infection. If using a refillable nebulizer, do not place more than a day's supply of drug in nebulizer. Change solution daily.

Clients with asthma benefit greatly from the use of sympathomimetic inhalers; however, they should be discouraged from using over-the-counter inhalers because of the non-selective beta-agonist drug effect of the epinephrine base. The nurse needs to recognize the possibility of misuse and the consequences of abuse in order to successfully help the client with inhalant drug therapy.

Cleaning
1. Once a day clean the inhaler and cap by rinsing it in warm running water. Let it dry before you use it again. Have another inhaler to use while it is drying.
2. Twice a week wash the plastic mouthpiece with mild dishwashing soap and warm water. Rinse and dry well before putting it back.

Checking how much medicine is left in the canister

1. If the canister is new, it is full.
2. An easy way to check the amount of medicine left in your metered dose inhaler is to place the canister in a container of water and observe the position it takes in the water (Figure 79). *Note:* This method does not work for all inhalers. Please ask your doctor if you can check *your* inhaler this way.

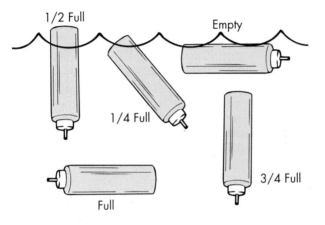

1/2 Full

Empty

1/4 Full

Full

3/4 Full

Figure 79

Notes

Guidelines for Instillation of Eyedrops and Ointments

Education

Instruct the client and/or home caregiver in proper administration of eye medications (Figure 80). Caution the client to always check the bottle label for correct medication and concentration, such as 0.1% or 1%. Checking labels is increasingly important because many beauty aids and home products (glues) are now packaged in similar containers. Discard solutions that have become cloudy or darkened.

Store medications as directed on the label; some may need refrigeration. Once opened, most medications have a limited life (3 months or the end of the current illness). If stored longer, the medication is more likely to become contaminated and lead to an infection of the eye. To avoid such contamination from the outset, the sterility of the preparation and/or dropper must be maintained. Do not allow the tube tip or dropper to touch anything, including the skin. Hold the

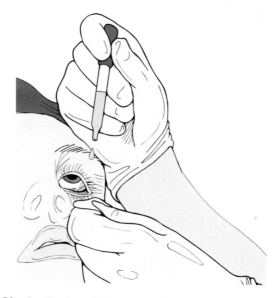

Figure 80   Instillation of drops into the conjunctiva of the lower lid of the eye.

From McKenry LM, Salerno E: *Mosby's pharmacology in nursing,* ed 20, St. Louis, 1998, Mosby.

dropper with the tip down. Never allow medication to flow into the bulb of the dropper. Keep the container closed when not in use. If two or more family members are using eye medications, each should have a separate vial to prevent cross-contamination. Inform the client of signs of side effects/adverse reactions, as well as signs of progress. Advise the client when to contact or return to the prescriber for assessment.

To instill eyedrops

Wash your hands and put on gloves, if necessary.

Gently cleanse exudate from the eye, if necessary.

Ask the client to tilt the head toward the side of the affected eye.

Gently pull the lower eyelid down and ask the client to look up.

Instill the correct number of drops in the sac formed by the lower eyelid (See Figure 80).

Take care not to touch the dropper to the eye or eyelashes.

Gently apply pressure for 30 seconds to 1 minute over the inner canthus next to the nose to prevent absorption through the tear duct and premature drainage of the medication away from the eye.

Ask the client to gently close the eye, which distributes the solution. Warn against squeezing the eye tightly, which will force out the medication.

Wipe away any excess medication.

If both eyes are to be medicated, do the second instillation quickly before the patient begins to blink and tear as a reaction to the burning sensation occurring in the first eye medicated.

To instill eye ointment

The procedure is the same except the ointment is expressed directly onto the exposed conjunctival sac from inner to outer canthus with a small individual tube and close eye; gently massage to distribute the medication.

Eyedrops and Look Alikes

Containers that are facsimiles are the culprits behind many ophthalmic emergencies. Thinking they are instilling eyedrops, adults and children have instead dropped in superglue, contact lens cleaners, ear drops, and perfumes. These products are often sold in bottles that are similar in shape, size, and color. The elderly who may have poor eyesight are particularly at risk for mistaking one product for another.

In most cases, the injured eye responds to copious flushing to dilute and wash out the offending agent, followed by topical antibiotics, lubricants, or cycloplegics, and patching, if needed. If the client has instilled glue in the eye and has no significant pain, irrigation and a sterile eyepatch soaked in tap water and left overnight are sufficient. The solvents to dissolve the glue are too toxic for the eye, so if the conservative approach does not work, the client may need to be referred to an ophthalmologist, who may cut the eyelids apart to prevent corneal abrasion.

Advise all clients to keep their eyedrops in one particular place away from other chemicals. Recommend that they check the labels on the container while still wearing their glasses or contact lenses to ensure they have the right medicine before administering their eyedrops.

From O'Boyle JE, Enzenaur RW: "Super glue" in the eye, *Emerg Med* 24(6):59-60, 62, 1992.

Instructions for Use of Ear Wash and Drops

You have been given a prescription that you should have filled at your own drugstore. You will also need a 2- or 3-ounce ear syringe, which you can buy at a drugstore if you do not have one. Someone else should wash your ear for you; you cannot do it as well yourself. The instructions below should be followed carefully:

1. Wash hands before and after this procedure.
2. Fill the ear syringe with the solution.
3. The solution must be at body temperature. If the solution is too warm or too cool, you will feel dizzy. Warm the solution by placing the syringe in a pan of hot water. Do *not* warm the solution on the stove.

From *Mosby's patient teaching guides,* St. Louis, 1995, Mosby.

4. Lie down with the ear to be washed facing up and pull up and out on the external ear. Place the tip of the ear syringe into the ear canal. Do not be afraid to push it down into the ear. However, you should get a return flow. If you do not, you have it in too far. Pull the syringe out slightly.

5. Pump the warmed solution from the syringe back and forth into the ear by squeezing and releasing the bulb of the syringe. Do this vigorously and repeatedly. The ear wash must be forced back and forth, in and out of the ear canal.

6. Lean over and let the solution run out of the ear.

7. Pull the ear up, back, and out to straighten the ear canal.

8. Put three to five warmed drops into the ear.

9. If the solution burns too much at first, you may dilute the solution. Mix 2 ounces of water with 2 ounces of the solution. Later, decrease the amount of water used with each irrigation.

10. Use the solution and drops twice a day for 2 weeks and then until the ear stops running or becomes dry. If you are not sure that the ear is dry, check it by putting a cotton swab down into the ear canal. If the cotton swab comes out dry, stop using the solution and drops. If the cotton swab is wet or there is an odor, continue using the solution and drops for 4 days.

11. Do not use the solution and drops as long as the ear remains dry and is not running, and as long as there is no odor. Should the ear start to run after being dry for a period of time, start using the ear solution and drops until the ear is dry again.

12. **Do not get any water in your ears.** You should not go swimming until you are told you may do so. Whenever there is a chance of getting water in your ears, such as when you shower or wash your hair, use cotton in the ear. First, place a dry piece of cotton in the ear and then a second piece that has been saturated with petroleum jelly.

13. If you have any questions, call your doctor.

Administration of Ear Drops

The infant or child is positioned on the unaffected ear. The nurse pulls the pinna down and back to administer ear drops to infants and children under 3 years of age.

When administering ear drops to children older than 3 years and adults, the nurse gently pulls the pinna up and back. The nurse should stabilize his or her hand on the client's head for safety and instill the prescribed number of drops. The drops are directed toward the ear canal to avoid hitting the tympanic membrane, which can cause pain. The client should remain in the position for 5 to 10 minutes. Otic drops should be warmed before they are instilled, to prevent nausea or vertigo.

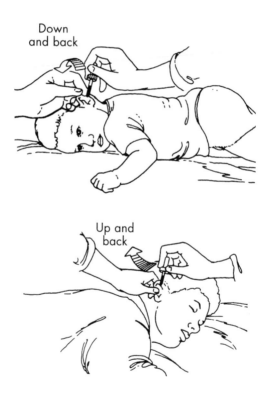

From Myers J: *Quick medication administration reference*, ed 3, St. Louis, 1998, Mosby.

Sublingual Administration

The client places the tablet under the tongue, where it dissolves and is rapidly absorbed through the blood vessels and enters the systemic circulation. This site is used for nitroglycerin tablets to relieve chest pain.

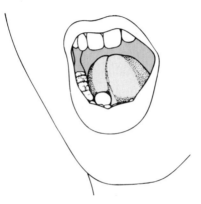

From Myers J: *Quick medication administration reference,* ed 3, St. Louis, 1998, Mosby.

Administering a Rectal Suppository

Position client on side and drape. Unwrap suppository and remove from package. Apply water-soluble lubricant. Gently insert suppository about an inch past the internal sphincter.

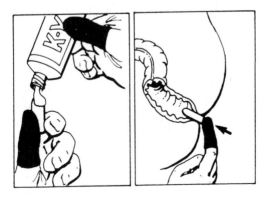

From Myers J: *Quick medication administration reference,* ed 3, St. Louis, 1998, Mosby.

Administration of Vaginal Medication

Gently insert the vaginal applicator as far as possible into the vagina and push plunger to deposit the medication.

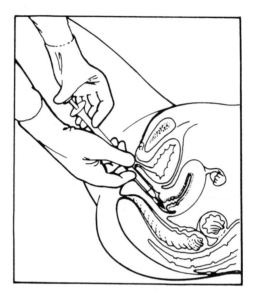

From Myers J: *Quick medication administration reference,* ed 3, St. Louis, 1998, Mosby.

Using Oxygen at Home Teaching Guide

Your doctor has prescribed extra oxygen at a flow rate of _____ liters per minute for _____ hours every day. The medical supply company will show you how to set the flow rate and how to care for the equipment. Keep the supplier's phone number handy so that you can call if the system doesn't work properly.

You will be using a liquid oxygen unit, an oxygen tank, or an oxygen concentrator. You will breathe the oxygen through either a mask or a nasal cannulae (two short prongs that fit just inside your nostrils). The system will also have a humidifier to warm and moisturize the oxygen.

From *Mosby's patient teaching guides,* St. Louis, 1995, Mosby.

It is a good idea to also have a small portable oxygen tank for an emergency backup system in case of power failure.

Here are some general guidelines and safety tips for using oxygen equipment.

General guidelines

Always keep your oxygen flow rate where your doctor prescribes.

Sometimes it is hard to tell whether oxygen is flowing through the tubes. If you have doubts, check to be sure that the system is turned on and there are no kinks in the tubing. If you still are not sure, place the nasal cannulae in a glass of water with the prongs up and watch for bubbles. (Always shake the water off before inserting the cannulae into your nostrils.) If no bubbles appear, oxygen is not flowing through the tubes and you need to call your supplier.

Each time before using your oxygen, check the humidifier bottle. If it is near the fill line, empty the bottle and refill it with sterile or bottled water.

Even with the humidifier, oxygen can dry the inside of your nose. A water-soluble lubricant (such as K-Y Jelly) helps ease dryness and cracking. Do not use petroleum-based products such as Vaseline because this will make the dryness worse.

To avoid running out of oxygen, reorder your new supply when the register reads ¼ full—2 or 3 days before you need a new tank.

Safety first

Oxygen is highly combustible. By following these rules, you can be confident that your oxygen system is not posing a serious fire hazard:

- Keep your oxygen unit away from open flames and heat. This includes smoking—do not smoke and do not allow others to smoke around you. If you have a gas stove, gas space heater, or kerosene heater or lamp, stay out of the room while it is on.
- To prevent leakage, always keep your oxygen system upright, and make sure the system is turned off when not in use. Do not place carpets, bed clothes, or furniture over the tubing, since this may cause a leak.
- Keep an all-purpose fire extinguisher close by.
- If a fire should occur, turn off the oxygen and leave the house at once.
- Notify your local fire department that you have oxygen in the house. In most areas, the fire department offers free safety inspections, which can help make your home even safer for using oxygen.

Call your doctor immediately if:

- Your breathing is difficult, irregular, shallow, or slow.
- You become restless or anxious.
- You are tired, drowsy, or have trouble waking up.
- You have a persistent headache.
- Your speech becomes slurred, you cannot concentrate, or you feel confused.
- Your fingernails or lips are bluish.

These symptoms may arise when you are not getting enough oxygen or when you are getting too much oxygen. Only your doctor can determine how much oxygen you need. Therefore, you must never change the flow rate without instructions from your doctor.

Chest Physiotherapy

In some lung conditions, such as chronic bronchitis, emphysema, and cystic fibrosis, thick mucus collects in the lungs. This makes breathing more difficult and increases the chance of getting pneumonia or other infections. To help loosen the mucus and move it out of the lungs, your doctor has suggested that you perform chest physiotherapy. This consists of postural drainage, chest percussion, and coughing.

You should do chest physiotherapy twice a day (unless your doctor tells you otherwise)—once when you first get up in the morning and once in the evening before you go to bed. Whenever you have more mucus than usual, you should do chest physiotherapy more often.

Remember that drinking a lot of fluids (at least 2 quarts daily) will also help thin the mucus.

You can do the postural drainage and coughing by yourself. Someone will need to help you with chest percussion.

Postural drainage

1. Place pillows on the floor beside the bed and a box of tissues close by.
2. Lie on the bed with your trunk over the side, head and arms resting on the pillows. You will lie on your stomach and on each side. Stay in each position 10 to 20 minutes.

From *Mosby's patient teaching guides,* St. Louis, 1995, Mosby.

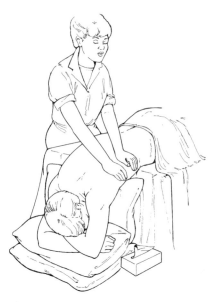

Chest percussion

Here is where a friend or family member will have to help you. You will stay in the postural drainage position for percussion.

1. The helper should make a cup with his or her hands. This is done by keeping fingers together, flexing the fingers, and tucking the thumb tightly against the index finger.
2. The helper firmly pats your back rhythmically, alternating the cupped hands, for 3 to 5 minutes. When done correctly, this will make a sound like a galloping horse. (With just a little practice, this technique is easy to master.)

Coughing

Stay in the postural drainage position.

1. Take a slow, deep breath through your nose. Hold your breath for 3 seconds. (Counting one 100, two 100, three 100 will help you hold your breath long enough.)
2. Open your mouth slightly, coughing three times as you breathe out. A good cough that helps bring up mucus sounds hollow, deep, and low. (A high-pitched cough is not effective.)
3. Take a slow, deep breath through your nose and breathe normally for a few minutes. Then repeat the coughing procedure several more times.
4. Be sure you spit the mucus into a tissue. (Do not swallow it, since this can cause nausea.)

Guidelines for Women With Lymphedema

Lymphedema

Swelling of the arm may occur in women who have had a mastectomy and removal of lymph glands under the arm and after other operations or radiation therapy that involves these glands.

Precautions to observe

- Care for simple cuts, scratches, or burns by careful washing and covering them with a protective dressing. Be sure to change plastic Band-Aids or bandages often to avoid infection.
- Wear loose-fitting gloves and avoid wearing anything that will constrict the hand or arm, such as tight sleeves or jewelry.
- Let technicians, nurses, and doctors know of the surgery and the need for care in taking blood pressure and giving vaccinations and injections on the operated side.
- Manicure nails carefully. Avoid cutting or tearing cuticles. Cuticles can be kept soft with a lanolin-based cream.
- Protect fingers from punctures by sharp objects such as needles and pins.
- Protect hand and arm when gardening by wearing gloves. This avoids punctures from thorns of roses or other plants or tools.
- Protect arm and chest from overexposure to the sun, particularly if the client has received radiation therapy. Apply a sunscreen liberally to exposed areas.
- Think through a task before starting it to see if there are precautions that should be taken to protect hands and arms.

Swelling (lymphedema)

Swelling does not mean a recurrence of cancer, but it is a side effect that occurs in some women following surgery or radiation. Swelling can occur immediately after surgery (may be only temporary), or months, or even years later. If the hand and arm swell, contact physician. The physician may refer the client to a specialist in physical medicine or to the physical therapy department of a hospital.

Corrective measures to use for swelling

The physician may prescribe antibiotics if there is evidence of infection or the physician may recommend treatment with a compression unit. A compression unit with a lymphedema sleeve is a sleevelike ap-

Modified from *Reach to recovery: an ounce of prevention: suggestions on hand and arm care,* Pamphlet No 4605-PS, Z-86.

paratus into which the affected arm is placed while the sleeve inflates and forces the fluids back into the lymph system to attempt to reduce the swelling. The physician will prescribe the length of time to leave the affected arm in the compression unit and the correct pressure setting. The sleeve will help control the swelling with regular use, but the technique is usually not curative. Some physicians advise clients to use the unit once or twice a day, or suggest treatments at the hospital as an outpatient. Ask the physician to write a prescription detailing the need, and check with the insurance company to see if payment or partial payment will be made for treatments or for the purchase of a portable unit. Some units are portable and can be used at home. The unit should be taken to the physiatrist (doctor of physical medicine) or physical therapy department at a hospital for setting and instruction.

Postmastectomy Exercises

Surgical treatment for breast cancer ranges from a lumpectomy (a limited removal of cancerous breast tissue and surrounding tissue) to a radical mastectomy (the removal of the breast, chest wall muscles, lymph nodes, and lymphatic structures beneath the armpit).

After breast surgery, your physician will tell you when you are able to do specific exercises to help keep your arm and shoulder active. Progressive exercises will help you gain full motion and strength in your arm and shoulder. Normal shoulder motion is achieved when you can reach across the top of your head and touch your opposite ear with your hand while keeping your head straight up. You should recover full motion in approximately 2 to 3 months.

Exercises should begin within 24 hours of your surgery. You may be instructed to limit the movement of your upper arm sideways from your body for a period of 1 week to 10 days after your surgery. However, you should actively move your wrist and elbow on the operated side as soon as possible. Combing your hair, brushing your teeth, and moving your arm to feed yourself are the first important steps to recovery.

Also practice deep breathing exercises during the first 24 to 48 hours. Lie flat on your back and take a deep breath. You should feel the expansion of your chest. Let your air out slowly and feel the downward chest movement. Repeat this three or four times. You may feel stiffness and tightness in your chest and arm when you are doing progressive exercise. This will come and go for a while. Continue to work to im-

From Mosby: *Mosby's patient teaching guides,* St. Louis, 1998, Mosby.

prove your motion at least three times a day until you no longer have that discomfort.

You can begin range-of-motion exercises when the wound is healed (about 10 to 12 days after surgery). The type of exercises you need depends on the type of breast surgery you had (radical mastectomy, modified radical mastectomy, or lumpectomy). Ask your physician what type of exercises you need.

As a general guideline, begin with 5 repetitions of an exercise and work up to 20, unless directed otherwise by your physician or therapist. The number of times you do an exercise will depend on your pain and your presurgery condition. Doing the very best you can is what counts. Whether you do 5 or 20 repetitions of exercises per day, you should set goals to increase this number a little bit each day. Listed below are a few common postmastectomy exercises.

1. Begin with "pendulum" exercises. Bend forward to let your shoulder hang forward. Move your arm forwards and backwards (Figure 81), then side to side. This will improve the movement and strength of your shoulder.
2. While standing straight, raise your arm forward toward the ceiling (Figure 82, *A*), then lower your arm to your side. Then raise your arm outward from your side and up, as close to being even with your shoulders as possible. When you reach the goal of raising your arm from your side to shoulder height, begin to reach your arm toward the ceiling until you are able to touch your head with the inside of your extended arm (Figure 82, *B*).
3. Another beginning exercise is to do "wall push-ups" (Figure 83). Stand in front of a wall with your arms outstretched and the palms of your hands touching the wall. Slowly bend your elbows and, without moving your feet, do body push-ups against the wall.

The following activities, which include housework, hobbies, and sports, can also help improve your strength and motion: vacuuming, mopping the floor, pulling out and pushing in drawers, playing golf, kneading bread, swimming the breast stroke, raising windows, lifting yourself out of the bathtub, reaching to an upper shelf, pulling up a dress zipper, washing your back, drying your back with a bath towel, knitting, typing, and playing the piano. It is important to seek activities that challenge your strength and motion. Exercise is good for your body and helps you to keep a positive attitude.

If you are having problems with exercising or regaining motion, ask your physician for a referral to an occupational therapist who can prescribe exercises specifically for you. Another good resource before and immediately after surgery is Reach To Recovery, offered through the American Cancer Society (1-800-ACS-2345).

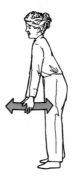

Figure 81

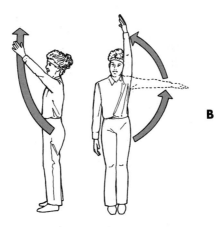

A   B

Figure 82

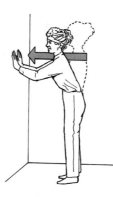

Figure 83

PHARMACOLOGICAL ISSUES

In working with individuals in the home and community, the nurse often finds that medications present major issues for clients. To properly comply with taking medications, clients want to understand the importance of the medicine to their overall care and how they will be affected. The following information will give the nurse cues to medication interactions with other drugs, foods, and physiological responses of clients to certain pharmacological agents. The use of proper agents is emphasized.

Summary of Essential Equivalents

Household/metric   Apothecary/household

2 tbs	30 mL
5 tsp	25 mL
4 tsp	20 mL
1 tbs	15 mL
2 tsp	10 mL
1 tsp	5 mL
½ tsp	

8 dr	1 oz
6 dr	¾ oz
4 dr	½ oz
2 dr	¼ oz
1 dr	⅛ oz

One Ounce Medicine Cups (30 mL)

Medicine cups showing household/metric and apothecaries'/household measurements.

Approximate equivalents of metric, apothecaries', and household measures

Household	Apothecaries'	Metric
60 drops (gtt)	1 teaspoon (tsp)	5 mL (or cc)*
1 teaspoon (tsp)	1 fluidram (f℥)	5 mL
1 tablespoon (tbs)	4 fluidrams	15 mL
2 tablespoons (tbs)	8 fluidrams = 1 ounce (℥)	30 mL
1 measuring cup	8 ounces	240 mL
1 pint	16 ounces	500 mL
1 quart	32 ounces	1000 mL

*The abbreviations *mL* and *cc* are used interchangeably; however, *mL* is generally used for liquids, *cc* for solids and gases, and *g* for solids.

Approximate equivalents from Brown M, Mulholland J: *Drug calculations: process and problems for clinical practice,* ed 5, St. Louis, 1995, Mosby.

Particulars of the household system

1. Some of the units for liquid measures are the same as those in the apothecaries' system, for example, pint and quart.
2. There are no standard rules for expressing household measures, which accounts for variety in their use.
3. Standard cookbook abbreviations are used in this system.
4. Arabic numerals and fractions are used to express quantities.
5. The basic unit in the household system is the **drop (gtt). Note: Drops should never be used as a measure for medications since the size of drops varies and therefore can be inaccurate. When drops are used as a measure for medications, they should be calibrated or used only when associated with a dropper size, as in intravenous (IV) flow rates.**
6. Common household measures and conversions within this system are as follows.

   Drop (gtt)
   Teaspoon (t, tsp) (60 gtt = 1 tsp)
   Tablespoon (T, tbs) (3 tsp = 1 tbs)
   Cup (C) (16 tbs = 1 C)
   Pint (pt) (2 C = 1 pt)
   Quart (qt) (2 pt = 1 qt)

Points to remember

In the apothecaries' system, the abbreviation or symbol is placed before the quantity.

Apothecaries' measures are approximate.

The apothecaries' system uses fractions, Roman numerals, and Arabic numerals.

Teaspoon, tablespoon, and drop are common measures used in the household system.

There are no rules for stating household measures.

The household system uses fractions and Arabic numerals.

Conversions between metric, apothecaries', and household are not equal measures.

From Gray D: *Calculate with confidence,* ed 2, St. Louis, 1998, Mosby.

Calculating Pediatric Dosage

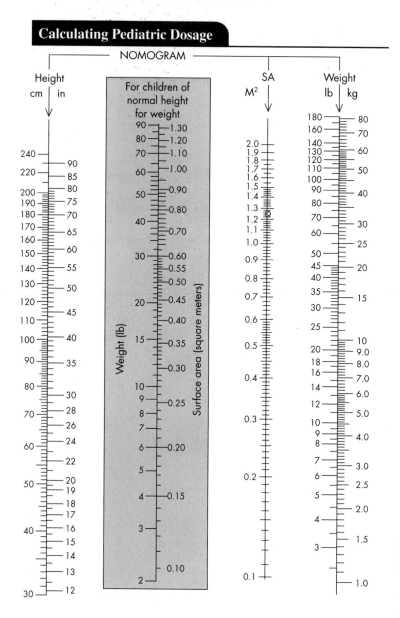

West nomogram (for estimation of surface areas). Surface area is indicated where a straight line connecting height and weight intersects surface area (SA) column or, if client is approximately of normal proportion, from weight alone (enclosed area). (From Behrman RE, Vaughan VC, editors: *Nelson textbook of pediatrics,* ed 14, Philadelphia, 1992, WB Saunders; modified from data of E Boyd by CD West.)

Clark's rule

Because this formula is based on weight alone, it is often considered an imprecise calculation for children.

$$\frac{\text{Average adult dose} \times \text{Weight of child in pounds}}{150} = \text{Estimated safe dose}$$

Example: How much acetaminophen (Tylenol) should a 1-year-old child weighing 21 pounds receive if the average adult dose is 10 grains?

Answer:

$$\frac{10 \text{ (grains)} \times 21 \text{ (weight in pounds)}}{150} = \text{gr } 1\frac{2}{5}$$

$$\frac{\text{BSA of child}}{\text{BSA of adult}} \times \text{Adult dose} = \text{Estimated child's dose}$$

$$\text{BSA of child (m}^2) \times \text{Dose/m}^2 = \text{Estimated child's dose}$$

From McKenry L, Salerno E: *Mosby's pharmacology in nursing,* ed 20, St. Louis, 1998, Mosby; Wong D: *Whaley and Wong's nursing care of infants and children,* ed 6, St. Louis, 1999, Mosby.

Calculation of IV Rates

1. *Flow rate*

    (must know amount of solution ordered and amount of time of infusion)

    EXAMPLE: infuse D5NS, 1000 ml, over 8 hours using a macro drip set (15 gtt/ml)

    A. Calculate amount of solution per hour:

    $$\frac{1000 \text{ ml}}{8 \text{ hr}} = 125 \text{ ml/hr}$$

    B. Calculate gtt/min:

    $$\frac{\text{gtt/ml of tubing}}{60 \text{ min/hr}} \times \frac{\text{Amount of fluid}}{1}$$

    $$\frac{15}{60} \times \frac{125}{1} = \frac{1875}{60} = 31 \text{ gtt/min}$$

From Hermey C: *Quick reference for IV therapy,* St. Louis, 1995, Mosby.

2. *Flow rate in mg*

(must know amount of solution, amount of drug, gtt factor/ml, and amount of drug to be administered)

EXAMPLE: lidocaine drip, 2 g, in D5W, 500 ml, to infuse at 2 mg/min

A. Calculate amount of drug/ml in mg:

$$2 \text{ g} = 2000 \text{ mg}$$

$$\frac{2000 \text{ mg}}{500 \text{ ml}} = 4 \text{ mg/ml}$$

B. Calculate number of gtt for 1 mg:

$$\frac{4 \text{ mg}}{1 \text{ ml}} \times \frac{4 \text{ mg}}{60 \text{ gtt}} = \frac{1 \text{ mg}}{15 \text{ gtt}}$$

C. Calculate number of desired mg:

$$\frac{1 \text{ mg}}{15 \text{ gtt}} = \frac{2 \text{ mg}}{X}$$

$$X = 30 \text{ ml}$$

3. *μg/kg/min*

(to determine number of μg/kg/min when drip factor is known, must know client weight, amount of drug, amount of solution, gtt factor/ml, and gtt being administered)

EXAMPLE: client weighing 154 lb is receiving dopamine, 400 mg, in D5W, 500 ml, at 30 gtt/min

A. Convert pounds to kg:

$$\frac{154}{2.2} = 70 \text{ kg}$$

B. Calculate number of mg in 1 ml of solution:

$$\frac{400 \text{ mg}}{500 \text{ ml}} = 0.8 \text{ mg/ml}$$

C. Convert mg to μg:

$$0.8 \text{ mg} \times 1000 = 800 \text{ μg}$$

D. Divide μg by weight to obtain μg/kg/ml:

$$\frac{800 \text{ μg}}{70 \text{ kg}} = 11.4 \text{ μg/kg/ml}$$

E. Find μg/kg/gtt:

$$\frac{11.4 \text{ μg/kg}}{60 \text{ gtt}} = \frac{X}{1 \text{ gtt}}$$

$$X = 0.19 \text{ μg/kg/gtt}$$

F. Multiply current drip rate by number calculated to obtain μg/kg/min:

$$0.19 \times 30 = 5.70 \text{ μg/kg/min}$$

4. *gtt/min*

(to determine number of gtt/min when μg/kg/min is ordered, must know client weight, amount of drug, amount of solution, gtt factor/ml, and dosage to be administered)

EXAMPLE: client weighs 154 lb; MD orders 5 μg/kg/min of dopamine, 400 mg, in D5W, 500 ml

A. Convert lb to kg:

$$\frac{154}{2.2} = 70 \text{ kg}$$

B. Calculate number of mg in 1 ml of solution:

$$\frac{400 \text{ mg}}{500 \text{ ml}} = 0.8 \text{ mg/ml}$$

C. Convert mg to μg:

$$0.8 \times 1000 = 800 \text{ μg}$$

D. Divide μg by weight to obtain μg/kg/ml:

$$\frac{800 \text{ μg}}{70 \text{ kg}} = 11.4 \text{ μg/kg/ml}$$

E. Calculate rate needed to administer ordered dose of drug:

$$\frac{11.4 \text{ μg/kg/ml}}{60} = \frac{5 \text{ μg/kg/min}}{X}$$

$$X = 26 \text{ gtt/min}$$

5. *Pediatric dosage*

$$\frac{\text{BSA of child}}{\text{BSA of adult}} \times \text{Adult dose} = \text{Pediatric dose}$$

Diagnosis of Tuberculosis Infection: Tuberculin Skin Test

The tuberculin skin test is used to determine whether a person is infected with *Mycobacterium tuberculosis.* Tuberculin skin testing is contraindicated only for persons who have had a necrotic reaction to a previous tuberculin skin test. It is *not* contraindicated for any other persons, including infants, children, pregnant women, persons who are HIV infected, or persons who have been vaccinated with BCG.

Administering the tuberculin skin test

The Mantoux test is the intradermal injection of 0.1 milliliters of purified protein derivative tuberculin containing 5 tuberculin units into the volar surface of the forearm. The injection should be made just beneath the surface of the skin, with the needle bevel facing upward to produce a discrete, pale elevation of the skin that is 6 millimeters to 10 millimeters in diameter.

Interpreting skin test results

The reaction to the Mantoux test should be read 48 to 72 hours after the injection. The reading should be based on a measurement of induration (swelling), not on erythema, or redness. The diameter of induration should be measured perpendicularly to the long axis of the forearm. All reactions, even those classified as negative, should be recorded in millimeters.

Classification of the tuberculin skin test reaction

An induration of **5 mm or more** is considered positive for
- HIV-infected persons
- close contacts of a person with infectious TB
- persons who have abnormal chest radiographs
- persons who inject drugs and whose HIV status is unknown

An induration of **10 mm or more** is considered positive for

- foreign-born persons
- HIV-negative persons who inject drugs
- medically underserved, low-income populations
- residents of long-term care facilities

From Centers for Disease Control and Prevention: *Tuberculosis information: diagnosis of TB infection and TB disease,* Document #250102, Atlanta, March 1996.

- persons with certain medical conditions*
- children less than 4 years old without any other risk factors
- staff of long-term care facilities and health care facilities

An induration of **15 mm or more** is considered positive for persons who do not have any risk factors for TB.

Some persons who have positive skin test results may have TB disease. The possibility of TB disease must be ruled out before preventive therapy is used.

---

*e.g., diabetes mellitus, prolonged corticosteroid therapy, immunosuppressive therapy, gastrectomy, some hematological and reticuloendothelial diseases, end-stage renal disease, silicosis, and body weight *that is 10% or more below* ideal.

Biological Agents for Diagnostic Tests

Biological product	Indication/adult dose
Tuberculin (purified protein derivative, PPD, Mantoux Test) (Aplitest, Tuberculin Tine Test)	Diagnostic: tuberculosis Adult dose: 5 U.S. units, intradermal. Special instructions for application of Tine test should be followed.
Tuberculin (PPD) (Aplisol, Tubersol)	Diagnostic: tuberculosis Adult dose: 5 U.S. units, intradermal following specific instructions as noted by manufacturer or *USP DI*.
Allergenic extracts	Several hundred individual purified fluid allergens available for diagnosis and hyposensitization of allergies: pollens, poison ivy, foods, dusts, yeast, and other allergens. Treatment: periodic subcutaneous injection of gradually increasing potent dilutions of specific allergen.

From McKenry LM, Salerno E: *Mosby's pharmacology in nursing,* ed 20, St. Louis, 1998, Mosby.

Common Tests for Screening Selected Conditions

Identifies/detects	Test(s)	Available
Ketones in blood or urine	Acetone tests: Acetest, Ketostix	Tablets, strips
Protein in urine	Albumin tests: Albustix	Strips
Nitrate, uropathogens, bacteria	Microstix-3, Uricult	Culture paddle, strips
Bilirubin in urine	Ictotest	Tablets
Urea nitrogen in blood	Azostix	Strips
Candida albicans, vaginal	Isocult for Candida, CandidaSure	Culture paddle Reagent slides
Chlamydia trachomatis	Chlamydiazyme, Sure Cell Chlamydia	Kits
Cholesterol	Advanced Care Cholesterol Test- for home use	Kit
Cryptococcal neoformans in CSF and serum	Crypto-LA	Slide tests
Gastrointestinal duodenal fluid stomach acid	Entero-Test Gastro-Test	String capsules String capsules
Glucose in blood	Chemstrip bG, Dextrostix, Diascan, Glucometer Encore, and others	Strips
Glucose in urine	Clinitest, Chemstrip bG, Clinistix, Tes-Tape	Tablets, strips
Gonorrhea	Biocult-GC, Gonozyme Diagnostic, others	Kits

From McKenry LM, Salerno E: *Mosby's pharmacology in nursing,* ed 20, St. Louis, 1998, Mosby.

Common Tests for Screening Selected Conditions—cont'd

Identifies/detects	Test(s)	Available
Human immunodeficiency virus (HIV) tests	HIV-1 LA Recombigen, HIV-1 Latex Agglutination test, HIVAB HIV-1 EIA, others	Kits
Meningitis	Bactigen N Meningitidis	Slide tests
Mononucleosis	Mono-Diff, Mono-Latex, others	Kits
Occult blood screening	ColoCare, Colo-Screen, others	Kits
Ovulation tests	Answer Ovulation, Clearplan Easy, Ovu-Quick Self-Test, others	Kits
Human chorionic gonadotropin pregnancy tests	Advance, Answer Plus, Answer Quick & Simple, Fact Plus, others	Kits
Rheumatoid factor	Rheumatex, Rheumaton	Slide tests
Hemoglobin S sickle cell test	Sickledex	Kit
Staphylococcus aureus	Isocult for Staphylococcus	Culture paddles
Streptococci tests	Sure Cell Streptococci, Bactigen Strep B, others	Kits
Virus tests, miscellaneous	Human T-Lymphotropic Virus Type, Sure Cell Herpes, Rubazyme for Rubella, others	Kits

Food-Drug Interactions

Drug category/medication	Foods to avoid	Rationale
Antacids		
Calcium carbonate (Tums)	Avoid large amounts of dairy products If used as a calcium supplement, avoid concurrent administration of bran and whole grain breads or cereals	Milk or cream may increase acid secretion. Reduces absorption of calcium.
Antibiotics		
Erythromycin, penicillins*	Meals, acidic fruit juices, citrus fruits, or acidic beverages, such as cola drinks	The antibiotics are acid labile (reduced absorption). Take medication 1 hour before meals or apart from acidic foods or 2 hours after meals.
Tetracyclines	Calcium-containing foods: milk, ice cream, yogurt, cheeses, and others	Calcium may complex with tetracycline, resulting in reduced absorption of the antibiotic. Most tetracyclines, with the exception of doxycycline and minocycline, should be administered 1 hour before or 2 hours after meals.
Anticoagulants		
Warfarin (Coumadin), dicumarol, heparin	Beef liver and green leafy vegetables contain vitamin K (spinach, cabbage, brussels sprouts)	Vitamin K can counteract therapeutic action of anticoagulants. A normal, balanced diet will not interfere with this medication. Fad or extreme diets with foods high in vitamin K can affect anticoagulant activity.

Laxative

Mineral oil (Agoral plain, Mineral Oil)

Take 2 hours apart from food

Do not administer at bedtime

May decrease absorption of vitamins A, D, E, and K. Also reduces absorption of calcium. Aspiration of mineral oil may induce lipid pneumonitis.

MAO inhibitors

Phenelzine (Nardil), tranylcypromine (Parnate)

Foods with high tyramine content, such as aged cheese (brie, cheddar, processed American, camembert, and others), aged meat, sour cream, yogurt, pickled herring, chicken liver, canned figs, raisins, bananas, avocados, soy sauce, yeast extract, meat tenderizers, alcoholic beverages such as beer and wine (chianti, sherry, or hearty red wines), sausages, chocolate, anchovies

Concurrent use may result in severe headache, nosebleed, chest pain, eyes sensitive to light, or severe hypertension, which may result in a hypertensive crisis.

From McKenry LM, Salerno E: *Mosby's pharmacology in nursing,* ed 20, St. Louis, 1998, Mosby.

*Erythromycin base (E-Mycin, Ery-Tab, E-Mycin Eryc) or stearates (Erypar, Erythrocin Stearate, Ethril, Wyamycin S) are best absorbed in the fasting state. Erythromycin ethylsuccinate (E.E.S.), estolate (Ilosone), and enteric-coated erythromycin may be given before or with meals. Penicillin, such as penicillin G, ampicillin, cloxacillin, cyclacillin, dicloxacillin, mafcillin, and oxacillin may have decreased absorption if given with food or acidic-type products.

Drugs That Change Urine or Stool Color

Medications that may alter urine color

Drug	Possible color changes
Amitriptyline (Elavil)	Blue-green
Anticoagulants (coumarin and others)	Pink, red, or dark brown (indicative of systemic bleeding)
Cascara sagrada	In acid urine, brown; basic urine, yellow to pink; on standing, black
Iron salts, dextran, and others	Brown to black
Laxatives (danthron, senna)	Pink to red or brown
Laxatives (phenolphthalein)	Pink to red
Levodopa (Laradopa, Dopar)	May cause dark urine and sweat
Methyldopa (Aldomet)	Pink, amber to dark urine
Metronidazole (Flagyl)	Dark urine
Nitrofurantoins (Furadantin, Macrodantin)	Yellow to rusty brown urine
Phenazopyridine (Pyridium)	Orange red urine; may stain clothing
Phenytoin (Dilantin)	Red-brown or darkening of urine
Phenothiazines (chlorpromazine, or Thorazine, and others)	Pink, red, or orange urine
Rifampin (Rifadin)	Red, orange, or brown urine, stool, saliva, sweat, and tears

Medications that may alter stool color

Drug	Possible color changes
Antacids with aluminum salts (Maalox, Mylanta, and others)	White specks or discoloration of stools
Anticoagulants (coumarin and others)	Red, orange, to black because of internal bleeding
Bismuth or iron salts	Black
Laxative (phenolphthalein)	Red
Laxative (senna)	Yellow, orange to brown
Phenazopyridine (Pyridium and others)	Orange, red

From McKenry LM, Salerno E: *Mosby's pharmacology in nursing,* ed 20, St. Louis, 1998, Mosby.

Drug-Nutrient Interactions

Drugs Affecting Appetite

Appetite depressants

Amphetamines and related compounds
Benzphetamine (Didrex)
Fenfluramine (Pondimin)
Phenylpropanolamine
   (Dexatrim, Dimetapp, Triaminic)

Antibiotics
Amphotericin B (Fungizone)
Gentamicin (Garamycin)
Metronidazole (Flagyl)
Zidovudine (AZT)

Carbonic anhydrase inhibitors
Acetazolamide (Diamox)
Dichlorphenamide (Daranide)

Digitalis preparations
Methylphenidate (Ritalin)

Appetite stimulants

Antidepressants
Amitriptyline (Elavil)

Antihistamines
Astemizole (Hismanal)
Cyproheptadine (Periactin)

Tranquilizers
Lithium carbonate (Lithane)
Benzodiazepines: all, including
Prazepam (Centrax)
Diazepam (Valium)
Phenothiazines: all, including
Chlorpromazine (Thorazine)
Promethazine (Phenergan)

From Moore M: *Nutritional care,* ed 3, St. Louis, 1997, Mosby.

Steroids
Anabolic steroids
Oxandrolone (Anavar)
Glucocorticoids
Dexamethasone (Decadron)
Methylprednisolone (Medrol)
Tetrahydrocannabinol (marijuana)

Drugs whose absorption is affected by food

Absorption increased
Carbamazepine (Tegretol)
Griseofulvin (Fulvicin)
Hydralazine (Apresoline)
Metoprolol (Lopressor)
Nitrofurantoin (Macrodantin)
Propoxyphene (Darvon)
Propranolol (Inderal)
Spironolactone (Aldactone)

Absorption reduced
Amoxicillin (Amoxil)
Ampicillin (Polycillin)
Aspirin
Astemizole (Hismanal)
Demeclocycline (Declomycin)
Doxycycline (Vibramycin)
Dipyridamole (Persantine)
Levodopa (Dopar)
Methotrexate
Oxytetracycline (Terramycin)
Penicillin G
Penicillin V (K)
Phenobarbital (Luminal)
Phenytoin (Dilantin)
Propantheline (Pro-Banthine)
Tetracycline (especially affected by dairy products)

Some drugs that affect taste sensitivity*
Amphetamines ($\downarrow$ sweet, $\uparrow$ bitter)
Ampicillin
Amphotericin B
Aspirin
Captopril
Chlorpheniramine maleate[†]
Clindamycin (bitter aftertaste)
Clofibrate ($\downarrow$ sensitivity, aftertaste)
Diazoxide
Ethacrynic acid
Griseofulvin
Insulin
Lincomycin
Lithium carbonate (strange, unpleasant taste)
Meprobamate
Methicillin (aftertaste)
Metronidazole
Oxyfedrine
Penicillamine
Phendimetrazine tartrate
Phenytoin
Propantheline
Sodium lauryl sulfate[‡]
Streptomycin
Tetracyclines
Zidovudine

---

*Sensitivity decreased unless otherwise noted.

[†]Antihistamine found in many over-the-counter cold/allergy products.

[‡]Toothpaste ingredient.

Nutritional effects of selected drugs

Drug	Effect on nutrition
Alcohol	↑ Excretion of Mg, K^+, Zn; impaired folic acid utilization
Antacids	
All	↓ Fe absorption caused by ↑ gastric pH
Aluminum hydroxide	↓ Phosphate absorption
Antibiotics/antifungals/ Antitubercular agents	
Amphotericin B	Hypokalemia; ↑ urinary excretion of Mg
Cephalosporins	False positive urine glucose by Clinitest (enzyme-based tests such as Tes-Tape or Clinistix not affected)
Chloramphenicol	↓ Hgb synthesis (interferes with response to Fe, folic acid, or vitamin B_{12} therapy)
Cycloserine	↓ Serum levels of vitamins B_{12}, B_6, folic acid
Gentamicin	↑ Urinary excretion of Mg, K^+, Ca (>10 g cumulative dose)
Isoniazid	Depletion of vitamin B_6; supplement should be given
Neomycin	Diarrhea and mucosal injury; ↓ absorption of fat, lactose, protein, vitamins A, D, K, B_{12}, Ca, Fe, K^+
Paraaminosalicylic acid	↓ Absorption of fat, folic acid, vitamin B_{12}
Anticonvulsants	
Phenytoin	↓ Absorption of Ca
Phenobarbital	↓ Absorption of Ca
Primidone	↓ Absorption of Ca
Antidiarrheal agent	
Sulfasalazine	↓ Absorption of folic acid; megaloblastic anemia
Antihypertensive agents	
Diazoxide	Hyperglycemia
Hydralazine	↑ Excretion of vitamin B_6
Nitroprusside	↓ Serum vitamin B_{12}
Antiinflammatory agents	
Aspirin	↑ Urinary loss of vitamin C; Fe deficiency caused by GI blood loss
Colchicine	↓ Absorption of vitamin B_{12}, fat, carotene, lactose, protein, Na, K^+
Indomethacin	↑ Urinary loss of vitamin C; Fe deficiency caused by GI blood loss

Nutritional effects of selected drugs—cont'd

Drug	Effect on nutrition
Carbonic anhydrase inhibitors	
All	Hyperglycemia; $\uparrow$ excretion of K^+
Cardiac drugs	
Digitalis, digoxin, digitoxin, etc.	Diarrhea, malabsorption of all nutrients
Chelating agents	
Penicillamine	$\downarrow$ Absorption of Cu, Zn, Fe
Corticosteroids	
All	$\uparrow$ Protein catabolism; $\downarrow$ protein synthesis; hyperglycemia; $\uparrow$ serum triglycerides and cholesterol; $\downarrow$ absorption of Ca, P, K^+; $\uparrow$ requirement for vitamins C, B_6, D, folic acid, Zn; osteopenia
Diuretics	
All	$\uparrow$ Urinary excretion of Mg, Zn, K^+, thiamin (some greater than others)
Ethacrynic acid	Hypomagnesemia, hypokalemia; $\uparrow$ loss of urinary Ca
Furosemide	$\downarrow$ Glucose tolerance; hyperglycemia; $\uparrow$ loss of urinary Ca
Thiazides	$\downarrow$ Glucose tolerance; hyperglycemia; hypokalemia
H_2 Receptor antagonists	
All (cimetidine, famotidine, nizatidine, ranitidine)	$\downarrow$ Fe and Ca absorption caused by $\uparrow$ gastric pH
Hypocholesterolemics	
Cholestyramine	$\downarrow$ Absorption of fat, vitamins A, E, D, K, B_{12}, Fe
Clofibrate	$\downarrow$ Absorption of carotene, Fe, vitamin B_{12}, fat
Colestipol	$\downarrow$ Absorption of fat, vitamins A, D, E, K
Laxatives	
Cathartics (e.g., senna, cascara, phenolphthalein	$\uparrow$ Fecal loss of Ca and K^+ (clinically significant only with laxative abuse)
Mineral oil	Potential for $\downarrow$ absorption of vitamins A, D, E, K, Ca^{2+}; recent evidence indicates that effects on vitamin absorption are probably not clinically significant

Continued.

Nutritional effects of selected drugs—cont'd

Drug	Effect on nutrition
Laxatives—cont'd	
Levodopa	$\uparrow$ Requirement for vitamin B_6
Lipid emulsions	$\uparrow$ Requirement for vitamin E
Opiates	
Heroin	$\downarrow$ Glucose tolerance, $\downarrow$ K^+
Oral contraceptive agents	$\uparrow$ Serum vitamin C; possible $\downarrow$ serum vitamin B_{12}, B_6, B_2, folic acid, Mg, Zn; $\uparrow$ Hct, Hgb, serum Fe, Cu, vitamins A, E
Parasympatholytic agents	
Atropine	$\downarrow$ Fe absorption caused by $\uparrow$ gastric pH
Potassium supplements	$\downarrow$ Vitamin B_{12} absorption
Sedatives-hypnotics	
Glutethimide	$\uparrow$ Absorption of Ca
Uricosuric agents*	$\uparrow$ Excretion of Ca, Mg, Na, K^+, P, Cl, vitamin B_2, amino acids
Urinary antiseptics	
Nitrofurantoin	$\downarrow$ Serum folic acid: megaloblastic anemia

*Used in treatment of gout.

Foods, food components, or nutrients with specific effects on drug action

Food, food component, or nutrient	Drugs affected (examples); common usage
Diet factors that decrease drug effectiveness	
Vitamin K sources: liver, cabbage, spinach, kale	Coumarin (Warfarin) (Coumadin); anticoagulant
Caffeine	Guanadrel (Hylorel); antihypertensive
Folic acid supplement	Methotrexate; cancer chemotherapy
High-protein diet	Levodopa (Dopar, Larodopa); anti-Parkinson's agent
Pyridoxine (vitamin B_6) supplement	Levodopa; anti-Parkinson's agent
Diet factors that increase risk of drug toxicity	
Caffeine	Lithium (Lithane, Lithobid); antimanic
Sodium-restricted diet	Lithium; antimanic
Folic acid deficiency	Methotrexate; cancer chemotherapy
Potassium deficit	Digitalis and related drugs, antiarrhythmics
Diet factors with other drug interactions	
Imported (natural) licorice—can cause excessive potassium losses, cardiac dysrhythmia, sodium and water retention	Thiazide: chlorothiazide (Diuril), hydrochlorothiazide (Hydrodiuril), chlorthalidone (Hygroton); diuretics
Tyramine and dopamine sources: liver, hard salami and other dry sausages; any pickled, aged, fermented, or smoked protein foods such as pickled herring, aged cheese, yogurt; commercial gravies; meat extracts; alcoholic beverages; sour cream; soy sauce; Italian broad (fava) beans; raisins; figs; bananas—can cause headache, hypertensive crisis, potential intracranial hemorrhage	Monoamine oxidase (MAO) inhibitors: phenelzine (Nardil), isocarboxazid (Marplan), tranylcypromine (Parnate), procarbazine (Matulane); antidepressants except procarbazine, which is antineoplastic

Drug Interactions With Antibiotics

Drug	Possible effect and management
Anticoagulants, oral coumarin or indanedione, heparin or thrombolytic agents	Increased risk of bleeding when given with high doses of parenteral carbenicillin or ticarcillin, as these drugs inhibit platelet aggregation. Monitor closely for signs of bleeding. Concurrent use of these penicillins with thrombolytic agents also increases the risk for severe bleeding; thus concurrent drug administration is not recommended.
Antiinflammatory nonsteroidal analgesics, platelet aggregation inhibitors (such as salicylates, dextran, dipyridamole, valproic acid), and sulfinpyrazone	With high doses of carbenicillin or ticarcillin (parenteral dosage forms), an increased risk for bleeding or hemorrhage exists. These drugs inhibit platelet function and large doses of salicylates may induce hypoprothrombinemia and also gastrointestinal ulcers (from NSAIDs, salicylates, or sulfinpyrazone), all adding to the potential risk of hemorrhage.
Captopril, potassium-sparing diuretics, enalapril, lisinopril, potassium-containing drugs, or potassium supplements	If given concurrently with parenteral penicillin G potassium, serum potassium levels may increase, causing hyperkalemia. Monitor closely; dosage adjustments may be necessary.
Cholestyramine or colestipol	May decrease absorption of oral penicillin G if given concurrently. Advise clients to take antibiotic first and other medications 3 hours later.
Estrogen-containing contraceptives	When used concurrently with ampicillin, bacampicillin, or penicillin V, the effectiveness of the oral contraceptives may be decreased because of increase in estrogen metabolism or reduction in enterohepatic circulation of estrogens. Advise clients to use an alternate method of contraception while taking these antibiotics.
Probenecid	Decreases renal tubular secretion of penicillins, resulting in elevated serum levels and an increase in half-life. It may also increase toxicity. Several combinations of penicillin and probenecid are marketed to take advantage of this effect.

From McKenry L, Salerno E: *Mosby's pharmacology in nursing,* ed 19, St. Louis, 1995, Mosby.

Selected Types of Laxatives

- **Saline laxatives**—retain and increase water content of feces by virtue of osmotic qualities.
- **Stimulant laxatives**—increase peristalsis in the colon by irritating intramural sensory nerve plexi endings in the mucosa
- **Bulk laxatives**—absorb water and increase the volume, bulk, and moisture of nonabsorbable intestinal contents, thereby distending the bowel and initiating reflex bowel activity
- **Intestinal lubricants**—mechanically lubricate feces to facilitate defecation
- **Emollients, or fecal softening agents**—act as dispersing wetting agents, facilitating nature of water and fatty substances within the fecal mass; when a homogeneous mixture is produced, the feces become soft
- **Hyperosmotic agents**—increase the introluminal osmotic pressure in the bowel; because they are not absorbed, they draw water into the intestine, resulting in an increased volume that stimulates peristalsis

From McKenry L, Salerno E: *Mosby's pharmacology in nursing,* ed 19, St. Louis, 1995, Mosby.

Over-the-Counter Varieties of Laxatives

	Stimulant (contact)	Osmotic saline	Stool softener surfactant or wetting agent	High-fiber and bulk-forming	Lubricant
Disadvantages with repeated frequent (long-term) administration	Watery stools, gripping	Watery stools, cramps	Unreliable results, may contribute to liver toxicity	Obstruction of narrowed lumen, some difficulty in chewing and swallowing	Anal leakage, lipid pneumonia
Increases rates of transit in small bowel	Yes	Yes	Yes	Yes	Unknown
Causes net secretion of water and electrolytes in small bowel	Yes	Yes	Yes	Yes	No
Inhibits absorption in small bowel	Yes	Yes	Yes	Yes	Yes
Increases mucosal permeability in small bowel	Yes	Not studied	Yes	Not reported	Not reported
Causes mucosal damage in small bowel	Yes	Not studied	Yes	Not reported	Not reported

	Mucosal surface irritation to stimulate or increase intestinal motor function or activity	Hyperosmolar ingredients trap water in intestinal lumen, hypertonicity of colon increases liquid in colon; hyperosmotic or saline	Changes surface tension of fecal mass, provides increased penetration of colonic water; penetrates and softens fecal mass by wetting agents	Absorbs water on surface, increases soft fecal mass, adds bulk and moisture to feces causing distention and elimination	Coats over fecal mass, passes with ease, lubricates gastrointestinal tract and softens feces
Acts only in colon (not small bowel)	No	No	No	No	Yes
Indicated for long-term treatment	No	No	No	Probably	No
Examples of type	Anthraquinone, bisacodyl, phenolphthalein, castor oil, danthron	Magnesium salts, MOM, sodium salts, glycerin	DSS, DCS Poloxamer 188	Methylcellulose, karaya gum, sodium CMC, malt soup extract, psyllium seed, agar, plantago bran (unprocessed), polycarbophil	Mineral oil
Physical or chemical property responsible for action	Mucosal surface irritation to stimulate or increase intestinal motor function or activity	Hyperosmolar ingredients trap water in intestinal lumen, hypertonicity of colon increases liquid in colon; hyperosmotic or saline	Changes surface tension of fecal mass, provides increased penetration of colonic water; penetrates and softens fecal mass by wetting agents	Absorbs water on surface, increases soft fecal mass, adds bulk and moisture to feces causing distention and elimination	Coats over fecal mass, passes with ease, lubricates gastrointestinal tract and softens feces

From McKenry LM, Salerno E: *Mosby's pharmacology in nursing*, ed 20. St. Louis, 1998, Mosby.

Site and Mechanism of Action of Laxatives Within the Intestines

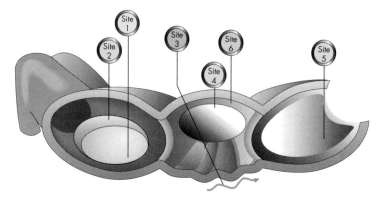

Site 1 Stool softener
Mechanism: Wetting agent used to soften fecal mass
Example: Docusate
Onset of action: 1 to 3 days
Precaution: Liquid dosage form may cause throat irritation; dilute in fruit juice or milk before administration.

Site 2 Bulk forming (high fiber)
Example: Psyllium hydrophilic
Mechanism: Absorbs water to increase bulk, distending bowel to initiate reflex bowel activity
Onset of action: 12 hours to 3 days
Precaution: Contraindicated in patients with dysphagia because esophageal obstruction may result. Avoid in dehydrated persons or individuals with limited or restricted fluid intake.

Site 3 Stimulant
Example: Senna
Mechanism: Increase peristalsis via nerve stimulation in colon
Onset of action: 6 to 12 hours
Precaution: May cause discoloration of feces and urine (alkaline urine from pink, red to brown; acid urine from yellow to brown)

Site 4 Osmotic saline
Example: Magnesium citrate
Mechanism: Increases water content of feces, resulting in distention, peristalsis, and evacuation. Laxation may be enhanced by release of cholecystokinin.
Onset of action: 1 to 3 hours
Precaution: Avoid use in patients who are dehydrated or whose renal function is impaired and in those with a colostomy or ileostomy. Ensure adequate fluid intake of at least 8 ounces of fluid with each dose to prevent dehydration.

Site 5 Lubricant
Example: Mineral oil
Mechanism: Coats surface of feces and colon to ease passage of stool; also softens fecal mass.
Onset of action: 6 to 8 hours
Precaution: Avoid administration within 2 hours of meals because it may reduce absorption of vitamins A, D, E, and K. Avoid use in dysphagic and bedridden patients because aspiration of mineral oil may result in lipid pneumonitis.

Site 6 Combination of stool softener and stimulant
Example: Docusate and senna
Mechanism: Stool softener and stimulant
Onset of action: 6 to 12 hours
Precaution: As noted for individual laxatives

From Lilley LL, Aucker RS: *Pharmacology and the nursing process,* ed 2, St. Louis, 1999, Mosby.

Drug Effects of Laxatives

Drug effect	Bulk	Emollient	Hyperosmotic	Saline	Stimulant
Increases peristalsis	Y	Y	Y	Y	Y
Causes increased secretion of water and electrolytes in small bowel	Y	Y	N	Y	Y
Inhibits absorption of water in small bowel	Y	Y	N	Y	Y
Increases wall permeability in small bowel	N	Y	N	N	Y
Causes wall damage in small bowel	N	Y	N	N	Y
Acts only in large bowel	N	N	Y	N	N
Increases fecal mass water	Y	Y	Y	Y	Y
Softens fecal mass	Y	Y	Y	Y	Y

From Lilley LL, Aucker RS: *Pharmacology and the nursing process*, ed 2, St. Louis, 1999, Mosby.

Y, Yes, *N*, no

Therapeutic Effects of Laxatives

Laxative group	Therapeutic effect
Bulk-forming	Acute and chronic constipation, irritable bowel syndrome, diverticulosis
Emollient	Acute and chronic constipation, softens fecal impacts, facilitates bowel movements in anorectal conditions
Hyperosmotic	Chronic constipation, diagnostic and surgical preparations
Saline	Constipation, removal of anthelmintics and parasites, diagnostic and surgical preparations
Stimulant	Acute constipation, diagnostic and surgical bowel preparations

From Lilley LL, Aucker RS: *Pharmacology and the nursing process,* ed 2, St. Louis, 1999, Mosby.

Adverse Effects of Laxatives

Laxative group	Side/adverse effect
Bulk-forming	Impaction above strictures, fluid overload
Emollient	Skin, rashes, decreases absorption of vitamins, lipid pneumonia
Hyperosmotic	Abdominal bloating, rectal irritation
Saline	Magnesium toxicity (with renal insufficiency)
Stimulant	Nutrient malabsorption, skin rashes, gastric irritation, rectal stimulation

From Lilley LL, Aucker RS: *Pharmacology and the nursing process,* ed 2, St. Louis, 1999, Mosby.

Drug Interactions of Laxatives

Laxative group	Interacting drug	Result
Bulk-forming	Antibiotics, digoxin, nitrofurantoin, salicylates, tetracyclines, oral anticoagulants	Decreased absorption
Emollient (mineral oil)	Oral anticoagulants	Increased or decreased effect of anticoagulant
	Fat-soluble vitamins (A, D, E, and K)	Decreased absorption
Hyperosmotic	Oral antibiotics	Decreased effects of lactulose
Saline	Barbiturates, general anesthetics, opioids, antipsychotics	Increased CNS depression
	Neuromuscular blockers	Increased effects
Stimulant	Antacids, H$_2$ blockers*	Gastric irritation
	Antibiotics, digoxin, nitrofurantoin, salicylates, tetracyclines, oral anticoagulants†	Decreased absorption

From Lilley LL, Aucker RS: *Pharmacology and the nursing process*, ed 2, St. Louis, 1999, Mosby.
*With bisacodyl.
†With bascara.

Dosages of Selected Laxative Agents

Agent	Pharmacologic class	Dosage range	Purpose
Methylcellulose (Citrucel)	Bulk-forming laxative	*Adult/Pediatric >12 y/o* PO: 1 tbs in 8 oz of water 1-3 times/day *Pediatric 6 to ≤12 y/o* PO: ½ adult dose in 4 oz of water 1-3 times/day	Constipation
Psyllium (Metamucil, Fiberall)	Bulk-forming laxative	*Adult/Pediatric ≥12 y/o* PO: 1-2 tsp in 8 oz of water 1-3 times/day *Pediatric 6 to ≤12 y/o* PO: ½ the adult dose in 4 oz of water at bedtime 1-3 times/day	Constipation
Mineral oil (Agoral Plain, Mineral Oil Enema, Kondremul, Zymenol)	Emollient laxative	*Adult/Pediatric ≤12 y/o* PO: 15-45 ml as a single daily dose *Pediatric 6-11 y/o* PO: 5-10 ml/day at bedtime *Adult/Pediatric ≥12 y/o* PO: 5-45 ml as a single daily dose at bedtime *Pediatric 2-11 y/o* PO: 30-60 ml/day	Constipation Enema
Glycerin (Fleet Babylax, Glycerin, Sani-Supp)	Hyperosmotic laxative	*Rectal:* Insert one adult, child, or infant suppository into rectum	Constipation
Magnesium salts	Saline laxative	*Citrate—Adult/Pediatric ≥12 y/o* PO: 11-25 g/day 6-11 y/o: 5.5-12.5 g/day 2-5 y/o: 2.7-6.25 g/day	Constipation

	Saline laxative—cont'd	*Sulfate—Adult/Pediatric* PO: ≥12 y/o: 10-30 g/day 6-11 y/o: 5-10 g/day 2-5 y/o: 2.5-5 g/day	Constipation
Senna (Black Draught, Dr. Caldwell Senna Laxative, Fletcher's Castoria, Senokot, Senolax)	Stimulant/irritant laxative	*Pediatric >27 kg* PO: ½ adult dose; *(do not use Black Draught for Children)* *Pediatric 1 mo-1 yr* PO: 1.25-2.5 ml at bedtime (syrup) *Adult* PO: 1-8 tabs (Senokot)/day PO: ½ to 4 tsp of granules added to liquid PR: 1-2 supp at bedtime	
Docusate (Calcium, potassium, and sodium salts)	Fecal softener	*Adult/Pediatric >12 y/o* PO: 50-360 mg/day *Pediatric 2-12 y/o* PO: 50-150 mg/day *Pediatric <2 y/o* PO: 25 mg/day	Stool softener
Polyethylene glycol (CoLyte, GoLytely, OCL)	Bowel evacuant	*Adult* PO: 4 L daily administered in 240-ml doses q10min	Bowel cleansing before examination
Lactulose (Chronulac, Constilac, Duphalac)	Disaccharide laxative	*Adult* PO: 15-30 ml/day	Constipation

From Lilley LL, Aucker RS: *Pharmacology and the nursing process*, ed 2, St. Louis, 1999, Mosby.

Pharmacology of Antidepressants

Drug	Therapeutic dosage range (mg/day)	Average (range) of elimination half-lives (hr)*	Potentially fatal drug interactions
Tricyclics			
Amitriptyline (Elavil, Endep)	75-300	24 (16-46)	Antiarrhythmics, MAOIs
Clomipramine (Anafranil)	75-300	24 (20-40)	Antiarrhythmics, MAOIs
Desipramine (Norpramin, Pertofrane)	75-300	18 (12-50)	Antiarrhythmics, MAOIs
Doxepin (Adapin, Sinequan)	75-300	17 (10-47)	Antiarrhythmics, MAOIs
Imipramine (Janimine, Tofranil)	75-300	22 (12-34)	Antiarrhythmics, MAOIs
Nortriptyline (Aventyl, Pamelor)	40-200	26 (18-88)	Antiarrhythmics, MAOIs
Protriptyline (Vivactil)	20-60	76 (54-124)	Antiarrhythmics, MAOIs
Trimipramine (Surmontil)	75-300	12 (8-30)	Antiarrhythmics, MAOIs
Heterocyclics			
Amoxapine (Asendin)	100-600	10 (8-14)	MAOIs
Bupropion (Wellbutrin)	225-450	14 (8-24)	MAOIs (possibly)
Maprotiline (Ludiomil)	100-225	43 (27-58)	MAOIs
Trazodone (Desyrel)	150-600	8 (4-14)	—

Selected serotonin reuptake inhibitors (SSRIs)

Fluoxetine (Prozac)	10-40	168 (72-360)[†]	MAOIs
Paroxetine (Paxil)	20-50	24 (3-65)	MAOIs[‡]
Sertraline (Zoloft)	50-150	24 (10-30)	MAOIs[‡]

Monoamine oxidase inhibitors (MAOIs)[§]

Isocarboxazid (Marplan)	30-50	Unknown	For all 3 MAOIs:
Phenelzine (Nardil)	45-90	2 (1.5-4)	Vasoconstrictors[‖], decongestant
Tranylcypromine (Parnate)	20-60	2 (1.5-3)	meperidine, and possibly
			other narcotics

Adapted from Depression Guideline Panel. Depression in Primary Care: Volume 2. *Treatment of major depression.* Clinical Practice Guideline, Number 5. Rockville, MD: U.S. Department of Health and Human Services, Public Health Service, Agency for Health Care Policy and Research. AHCPR Pub. No. 93-0551, April 1993.

*Half-lives are affected by age, sex, race, concurrent medications, and length of drug exposure.

[†]Includes both fluoxetine and norfluoxetine.

[‡]By extrapolation from fluoxetine data.

[§]MAO inhibition lasts longer (7 days) than drug half-life.

[‖]Including pseudoephedrine, phenylephrine, phenylpropanolamine, epinephrine, and norepinephrine.

Side-Effect Profiles of Antidepressants

Drug	Anticholinergic	Central nervous system		Side effect	Cardiovascular		Other
		Drowsiness	Insomnia/agitation	Orthostatic-hypotension	Cardiac arrhythmia	Gastrointestinal distress	Weight gain (over 6 kg)
Amitriptyline	4+	4+	0	4+	3+	0	4+
Desipramine	1+	1+	1+	2+	2+	0	1+
Doxepin	3+	4+	0	2+	2+	0	3+
Imipramine	3+	3+	1+	4+	3+	1+	3+
Nortriptyline	1+	1+	0	2+	2+	0	1+
Protriptyline	2+	1+	1+	2+	2+	0	0
Trimipramine	1+	4+	0	2+	2+	0	3+
Amoxapine	2+	2+	2+	2+	3+	0	1+
Maprotiline	2+	4+	0	0	1+	0	2+

Trazodone	0	4+	0	1+	1+	1+	1+
Bupropion	0	0	2+	0	1+	1+	0
Fluoxetine	0	0	2+	0	0	3+	0
Paroxetine	0	0	2+	0	0	3+	0
Sertraline	0	0	2+	0	0	3+	0
Monoamine oxidase inhibitors (MAOIs)	1	1+	2+	2+	1+	1+	2+

Adapted from Depression Guideline Panel. Depression in Primary Care. Volume 2. *Treatment of major depression.* Clinical Practice Guideline, Number 5. Rockville, MD: U.S. Department of Health and Human Services, Public Health Service, Agency for Health Care Policy and Research. AHCPR Pub. No. 93-0551, April 1993.

*0 = absent or rare

1+

2+ = in between

3+

4+ = relatively common

†Dry mouth, blurred vision, urinary hesitancy, constipation

FDA-Approved Indications, Dosage, and Administration for Benzodiazepines

Drug	FDA approved indications*	Dosage and administration
Alprazolam (Xanax, generic)	Anxiety, panic.	*Adults:* antianxiety, 0.25-4 mg/day in divided doses. Antipanic, up to 10 mg/day. *Children up to 18 yrs old:* not recommended.
Chlordiazepoxide (Librium, generic)	Anxiety, sedative-hypnotic (alcohol withdrawal)	*Adults:* antianxiety, 5-25 mg PO 3 or 4 times a day. Alcohol withdrawal, 50-100 mg PO initially, repeat as needed up to 400 mg/day. Parenteral, 50-100 mg IM or IV 3 or 4 times/day. Preoperative, 50-100 mg IM 1 hr before surgery. *Children:* 6 yrs and older, 5-10 mg PO 2 to 3 times a day. Parenteral up to 12 yrs, not established; 12 and over, 25-50 mg IM or IV.
Clonazepam (Klonopin)	Seizures, panic	*Adults:* orally: initially 0.5 mg three times daily with increases of 0.5-1 mg every third day until seizures are controlled, side effects occur, or the maximum of 20 mg/day is reached.
Clorazepate (Tranxene, generic)	Anxiety, seizures, sedative-hypnotic (alcohol withdrawal)	*Adults:* antianxiety, 7.5-15 mg PO 2 to 4 times a day. Alcohol withdrawal, 30 mg initially, then 15 mg 2 to 4 times eventually reduced to 3.75 mg (see current reference for dosing guidelines). Anticonvulsant, 7.5-30 mg 3 times a day per recommended schedule (see current reference for dosing guidelines).
Diazepam (Valium, generic)	Anxiety, sedative-hypnotic, seizures, skeletal muscle relaxant	*Adults:* antianxiety, 2-10 mg PO 2 to 4 times a day. Sedative-hypnotic (alcohol withdrawal), 5-10 mg 3 or 4 times a day. Anticonvulsant or skeletal muscle relaxant (adjunct), 2-10 mg 3 or 4 times a day. Parenteral, IM or IV, individualized dose (usually 5 up to 20 mg depending on procedure). See current guidelines.
Estazolam (Prosom)	Sedative-hypnotic	*Adults:* 1-2 mg PO. *Children up to 18 yrs old:* not recommended.

Drug	Use	Dosage
Flurazepam (Dalmane, generic)	Sedative-hypnotic	*Adults:* 15-30 mg PO. *Children up to 15 yrs old:* not recommended.
Halazepam (Paxipam)	Anxiety	*Adults:* 20-40 mg 3 or 4 times a day. *Children up to 18 yrs old:* not recommended.
Lorazepam (Ativan, generic)	Anxiety, sedative-hypnotic	*Adults:* antianxiety, 1-3 mg 2 or 3 times a day. Sedative-hypnotic, 2-4 mg at bedtime. Parenteral, 0.5 mg/kg IM up to maximum of 4 mg or 0.044 mg/kg or total dose of 2 mg IV (whichever is less). *Children up to 12 years old:* PO not recommended. Parenteral not recommended for children up to 18 yrs old.
Midazolam (Versed)	Preoperative sedation and amnesia, conscious sedation	*Doses are individualized, generally adults:* 70-80 µg/kg 1/2 to 1 hr before surgery.
Oxazepam (Serax, generic)	Anxiety, sedative-hypnotic	*Adults:* antianxiety, 10-30 mg 3 or 4 times a day. Sedative-hypnotic (alcohol withdrawal), 15 or 30 mg 3 or 4 times a day. *Children up to 12 yrs old:* dosage not established.
Prazepam (Centrax, generic)	Anxiety	*Adults:* 10-20 mg PO 3 times a day or 20-40 mg at bedtime. *Children up to 18 yrs old:* dosage not established.
Quazepam (Doral)	Sedative-hypnotic	*Adults:* 7.5-15 mg at bedtime. *Children up to 18 yrs old:* dosage not established.
Temazepam (Restoril, generic)	Sedative-hypnotic	*Adults:* 7.5-15 mg at bedtime. *Children up to 18 yrs old:* dosage not established.
Triazolam (Halcion)	Sedative-hypnotic	*Adults:* 125-250 µg at bedtime. *Children up to 18 yrs old:* dosage not established.

From McKenry LM, Salerno E: *Mosby's pharmacology in nursing,* ed 20, St. Louis, 1998, Mosby.
*USP DI, 1996

Benzodiazepine Overdose

In conscious clients, administer an emetic followed by activated charcoal to adsorb the benzodiazepine. For unconscious clients, a gastric lavage with a cuffed endotracheal tube may be used.

Ensure maintenance of an adequate airway, closely monitor vital signs, administer oxygen for depressed respirations, and promote diuresis by the administration of intravenous fluids.

Medications that may be used include IV administration of flumazenil as a benzodiazepine antagonist and vasopressors such as norepinephrine, metaraminol, or dopamine to treat hypotension. Do not use barbiturates to treat excitation effects because they may exacerbate the condition.

Dialysis is of limited value in treating a benzodiazepine overdose.

From McKenry L, Salerno E: *Mosby's pharmacology in nursing,* ed 20, St. Louis, 1998, Mosby.

Notes

Lithium Dosage and Administration

	Adults	Elderly	Children
Lithium carbonate tablets/capsules/syrup	Acute mania: 300 to 600 mg orally 3 times daily; adjust dosage as necessary according to client's response and development of side effects/adverse reactions. Maintenance: 300 mg 3 or 4 times daily, adjusted as necessary. Maximum: 2.4 g/day	Usually require a lower dosage	Children up to 12 yr, 15 to 20 mg/kg of lithium per body weight daily, divided into 2 or 3 doses. Adjust dosage weekly as necessary
Lithium carbonate extended-release tablets	450 to 900 mg orally twice a day or 300 to 600 mg orally 3 times a day; adjust dosage as necessary. Maintenance: 450 mg orally twice daily or 300 mg 3 times daily; adjust dosage as necessary. Maximum daily dose: 2.4 g/day	Usually require a lower dosage	Children less than 12 yr, not established

From McKenry L, Salerno E: *Mosby's pharmacology in nursing*, ed 19, St. Louis, 1995, Mosby.

Client Teaching Tips for Psychotherapeutic Agents

Anxiolytics and antidepressants

- Take your medication exactly as prescribed by your physician. Do not skip or omit any doses and do not double up on the medication. If you remember you have not taken your medication and it is within an hour or 2 hours of the time you would have taken it, then go ahead and take the dose. If it is more than 2 hours after this time, skip that dose and take the medication at the next scheduled time.
- Keep medications out of reach of children.
- Change positions slowly to avoid fainting or dizziness.
- Call your physician immediately should you experience any fainting episodes while taking these medications.
- Do not suddenly stop taking this medication.
- If you experience drowsiness and sedating effects, do not operate heavy equipment or machinery.
- Avoid consuming alcohol and taking other CNS depressants.
- Do not take over-the-counter medication or any other medication without checking with your physician first to make sure this is okay.
- You may experience more drowsiness during the beginning of treatment. With the TCAs this should decrease after the first few weeks of therapy.
- You should contact your physician should you experience sores in the mouth, fever, sore throat, hallucinations, confusion, disorientation, shortness of breath, difficulty in breathing, yellow discoloration of the skin or eyes, or irritability.
- Caffeine and caffeinated beverages such as cola, tea, and coffee as well as cigarette smoking decrease the effectiveness of your medication.
- Keep all appointments and follow-up visits with your physician and other health care providers.
- Always carry or have about you a Medic-Alert tag or bracelet naming the medication you are taking.
- The therapeutic effects of MAOIs may not occur for up to 4 weeks. Therefore do not alter your dosing if you are not feeling better before this time. Remember a hypertensive crisis may occur if you consume foods high in tyramine, foods such as cheese, beer, wine, avocados, bananas, and liver. Caffeinated beverages should also be avoided. Remember that the drug will remain in the body for up to

From Lilley LL, Aucker RS: *Pharmacology and the nursing process,* ed 2, St. Louis, 1999, Mosby.

2 weeks after discontinuing the medication. Contact your physician should you experience chest pain, a severe throbbing headache, rapid pulse, or nausea.

Phenothiazines and haloperidol

- Take all medications exactly as prescribed. Do not double, omit, or skip doses. Remember, it may be several weeks before an improvement is experienced.
- Phenothiazines may cause drowsiness, dizziness, or fainting, so change positions slowly.
- You should wear sunscreen when taking phenothiazines because of the photosensitivity they cause.
- Avoid taking antacids or antidiarrheal preparations within 1 hour of a dose of a phenothiazine.
- Notify your physician immediately should you note fever, sore throat, yellow discoloration of the skin, or uncontrollable movements of the tongue while taking a phenothiazine.
- Do not take phenothiazines or haloperidol with alcohol or with any other CNS depressant.
- Long-term haloperidol therapy may result in tremors, nausea, vomiting, or uncontrollable shaking of small muscle groups, and any of these symptoms should be reported to your physician.
- You may take the oral forms of these medications with meals to decrease GI upset.

Lithium

- Take your medication exactly as prescribed. Do not double, skip, or omit doses.
- It may take several weeks before you notice any improvement related to the drug therapy.
- You may take your medicine with meals to decrease gastrointestinal upset.
- If you become ill with vomiting or diarrhea or are unable to eat or drink, it is important that you notify your physician of this immediately. Dehydration of any type, even as the result of excessive sweating, may result in drug toxicity.
- Many of the side effects of lithium will disappear with time; however, you should contact your physician should you experience any excessive vomiting, tremors, weakness, or any involuntary movements.
- Make sure to keep your appointments, especially ones when blood is drawn to determine the serum lithium levels.
- Always wear a Medic-Alert tag naming the agent you are taking.
- Keep the medication out of the reach of children.

Factors Affecting Lithium Serum Levels

Increased by: *Excretion:*
  Diarrhea
  Diuretics or dehydration
  Low-salt diets   Decreased
  High fevers or strenuous exercise
Decreased by:
  High salt intake
  High intake of sodium bicarbonate   Increased
  Pregnancy

From McKenry LM, Salerno E: *Mosby's pharmacology in nursing,* ed 20, St. Louis, 1998, Mosby.

Notes

Characteristics of Insulin Preparations After Subcutaneous Administration

Insulins*	Onset (hr)	Peak effect (hr)	Duration of action (hr)
Rapid acting			
Insulin injection (Regular Insulin, Humalin R)[†]	½-1	2-4	5-7
Intermediate acting			
Isophane insulin suspension (NPH Insulin)	3-4	6-12	18-28
Insulin zinc suspension (Lente Insulin)	1-3	8-12	18-28
Long acting			
Extended insulin zinc suspension (Ultralente)	4-6	18-24	36
Combinations			
Isophane human insulin (50%) & human insulin (50%) (Humalin 50/50)	½	3	22-24
Isophane human insulin (70%) & human insulin (30%) (Humalin 70/30, Novalin 70/30)	½	4-8	24

From McKenry LM, Salerno E: *Mosby's pharmacology in nursing*, ed 20, St. Louis, 1998, Mosby.

*Semilente insulin is available in Canada but is no longer available in the United States. Onset of action of Semilente insulin is 1-3 hr, peak effect is in 2-8 hours and duration of action is 12-16 hours.

[†]These insulins may be administered intravenously. Intravenously, the onset of action is within ¼ to ½ hour, peak effect within ¼ to ½ hour, and duration of action within ½ to 1 hour.

Pharmacokinetics and Usual Adult Dose of Hypoglycemic Agents

Generic (brand name)	Onset of action (hr)	Peak effect (hr)	Duration of action (hr)	Usual adult dose	
Sulfonylureas					
First generation					
Acetohexamide (Dymelor)	1	1.5-6*	8-24	250-1000 mg/day	Use with caution in elderly and clients with renal insufficiency
Chlorpropamide (Diabinese)	1	2-4	24-72	250-500 mg/day	Longest acting hypoglycemic. More reported side effects than other agents.
Tolazamide (Tolinase)	4-6	3-4	10-20	100-500 mg with breakfast	Active metabolites may be increased in renal impairment.
Tolbutamide (Orinase)	1	3-4	6-12	250-2000 mg daily in divided doses	Shortest acting agent. Rapidly metabolized to inactive metabolites.

Second generation					
Glipizide (Glucotrol)	1-1.5	1-3	12-24	5-40 mg before meals in divided doses	Dose 30 min before meals.
Glipizide extended release (Glucotrol XL)	—	6-12	24	5-20 mg with breakfast	Use with caution in elderly clients in renal failure.
Glyburide nonmicronized (Diabeta, Micronase)	2-4	4	24	1.25-20 mg with breakfast, divided dosages > 10 mg	
Glyburide micronized (Glynase PresTab)	1	3	24	0.75-12 mg/day. Doses over 6 mg divided and given with meals	Micronized formula has increase bioavailability, thus lower dose required.
Miscellaneous					
Acarbose (Precose)	Not absorbed			50-100 mg with meals	Most effective if given with high fiber diet.
Metformin (Glucophage)	—	2-3	6-12	500 mg or 850 mg bid or tid.	Take with food to reduce nausea & vomiting

From McKenry LM, Salerno E: *Mosby's pharmacology in nursing*, ed 20, St. Louis, 1998, Mosby.
*Includes active metabolite, hydroxyhexamide.

Hypoglycemic Oral Agents: Side Effects/Adverse Reactions

Side effects*	Adverse reactions†
Most frequent: diarrhea or constipation, dizziness, gas anorexia, headache, nausea, vomiting, abdominal distress	Less frequent: chlorpropamide only— respiratory difficulties (CHF in persons with cardiac problems). Sedation; cramping of muscles; convulsions; edema of face, hands, or ankles; comatose, increased weakness (antidiuretic effect)
Less frequent/rare: photosensitivity, rash	Rare: pruritus, jaundice, light-colored stools, dark urine (impairment of liver function). Increased fatigue, sore throat, increased temperature, increased bleeding or bruising (blood dyscrasias)
	Overdosage: symptoms of hypoglycemia

From McKenry L, Salerno E: *Mosby's pharmacology in nursing,* ed 20, St. Louis, 1998, Mosby.

*If side effects continue, increase, or disturb the client, inform the physician.

†If adverse reactions occur, contact the physician because medical intervention may be necessary.

Drugs With the Potential to Cause Intellectual Impairment

Alcohol
Analgesics
Anticholinergics
Antidepressants
Antipsychotics
Antihistamines
Antiparkinsonism agents

Cimetidine
Digitalis
Diuretics
Hypnotics
Sedatives
Sudden withdrawal of benzodiazepines

From Ebersole P, Hess P: *Toward healthy aging: human needs and nursing response,* ed 5, St. Louis, 1998, Mosby.

Some Preventable Drug Interactions Through Proper Administration

Drug	Take with food, milk, meals	Do not take with milk or its products	May impair nutrient and electrolyte uptake and use	Do not take with alcohol	Do not take with fruit juice	Take on empty stomach
Alcohol			X			
Aminophylline and derivatives	X					
Ampicillin					X	
Antacids						X
Antihistamines				X		
Antiinfectives			X	X		
Atropine			X			
Belladonna and associated alkaloids						X
Benzathine penicillin G					X	X
Bisacodyl (Dulcolax)		X	X	X		

From Ebersole P, Hess P: *Toward healthy aging: human needs and nursing response*, ed 5, St. Louis, 1998, Mosby.
Data from Knoben JE, Anderson PO: *Handbook of clinical data*, ed 7, Hamilton, Ill, 1993, Drug Intelligence Publications.

Continued.

Some Preventable Drug Interactions Through Proper Administration—cont'd

Drug	Take with food, milk, meals	Do not take with milk or its products	May impair nutrient and electrolyte uptake and use	Do not take with alcohol	Do not take with fruit juice	Take on empty stomach
Chloral hydrate				X		
Chlorpropamide (Diabinese)				X		
Cholestyramine (Questran)			X			
Clindamycin (Cleocin)			X			
Clofibrate (Atromid-S)			X			
Cloxacillin					X	X
Corticosteroids (oral)	X					
Diocytl sodium sulfosuccinate (Colace, Surfak)			X			
Diphenoxylate (Lomotil)			X			
Diuretics	X		X			
Donnatal						X

Erythromycin (oral)					X	X
Folic acid inhibitors			X			
Ibuprofen (Motrin)	X					
Indomethacin (Indocin)	X					
Iron salts						X
Monoamine oxidase inhibitors				X		
Methotrexate			X	X		
Methylphenidate (Ritalin)	X			X		X
Metronidazole (Flagyl)	X		X	X		
Mineral oil			X			
Narcotics			X	X		
Neomycin			X			
Nitrofurantoin (Furadantin)	X		X			

Continued.

Some Preventable Drug Interactions Through Proper Administration—cont'd

Drug	Take with food, milk, meals	Do not take with milk or its products	May impair nutrient and electrolyte uptake and use	Do not take with alcohol	Do not take with fruit juice	Take on empty stomach
Nitrofurantoin macrocrystals (Macrodantin)	X					
Penicillin (oral)						X
Phenazopyridine (Pyridium)						X
Phenylbutazone (Butazolidin)	X					
Phenytoin	X					
Potassium chloride solutions		X				
Rauwolfia derivatives	X			X		
Tetracyclines	X	X				
Tolbutamide (Orinase)				X		
Trimeprazine (Temaril)	X			X		

Effects of Systemic Drugs on Vision

Drug	Effect
Furosemide (Lasix)	Blurred vision, decreased tolerance to contact lenses, photophobia, allergic reactions to eyelids and conjunctivae
Propranolol (Inderal)	Transient blurred vision with diplopia, decreased accommodation
Dimetapp (antihistamine and anticholinergic effect)	Mydriasis (contraindicated in angle closure glaucoma), blurred vision, intolerance to contact lenses
Diazepam (Valium)	Allergic conjunctivitis
Digoxin (Lanoxin)	Diplopia, blurred vision, changes in color perception (warnings of toxicity)

Modified from Osis M: Drugs and vision, *Gerontion* 1(5):15, 1986.

General Physiological System Characteristics of Drug Toxicity

Cardiovascular
Arrhythmias
Tachycardias
Palpitations
Hypotension
Congestive heart failure
Hypertension
Bone marrow depression
Leukopenia
Thrombocytopenia
Anemia
Agranulocytosis

Central nervous system
Confusion
Gait changes
Insomnia
Drowsiness
Blurred vision or visual changes
Slurred speech
Ototoxicity
Tremors
Irritability
Problems with temperature control
Anticholinergic effects
Seizures

Hepatic changes
Jaundice
Clotting problems
Decreased liver function

Gastrointestinal
Anorexia
Nausea and vomiting
Diarrhea
GI bleeding
Pancreatitis

Renal
Electrolyte imbalance
Polyuria
Urinary retention
Fluid retention

Respiratory
Dyspnea
Asthmatic reactions

Skin
Rash
Urticaria
Pruritus
Photosensitivity

From Ebersole P, Hess P: *Toward healthy aging: human needs and nursing response,* ed 5, St. Louis, 1998, Mosby.

Common Useful Over-the-Counter Preparations

Medication (examples)	Use
Analgesic balm or ointment (Banalg, Ben-Gay)	Minor muscle aches and pain
Analgesic tablets (aspirin, acetaminophen)	Headaches, minor aches, pain, and fever
Antacids (Mylanta, Maalox)	Indigestion, upset stomach
Antidiarrheal (Kaopectate, Pepto Bismol)	Mild, uncomplicated diarrhea
Antihistamines (Benadryl, Chlortrimeton)	Allergies, allergic rhinitis
Antiseptics, liquid (hydrogen peroxide, isopropyl alcohol)	Hydrogen peroxide—minor cuts, scrapes and wounds; alcohol—sprains or muscle strain
Mouthwash (Gly-Oxide)	Oral wound cleansing product for minor dental inflammation or irritations
Throat lozenges (Cepacol)	Minor sore throat
Skin lotion (calamine lotion)	Insect bites, minor itching, poison ivy
Contraceptives (spermicides, condoms)	Prevention of unwanted pregnancy or sexually transmitted diseases
Ipecac syrup	Accidental poison treatment
Laxatives, mild (Milk of Magnesia)	Constipation
Motion or travel sickness preparations (Bonine, transdermal scopolamine)	Prevention of dizziness, nausea, vomiting
Nasal decongestants (Sudafed)	To reduce nasal stuffiness resulting from colds or allergies
Sunburn and other burn treatments (A&D ointment, Nupercainal cream or ointment)	To treat minor burns or prevent sunburn

From Myers J: *Quick medication administration reference,* ed 3, St. Louis, 1998, Mosby.

The client should read the container label carefully, and if there are any questions, the advice of the pharmacist or health care provider should be sought.

CONSIDERATIONS FOR THE ELDERLY

Medications That Should and Should Not Be Used by Older Adults

Category	Do not use	Limited use	Okay
Cardiovascular	Aldomet	Capoten	Inderal
	Catapres	Diazide	Lopressor
	Serpasil	Minipress	Tenormin
	Persantine	Lasix	Lanoxin
	Cyclospasmol		Nitrobid
	Pavabid		Coumadin
	Trental		K-Lor
Tranquilizers and hypnotics	Ativan	Serax	
	Dalmane		
	Halcion		
	Librium		
	Nembutal		
	Restoril		
	Valium		
	Xanax		
Antidepressants	Elavil		
	Triavil		
Antipsychotics		Desyrel	Norpramine
		Sinequan	Aventyl
		Tofranil	Pamelor
		Haldol	Lithium
		Mellaril	
		Navane	
		Prolixin	
		Stelazine	
		Thorazine	
Pain and anti-inflammatory	Bufferin		Advil
	Feldene		Aspirin
	Darvocet		Ecotrin
	Darvon		Empirin
	Demerol		Tylenol
	Talwin		Dilaudid
	Wygesic		Percodan
			Vicodin
Gastrointestinal	Mylanta	Antivert	Tagamet
	Tigan	Compazine	Zantac
	Colace	Phenergan	Pepcid
	Dialose Plus	Reglan	Maalox
	Doxidan	Milk of Magnesia	Metamucil
		Achromycin	

From Ebersole P, Hess P: *Toward healthy aging: human needs and nursing response,* ed 5, St. Louis, 1998, Mosby.

Continued.

Medications That Should and Should Not Be Used by Older Adults—cont'd

Category	Do not use	Limited use	Okay
Antinfectives			Bactrim
			Gantrisin
			Keflex
			Penicillin
			Septra
			Vibramycin
Neurological	Artane	Hydergine	Sinemet
	Cogentin		Dilantin
			Tegretol
Nutritional	Vitamin E		Calcium
Supplements			Feosol
			Fergon
			Niacin
			Vitamins
Others	Norflex	Premarin	Synthroid

Notes

Special Drug Considerations for the Elderly

Drug	Special considerations
Analgesic agents	
Acetaminophen (APAP) (Tylenol, Datril)	Acetaminophen is the preferred analgesic agent with noninflammatory pain and is as effective as propoxyphene and codeine. Chronic daily ingestion of more than 4 to 5 g can lead to liver damage.
Aspirin (ASA)	Aspirin is the least expensive and is preferred over acetaminophen in inflammatory pain. It is as effective as propoxyphene and codeine. Gastrointestinal blood loss occurs in three fourths who take it and is of concern to clients with borderline anemia; concomitant liquid antacid minimizes. Antiplatelet effect may be of benefit in prevention of recurrent myocardial infarction and transient ischemic attack.
Propoxyphene and propoxyphene combinations (Darvocet-N 100 and Darvon compounds)	Single-ingredient propoxyphene is not as effective as aspirin or acetaminophen alone, but a combination is as effective as aspirin or acetaminophen. Confusional reactions are increased. Avoid long-term full-dose use.
Codeine and codeine combinations (Tylenol No. 1-4)	Codeine has equal potency with aspirin and acetaminophen. Combination has greater potency. Nausea, vomiting, and constipation are more common.
Pentazocine (Talwin)	Pentazocine is less effective than aspirin and is prone to causing confusional reactions.
Phenacetin	Never use phenacetin chronically because both prescription and OTC medications will lead to analgesic nephropathy, especially in combination analgesics.
Meperidine (Demerol), morphine, hydromorphone (Dilaudid)	Use one third to one half usual adult dose, since much more potent. No side effect differences in equal analgesic doses, but incidence increases with age.

Continued.

Modified from Deverau MO, Andrus L, Scott C: *Elder care*, New York, 1981, Grune & Stratton.

Special Drug Considerations for the Elderly–cont'd

Drug	Special considerations
Antiinflammatory analgesic agents Phenylbutazone (Azolid, Butazolidin) and oxyphenbutazone (Tandearil)	Both have longer half-life and higher incidence of gastrointestinal upset and severe toxic reactions in older clients; therefore, give with meals or liquid antacid to minimize gastrointestinal effect. These are not recommended in those over 60 years of age by some authorities. Phenylbutazone and oxyphenylbutazone cause fluid retention, blood dyscrasias, and increased oral anticoagulant effect. Do not give full dose for more than 7 to 14 days.
Tolmetin (Tolectin), fenoprofen (Nalfon), sulindac (Clinoril), ibuprofen (Motrin), naproxen (Naprosyn)	All nonsteroidal antiinflammatory analgesics are less effective than aspirin in inflammatory disease but have lower incidence of gastrointestinal side effects. These are much more expensive than aspirin.
Antidiabetic agents	Weight reduction and dietary measures control up to 70% of maturity-onset diabetes. Oral agents may increase cardiovascular morbidity. Hypoglycemic signs of tremor, sweating, and tachycardia are not as readily discernible. Chlorpropamide (Diabense) and acetohexamide (Dymelor) have active metabolite and prolonged half-lives.
Cardiovascular drugs Digitalis preparations	Digoxin (Lanoxin) is the preferred glycoside. Avoid digitoxin and digitalis leaf (long hepatic and renal half-lives). Although beneficial in low output failure and atrial fibrillation, digitalis preparations are successfully withdrawn in up to three fourths of clients. Subacute toxicity of anorexia with weight loss is more common than initial signs of gastrointestinal or cardiovascular effects. Baseline and follow-up electrocardiograms are essential. Dose is based on lean body weight and creatinine clearance with attention to electrolyte and thyroid status. One third to one half of clients are noncompliant.

Cardiovascular drugs—cont'd

Quinidine

Quinidine has higher serum levels if used concurrently with both drugs and digoxin. Half-life is prolonged. Cinchonism (gastrointestinal effects, light-headedness, tinnitus) occurrence is more common with low body weight. Decrease loading dose by one third in clients with significant heart failure.

Propranolol (Inderal)

Toxic effects are more common, as is reduced beta-blocking responsiveness in older clients. Propranolol aggravates bronchospastic tendency in chronic obstructive pulmonary disease and can precipitate heart failure. Propranolol also affects diabetic control at higher doses, and there is increased tendency of "cold limb" effect in lower extremities in those with peripheral vascular or vasospastic diseases.

Nitroglycerin tablets (Nitrostat)

Nitrostat is the most stable form. Client must sit down before sublingual dose placement. Beware of orthostatic effect of all vasodilators.

Nitroglycerin ointment (Nitrol)

Never rub into skin. Headache may be relieved with aspirin or acetaminophen.

Long-acting nitrates (isosorbide [Isordil, Sorbitrate] and pentaerythritol tetranitrate [Peritrate])

Long-acting nitrates are variably effective. Be careful about blood pressure–lowering effect.

Antihypertensive agents

Diuretics

All diuretics increase incontinence.

Thiazides (many; no significant difference; use hydrochloriazide generic)

Start with lowest possible dose. Clients must drink sufficient liquids. Watch volume, serum electrolyte, urate, and glucose effect.

Continued.

Special Drug Considerations for the Elderly–cont'd

Drug	Special considerations
Furosemide (Lasix)	Furosemide is most potent diuretic and should be held until thiazides no longer effective. It promotes calcium excretion and profoundly depletes sodium, potassium, and chloride. Cautious use of potassium supplements and salt substitutes is necessary because the elderly tend to have lower total body potassium with decreased muscle mass.
Spironolactone (Aldactone)	Spironolactone is a potassium-sparing diuretic often used in combination with thiazide (Aldactazide). Special caution is necessary if concurrent potassium supplement or salt substitute is used. Fatal hyperkalemia has been reported.
Triemterene (Dyrenium)	Triamterene is a potassium-sparing diuretic most often used in combination with thiazide (Dyazide) with similar precaution as spironolactone.
Sympatholytic antihypertensive agents	
Methyldopa (Aldomet)	Beware of continued blood pressure below 120/70, orthostatic effects, impaired male sexual function, and drowsiness or sedation. Reduce dosage when methyldopa is given in combination with thiazide (Aldoril). Sodium retention is seen when diuretic is not used. Daily dose at bedtime may take advantage of sedative effect, with therapeutic effect equivalent to multiple daily doses.
Propranolol (Inderal)	Propranolol is the only sympatholytic agent not requiring diuretic to prevent sodium retention. See cardiovascular section. If pulse is less than 50 to 60 beats per minute, drug is poorly tolerated.
Guanethidine (Ismelin)	Guanethidine is a profound sympatholytic agent with long second phase half-life. Use in small doses. Tricyclic antidepressants can interfere with antihypertensive effect.
Reserpine	Avoid giving reserpine to those with depression, sinusitis, peptic ulcer disease, and history of breast cancer.

Anticoagulant agents

Heparin

Heparin increases risk of bleeding with age, especially in women over 60 years of age.

Warfarin (Coumadin)

Warfarin increases risk of bleeding with age because of altered sensitivity with genetic, nutritional, and liver factors. Carefully evaluate use, and do serial prothrombin times. Beware of risk of hemorrhage, especially with possible hemorrhagic stroke, peptic ulcer disease, hiatal hernia, and diverticulosis or any bleeding diathesis. Concurrent aspirin usage is not possible except with heart valve prostheses.

Sedative-hypnotics and minor tranquilizers

Barbiturates (Butisol, Nembutal), phenobarbital, secobarbital (Seconal), amobarbital (Amytal)

With the exception of phenobarbital as an anticonvulsant, continued use of other barbiturates is irrational because of prolonged half-lives, paradoxic excitation in some, and tolerance and sleep pattern aberrations in all.

Benzodiazepines, chlordiazepoxide (Librium), diazepam (Valium), clorazepate (Tranxene), lorazepam (Ativan), oxazepam (Serax), and flurazepam (Dalmane)

Prolonged half-lives and cumulation of benzodiazepines have been reported with all except Ativan and Serax. Prolonged daily sedative (1 to 3 months) or hypnotic (7 to 14 days) use is not recommended because of depression of normal sleep pattern and resultant confusion, delirium, and psychological changes. Serax is best choice because of short half-life. No hypnotic should be used nightly longer than 14 days; instead skip to every third night.

Chloral hydrate (Noctec)

Chloral hydrate is an excellent hypnotic in clients with no liver disease.

Continued.

Special Drug Considerations for the Elderly—cont'd

Drug	Special considerations
Antihistamines Diphenhydramine (Benadryl), hydroxyzine (Atarax, Visaril), phenylephrine (Dimetane), and chlorpheniramine (Chlor-Trimeton)	Antihistamines may be used for intercurrent use as needed for sedation and hypnotic effect. Beware of anticholinergic and tolerance effect with long-term use.
Nonbarbiturate hypnotic agents Ethinamate (Valmid), methaqualone (Quaalude), methyprylon (Noludar), glutethimide (Doriden), and ethchlorvynol (Placidyl)	None of these are recommended because of same types of problems as in barbiturates.
Major tranquilizers—antipsychotic agents Phenothiazines, thioridazone (Mellaril), trifluoperazine hydrochloride (Stelazine), triflupromazine (Vesprin), and fluphenazine (Prolixin)	Use lowest possible dose and titrate approximately. Increased incidence of extrapyramidal symptoms in elderly. Postural (orthostatic) hypotension is a problem. Temperature control and tardive dyskinesia are more common with higher doses.

Butyrophenone (Haldol) and thioxanthene (Navane)

Highest incidence of extrapyramidal symptoms occur with these drugs. These are potent antipsychotic agents with low order of side effects and create episodes of amnesia and confusion.

Antidepressant agents
Amitriptyline (Elavil), nortriptyline (Aventyl), imipramine (Tofranil), desipramine (Pertofrane), protriptyline (Vivactil), and doxepin (Sinequan)

Antidepressants are useful only in endogenous depression in up to one half usual dosage. These drugs can exacerbate tremors, psychosis, constipation, postural hypotension, benign prostatic hypertrophy, delayed micturition, and arrhythmias. Because of prolonged half-life, use caution in full-dose bedtime use, especially with Elavil and Tofranil.

Antiparkinsonian agents
Trihexyphenidyl (Artane), procyclidine (Kemadrin), benztropine (Cogentin), and diphenhydramine (Benadryl)

Prophylactic use with antipsychotic agents is generally not recommended. When extrapyramidal symptoms appear, 1 to 3 month use may be beneficial. Watch for constipation, tremors, and delirium resulting from prolonged use, especially with Cogentin.

Carbidopa-levodopa (Sinemet)

Carbidopa-levodopa is generally better tolerated than levodopa alone with less side effects (hypotension, syncope, anorexia, nausea, and emesis).

Side Effects of Drugs Used by the Elderly

Analgesic (mild)
ASA: gastric irritant, allergic rhinitis, anticoagulant, uric acid precipitation

Analgesic (strong)
Depress CNS, circulation, and respiration; some cause constipation, sedation

Antacids
Decrease nutrient absorption; interfere with absorption of some other drugs; decrease stomach acidity; decrease calcium metabolism and absorption

Antiarrhythmics
Procainamide may cause agranulocytosis, fever, chills, and hypersensitivity; lidocaine needs careful monitoring in persons with impaired liver function; quinidine can cause tinnitus, nausea, and arrhythmias; idiosyncrasies are common; propranolol (beta-adrenergic blocker), use cautiously with elderly

Antiarthritics
Phenylbutazone and oxyphenbutazone cause numerous side effects with high risk of severe or fatal toxic reactions; corticosteroids can cause gastrointestinal problems, depression, personality disturbance, irritability, and toxic psychoses

Anticholinergics
Blurred vision, dry mouth, urinary retention, intraocular pressure

Anticoagulants
Necessary to titrate to avoid internal bleeding; antibiotics and mineral oil decrease vitamin K production and thus potentiate anticoagulant effects

Anticonvulsants
Decrease folic acid activity, hypersensitivity; inhibit metabolism; primidone can cause anemia and visual hallucinations

Antidepressants
Imipramine, desipramine, amitryptyline, and nortriptyline all possess anticholinergic properties and must be used with caution in clients with glaucoma

Antihistamines
Drowsiness, blurred vision, and CNS depression, which is potentiated by alcohol

Antihypertensives
Thiazides and furosemide deplete potassium; triamterene or spironolactone may cause hyperkalemia; guanethidine and rauwolfia derivatives should be used together cautiously because they may cause excessive postural hypotension, bradycardia, and mental depression; hydralazine causes headaches, angina, and an arthritis-like syndrome

Antiinfectives
Hypersensitivity, gastrointestinal disturbance, pruritus, deafness, hepatic dysfunction, aplastic anemia; effects vary with the particular drug

Antiparkinsonians
Levodopa may cause nausea, hypotension, dyskinesia, agitation, restlessness and insomnia, cardiac and gastrointestinal effects; use with caution in clients with bronchial asthma or emphysema

From Ebersole P, Hess P: *Toward healthy aging: human needs and nursing response,* ed 5, St. Louis, 1998, Mosby.

Side Effects of Drugs Used by the Elderly—cont'd

Antipsychotics

In various degrees depending on the drug, all phenothiazines can cause photosensitivity, blood dyscrasias, agranulocytosis, and extra-pyramidal effects (seen in 90% of clients after 10 weeks of therapy); haloperidol causes lethargy, decreased thirst, and jaundice, dosage should be considerably reduced for geriatric client; lithium carbonate has toxic level close to therapeutic; side effects are diarrhea, vomiting, tremors, sodium depletion, and muscular weakness; adequate salt and water intake is essential

Cough and cold preparations

OTC cough and cold preparations contain antihistamines and adrenergic decongestants; drugs with anticholinergic effects can contribute to a variety of drug interactions when taken with prescription drugs

Digitalis

Therapeutic and toxic levels close; frequent toxicity producing nausea, arrhythmias, hazy, yellow vision, and weight loss; potassium depletion sensitizes myocardium to digitalis and may also prolong toxicity, resulting in confusion and hallucinations

Diuretics

Thiazides can cause photosensitivity, pancreatitis, sodium and potassium depletion, and precipitate uric acid; ethacrynic acid can cause potassium depletion, vertigo, gastrointestinal problems, and hearing impairment; furosemide has similar side effects and may also alter color vision; spironolactone is potassium sparing but may cause hyperkalemia and drowsiness

Estrogens

Titrate dosage; use for 3 weeks with 1-week rest

Hypnotics

Barbiturates cause daytime drowsiness and hangover, aggravate cerebral anoxia, hypotension, delirium, and depress respiratory function, may cause decrease in REM sleep and rebound on withdrawal; chloral hydrate causes gastrointestinal irritation; dalmane may cause an arthritic-like allergic reaction

Hypoglycemics

Action altered by other drugs; avoid alcohol; oral preparations have numerous adverse side effects; some persons allergic to pork or beef insulin

Laxatives

Phenolphthalein may cause cardiac and respiratory distress in susceptible individuals

Psychotropics

Antianxiety drugs cause CNS depression and ataxia and may be habit forming with a definite withdrawal syndrome; benzodiazepines cause drowsiness, vivid dreams, ataxia, and convulsions on withdrawal; alcohol should be avoided

Vitamins

Ascorbic acids in dose of 1 g/day can cause diarrhea and precipitation of oxalic and uric acid crystals; vitamin D in large doses produces hypercalcemia, weakness, fatigue, headache, nausea, vomiting, and diarrhea

How to Assess the "At-Risk" Geriatric Client

1. Interview client to obtain a complete drug history. Carefully question him or her about disease states, illnesses, current use of medications (prescribed, over-the-counter, home remedies, herbals, vitamins, etc.), drug allergies (obtain description of allergy, time it occurred, intervention used, outcome), and any troubling side or adverse effects.

2. Make list of name, strength, and directions of each medication (prescribed and OTC) the person takes. Include prn medications, especially if person reports taking them one or more times per week.

3. Identify all physicians prescribing for this client. This information may be obtained by client interview and should be verified by checking prescription labels.

4. Prescription bottles may also provide additional information to review, for example, check name(s) of pharmacy(ies) that have dispensed medications to the person. If more than one pharmacy is involved, determine the reason why.

5. Check all prescription and OTC drug containers for expiration dates. Ask the client for permission to destroy any expired medications because they have the potential of being ineffective or causing harm.

6. Question clients on their self-medication practices, that is, how do they remember to take their scheduled medications; do they ever forget to take a dose and if so, what do they do; have they ever deliberately stopped their medication—if yes, obtain an explanation why, etc. Such information will help in evaluating compliance (or noncompliance) and if the medications are being consumed safely, according to the prescribed schedule.

7. Discover whether the client has any limitations that may impair safe, self-administration of medication. Examples include physical impairment, memory loss, health or cultural beliefs, financial constraints, and lack of social support.

From McKenry L, Salerno E: *Mosby's pharmacology in nursing,* ed 20, St. Louis, 1998, Mosby.

Medications Most Commonly Prescribed for the Elderly

Medication	Common side/adverse effects
Aminoglycoside antibiotics (gentamycin, etc.)	Ototoxicity (hearing impairment or loss), renal impairment or failure
Analgesics, opioid	Confusion, constipation, urinary retention (morphine and others), nausea, vomiting, respiratory depression
Anticholinergics, antispasmodics, esp. antihistamines, antiparkinsonian drugs, atropine, etc.	Blurred vision, dry mouth, constipation, confusion, urinary retention, nausea, delirium
Anticoagulants (heparin, warfarin)	Bleeding episodes, hemorrhage, increase in drug-interaction potential
Antihypertensive medications	Sedation, orthostatic hypotension, sexual dysfunction, CNS alterations, nausea
Aspirin, aspirin-containing products	Tinnitus, gastric distress, ulcers, GI bleeding
Digoxin, digitalis preparations, especially at higher dosages	Nausea, vomiting, cardiac arrhythmias, visual disorders, mental-status changes, hallucinations
Diuretics (thiazides, furosemide, etc.)	Electrolyte disorders, rash, fatigue, leg cramps, dehydration
Hypnotics/sedatives (flurazepam, triazolam, etc.)	Confusion, daytime sedation, gait disturbances, lethargy, increased forgetfulness, depression, delirium
H_2 receptor antagonists (cimetidine, ranitidine, etc.)	Confusion, depression, mental status alterations
Nonsteroidal antiinflammatory agents (NSAIDs)	Gastric distress, GI bleeding, ulceration
Psychotropics (neuroleptic agents)	Sedation, confusion, hypotension, drug-induced parkinsonian effects, tardive dyskinesia
Tricyclic antidepressants (amitriptyline, doxepin, and others)	Confusion, cardiac arrhythmias, seizures, agitation, anticholinergic effects, tachycardia, etc.

From McKenry LM, Salerno E: *Mosby's pharmacology in nursing,* ed 20, St. Louis, 1998, Mosby.

Selected Problem Medications for the Elderly

Medication	Elderly response
Digoxin, digitalis preparations	Visual disorders, nausea, diarrhea, cardiac arrhythmias, hallucinations
Anticholinergics (antispasmodics)	Blurred vision, dry mouth, constipation, confusion, urinary retention, tachycardia
Phenothiazines	Hypotension, tremors, extrapyramidal side effects, restlessness
Analgesics, opioid	Confusion, constipation, urinary retention, nausea, vomiting, respiratory depression, addiction
Analgesics, nonnarcotic (aspirin)	Tinnitus, gastric distress, GI bleeding
Anticoagulant (heparin, warfarin)	Bleeding episodes, hemorrhage
Thiazide diuretics	Electrolyte imbalance (hypokalemia), rashes, fatigue, leg cramps, dehydration
Hypnotic-sedatives	Confusion, daytime sedation and ataxia, lethargy, increased forgetfulness
Antihypertensives (e.g., methyldopa)	Nausea, hypotension, diarrhea, bradycardia, heart failure
Antiarthritics (e.g., ibuprofen)	Edema, nausea, abdominal distress, gastric ulceration or bleeding

From McKenry L, Salerno E: *Mosby's pharmacology in nursing,* ed 19, St. Louis, 1995, Mosby.

Factors That May Complicate Drug Therapy in the Elderly

The elderly

- are living longer
- may have one or more chronic diseases
- may receive prescriptions from two or more prescribers
- undergo physiological changes that may result in:
  altered pharmacokinetics
  altered pharmacodynamics
- may have altered thought processes such as confusion, memory loss
- may have impaired physical mobility related to arthritis, fatigue

From McKenry LM, Salerno E: *Mosby's pharmacology in nursing,* ed 20, St. Louis, 1998, Mosby.

- may have sensory-perceptual alterations such as impaired vision or hearing
- may have limited income, which may affect continuity of drug therapy
- on an average use more prescription and OTC drugs than general population
- may experience polypharmacy, which has resulted in increase in reports of drug interactions, side effects, and adverse reactions

Inappropriate Drugs for the Elderly

Category	Drug examples
Analgesics	Propoxyphene (Darvon)
	Pentazocine (Talwin)
Antidiabetic	Chlorpropamide (Diabinese)
Antidepressant	Amitriptyline (Elavil)
Antiemetic	Trimethobenzamide (Tigan)
Antihypertensives	Propranolol (Inderal)
	Methyldopa (Aldomet)
	Reserpine (Serpasil)
Hypnotic/sedative	Diazepam (Valium)
	Chlordiazepoxide (Librium)
	Flurazepam (Dalmane)
	Meprobamate (Miltown)
	Pentobarbital (Nembutal)
	Secobarbital (Seconal)
Muscle relaxants	Cyclobenzaprine (Flexeril)
	Methocarbamol (Robaxin)
	Carisoprodol (Soma)
	Orphenadrine (Norflex)
Nonsteroidal antiinflammatory agents (NSAIDs)	Indomethacin (Indocin)
	Phenylbutazone (Butazolidin)
Platelet inhibitor	Dipyridamole (Persantine)
Peripheral vasodilators (dementia therapy)	Cyclandelate (Cyclospasmol)
	Isoxsuprine (Vasodilan)

From McKenry LM, Salerno E: *Mosby's pharmacology in nursing,* ed 20, St. Louis, 1998, Mosby.

Toxic Characteristics of Specific Drugs Prescribed for the Elderly

Drugs	Signs and symptoms

Benzodiazepines
  Diazepam (Valium)
  Flurazepam (Dalmane)
  Lorazepam (Atavan)
	Ataxia, restlessness, confusion, depression, anticholinergic effect

Cimetidine (Tagamet)	Confusion, depression
Digitalis	Confusion, headache, anorexia, vomiting, arrhythmias, blurred vision or other visual changes (halos, frost on objects, color blindness), paresthesia
Furosemide (Lasix)	Electrolyte imbalance, hepatic changes, pancreatitis, leukopenia, thrombocytopenia
Gentamycin (Garamycin)	Ototoxicity (impaired hearing or balance), nephrotoxicity
L-Dopa	Muscle and eye twitching, disorientation, asterixis, hallucinations, dyskinetic movements, grimacing, depression, delirium, ataxia
Lithium (Eskalith, Lithane)	Confusion, diarrhea, drowsiness, anorexia, slurred speech, tremors, blurred vision, unsteadiness, polyuria, seizures, muscle weakness
Methyldopa (Aldomet)	Hepatic changes, mental depression, fever, bradycardia, nightmares, tremors, edema
Nonsteroidal antiinflammatory agents (NSAIA) Ibuprofen (Advil, Motrin, Nuprin, Rufin)	Photosensitivity, fluid retention, anemia, nephrotoxicity, visual changes

Indomethacin (Indocin)
  Fenoprofen (Nalfon)
  Phenylbutazone (Butazolodin)
  Piroxicam (Feldene)
  Sulindac (Clinoril)
  Tolmetin (Tolectin)
	Confusion plus the above

Phenothiazide tranquilizers	Tachycardia, arrhythmias, dyspnea, hyperthermia, postural hypotension, restlessness, anticholinergic effects
Phenytoin (Dilantin)	Ataxia, slurred speech, confusion, nystagmus, diplopia, nausea and vomiting

From Ebersole P, Hess P: *Toward healthy aging: human needs and nursing response,* ed 5, St. Louis, 1998, Mosby.

Toxic Characteristics of Specific Drugs Prescribed for the Elderly–cont'd

Drugs	Signs and symptoms
Procainamide (pronestyl, Procan, Promine, Sub-Quin, Rhythin)	Arrhythmias, depression, hypotension, SLE syndrome, dyspnea, skin rash, nausea and vomiting
Ranitidine (Zantac)	Liver dysfunction, blood dyscrasias
Sulfonyurals—1st generation Chlorpropamide (Diabinese)	Hypoglycemia, hepatic changes, CHF
Tolbutamide (Orinase)	Bone marrow depression, jaundice
Theophylline (Bronkotabs, Elixophyllin, Quinibron)	Anorexia, nausea, vomiting, GI bleeding, tachycardia, arrhythmias, irritability, insomnia, seizures, muscle twitching
Tricyclic antidepressants Amitriptyline (Elavil, Endep, Amitril) Doxepin (Sinequan, Adapin) Imipramine (Tofranil)	Confusion, arrhythmias, seizures, agitation, tachycardia, jaundice, hallucinations, postural hypotension, anticholinergic effects

Notes

Notes

INDEX

Page numbers in italics indicate illustrations. Page numbers followed by a t
indicate tables.